Oxford Studies in Lexicography and Lexicology

Series Editors

Richard W. Bailey, Noel Osselton, and Gabriele Stein

Lexicography and Physicke

‘Ratifying of truthable and eligible English’

Gabriel Harvey, *Pierce’s Supererogation*, Z3[r]–Z3[v]

MA/DON

Lexicography and Physicke

The Record of Sixteenth-Century English Medical Terminology

R. W. McCONCHIE

CLARENDON PRESS · OXFORD
1997

Oxford University Press, Great Clarendon Street, Oxford OX2 6DP
Oxford New York
Athens Auckland Bangkok Bogota Bombay
Buenos Aires Calcutta Cape Town Dar es Salaam
Delhi Florence Hong Kong Istanbul Karachi
Kuala Lumpur Madras Madrid Melbourne
Mexico City Nairobi Paris Singapore
Taipei Tokyo Toronto Warsaw
and associated companies in
Berlin Ibadan

Oxford is a trade mark of Oxford University Press

Published in the United States
by Oxford University Press Inc., New York

British Library Cataloguing in Publication Data
Data available

Library of Congress Cataloging in Publication Data
Lexicography and physicke : the record of sixteenth-century English medical terminology / R. W. McConchie.
(Oxford studies in lexicography and lexicology)
Includes bibliographical references and index.
1. English language—Early modern, 1500–1700—Medical English.
2. Medicine—Lexicography. 3. Medicine—Terminology.
4. English language—Early modern, 1500–1700—Lexicography.
I. Title. II. Series.
R123.M359 1997 610′.14—dc21 97–12395
ISBN 0–19–823630–1

1 3 5 7 9 10 8 6 4 2

Typeset by Peter Kahrel, Lancaster
Printed in Great Britain on acid-free paper by
Biddles Ltd., Guildford and King's Lynn

Omistettu Ailille, Tainalle ja Arille

Acknowledgements

I wish to acknowledge both the intellectual debts and those less obvious but equally important debts incurred over the course of many years' work on this project. The University of Wollongong and its English Department has provided support in many forms, including research grants and other resources, over most of the period during which I was at work. Its Library and staff have patiently answered my every enquiry. Thanks are also due to my supervisors at Sydney University, Professor Robert Eagleson and Professor Alex Jones, for their help and sound advice. The State Library of New South Wales has provided me with access to the basic materials for this work. The Oxford Dictionaries and its Director, Mrs L. S. Burnett, and its staff, especially Miss Elizabeth Knowles, who has given me her valuable time and expertise freely in the midst of her labours on the *Shorter Oxford Dictionary*, must especially be thanked, as well as its archivist, Mrs Jenny McMorris. Mr John Simpson of the *OED* has also generously provided information and ready assistance. I am grateful to the Bodleian Library, especially the staff of Duke Humphrey's Library; the Wellcome Institute Libraries, both in London and Oxford; the late Professor Jürgen Schäfer; the University of Michigan Library at Ann Arbor for allowing me to consult the *OED* old slips; Professor Richard W. Bailey of the University of Michigan for his encouragement, advice, and support over a number of years; the Public Library of Melbourne; the Shakespeare Institute, then in Birmingham, and its Librarian, Susan Brock; Dr Vivian Salmon; the University of Helsinki English Department and the Helsinki University Library; Dr Juhani Norri; Brigitta Flick, Sally Vickers, and many others who have wittingly or unwittingly been of assistance, or have patiently listened to my tedious explanations. Whatever errors and misunderstandings remain are mine alone.

There are many other debts, some of which will have been overlooked with the passing of time, but which have none the less been greatly appreciated. Finally, my particular thanks and gratitude are due to Doreen Gillam, who has been mentor, colleague, and friend over many years.

I wish to acknowledge kind permission to quote from the following:

Barber, C. L. (1976), *Early modern English* (London: André Deutsch). By permission of André Deutsch Ltd.

Bennett, H. S. (1969), *English books and readers, 1475-1558* (Cambridge: Cambridge University Press). By permission of Cambridge University Press.

Eisenstein, Elizabeth L. (1979), *The printing press as an agent of social change* (Cambridge: Cambridge University Press). By permission of Cambridge University Press.

Hartmann, R. R. K. (1986), *The history of lexicography*. Amsterdam studies in the theory and history of linguistic science III (Amsterdam: John Benjamins). By permission of John Benjamins Publishing Company.

McLean, Antonia (1972), *Humanism and the rise of science in Tudor England* (London: Heinemann Educational). By permission of the author *per* Ruari McLean.

Sager, Juan C., Dungworth, D., and McDonald Peter F. (1980), *English special languages* (Wiesbaden: Brandstetter Verlag). By permission of Oscar Brandstetter Verlag GMBH & CO. KG.

Salmon, V. (1979), *The study of language in 17th-century England*. Studies in the history of the language sciences 40. (Amsterdam: John Benjamins). By permission of John Benjamins Publishing Company.

Slaughter, M. M. (1982), *Universal languages and scientific taxonomy in the seventeenth century* (Cambridge: Cambridge University Press). By permission of Cambridge University Press.

Starnes, De Witt T. *Renaissance dictionaries: English–Latin and Latin–English* ©1954, renewed 1982. By permission of the University of Texas Press.

Starnes, De Witt T. and Noyes, G. (1991), *The English dictionary from Cawdrey to Johnson 1604–1755*, new edition, ed. G. Stein,

(Amsterdam: John Benjamins). By permission of John Benjamins Publishing Company.

Vickers, B. (ed.) (1984), *Occult and scientific mentalities in the Renaissance* (Cambridge: Cambridge University Press). By permission of Cambridge University Press.

Webster, C. (ed.) (1979), *Health, medicine and mortality in the 16th century* (Cambridge: Cambridge University Press). By permission of Cambridge University Press.

Contents

Abbreviations

AOED	Archive of the Oxford Dictionaries, Oxford
Ath. Cant.	Cooper, C. H. and Cooper, T., *Athenae Cantabrigienses* 3 vols., Cambridge, 1858–1913
Ath. Ox.	Wood, Anthony, *Athenae Oxonienses, an exact History of all the writers and bishops . . . of Oxford*, London, 1691
BLC	*British Library Catalogue*
DNB	*Dictionary of National Biography*
EETS	Early English Text Society
EMED	Early Modern English Dictionary
IP	Langton, C., *An introduction into physyke, with an Vniversal dyet*, *c.*1550
MED	H. Kurath and M. Sherman Kuhn (eds.), *Middle English Dictionary*
NSSL	Sidgwick, Leonard W. and Power, H., *New Sydenham Society Lexicon*
OED	*Oxford English Dictionary*
OED-CD	*The Oxford English Dictionary on compact disc*
OED 2	*Oxford English Dictionary*, 2nd edn.
RCP	Royal College of Physicians
STC	Pollard, A. W., Redgrave, G. R., Jackson, W. A., Ferguson, F. S., and Panzer, Katherine F., *A Short-title Catalogue of Works Printed in England, Scotland and Ireland . . . 1475–1640*
VBT	Langton, C., *A uery brefe treatise, ordrely declaring the principal partes of phisick*, 1547

I
Introduction

The tendency to regard the lexicon as a part of the language with an existence independent of its other components or of the conceptual structure of the society of which that language is an expression should be resisted. The very existence of dictionaries may of course conduce to such a notion, but word and concept are, if not always coextensive, at least inextricably connected. Separating them leads to much fruitless historical speculation as to the 'adequacy' of the lexicon of the language, a linguistic phenomenon which is virtually as large as the capacity of its speakers to conceptualize, and practically as large as it needs to be at any one time; hence what is at stake is not the adequacy or the inadequacy of its wordstock, but the nature of the lexicalization of concepts, whether through metaphoric substitutions, description and periphrasis, the various forms of neologism, or through borrowing or calques. The limits to the process will be largely those consequent upon the pre-existing semantic webs already established in the language by its users.

Attention has frequently been drawn to a perceived lack of lexical resources in sixteenth-century English in the medical, technical, and scientific areas. The belief has been persistently repeated that the English language was inadequate for the expression of the higher matters of knowledge and science at the beginning of the sixteenth century, and that it gradually acquired the appropriate terminology as it limped along behind advances in knowledge in various areas of endeavour, and the writers and translators redoubled their efforts in advancing its resources. This view was repeated quite recently in the introduction to Jürgen Schäfer's splendid record of the glossaries of the sixteenth century and the new data for *OED* derived from them.

Around 1500 English was incapable of providing a linguistic medium for traditional scholarship and for the rapidly developing scientific disciplines since it lacked the necessary terminologies. This deficiency was remedied during the sixteenth century ... and by 1600 there was virtually no field of traditional or new learning which could not be studied in the vernacular. (Schäfer 1989: ii, 1)

Such claims do not usually attempt to discriminate between one science and another, or arise from a consideration of the special circumstances which might apply to one science but not to another. It has been more usual to contrast the language used in science generally with that of literature, or religion. In any case, more recent work has shown that Schäfer's chronological estimate of the process of vernacularization may be too late by at least a century (Voigts 1996). The first question with which this book is concerned is whether this inadequacy was real or perhaps merely perceived in sixteenth-century medical writing in English.

It must inevitably be true that on the whole the development of such areas of knowledge and the lexicon will advance in tandem. Conscious efforts to neologize or borrow have generally been made to meet a specific and immediate need—for example, William Turner's neologizing in the 1540s,[1] where the discovery of new botanical species required new, specific nomenclature—but to extrapolate from such evidence to the lexicon as a whole is fraught with dangers. It is perhaps too easy to suppose that in a discipline where the technology, the procedures, and the basic concepts are easily seen to be various, discrete, and in many cases unique that there should be clear correspondences between words and things, and that any discrepancies will be obvious. But that view is too simplistic. Semantic domains are reticular structures, not lists.

It is clear at the same time that the sixteenth century was a time of notable advance in the range and sophistication of scientific and medical terminology and the view has been put by Sarton and others that the scientific Renaissance (if such a label can for the moment be admitted) begins with, though is not necessarily caused by, the introduction in Europe of the crafts of printing and engraving.[2] The earliest text examined here postdates that momentous event by about three generations. The quantities of books published in medicine burgeoned as the century proceeded, and it is easy to suppose that the terminology expanded and developed with this process, but it must be remembered that the century and and a half which had gone before had already seen English claim a place alongside Latin as a language in which serious science and medicine could be written, and that the interrelationships, primarily between Latin and English, were complex (Voigts 1996, 1989*b*; Jones 1989). Neither was it a simple shift from a scribal to a print tradition with the spread of printing, the two remaining interlocked and intimately related in many respects (Blake 1989) perhaps well into the sixteenth century.[3] The question with which much of this book is concerned is which specialist medical terminology among those available eventually established a rightful place in English medical books, and what were the assumptions underlying the resolution of this problem.

Sixteenth-century English had available to it two large and respected lexicons from which to borrow, those of Latin and Greek, so that the web of native terminology was greatly complicated, as it still is, by the existence of competing and overlapping systems only partially assimilated into English. There was also the increasingly unfashionable but nevertheless extensive Arabic terminology still used in medicine, and still employed late into the sixteenth century. The craft of printing facilitated this growth by making a multiplicity of texts available at affordable prices, and by solving the age-old problem of the conservation of text,[4] although it was not in itself a cause of the growth in terminology. At the same time English was discovering a new freedom in word creation, again prompted by influences from outside the language, and in the transference of words from one grammatical class to another.

The general assumptions about the importance of Latin and Greek borrowings need some reassessment. It is often assumed that in some sense this put medicine at an advantage over the other emerging sciences, and it is not unusual to read that the macro-organization of the terminology of a science must be preceded by significant extensions and refinement of the discipline: 'Only when a sufficient body of knowledge has been accumulated, can an attempt be made to order it systematically and to reflect this ordering in regular patterns of designation. This was done for medicine and biology through the creation of a new quasi-artificial language based on Greek and Latin' (Sager et al. 1980: 239). But such assumptions are not always based upon careful examination of the historical evidence. My own investigations lead rather to the conclusion that the process referred to was in fact never accomplished for medicine, precisely because a substantial and highly prestigious terminology was already in existence, and this was borrowed wholesale. Further, its adoption by the medical profession might have hindered rather than assisted progress, since so much of the effort of humanist physicians was directed towards cleansing the terminology of its medieval accretions and corruptions, and since the terminology at hand was the tool of an already existing theoretical framework and of long-established assumptions and procedures. One can only imagine what would happen to, say, the terminology of anatomy now if it were to be completely rewritten, on the basis of the current understanding of anatomical classification and function. To take only one example, the pituitary gland would hardly be named now on the assumption that it discharged mucus into the nose.

There is a tendency to regard the relationship between word and object or concept as being like that between tool and product; the one assisting in the production of the other. But that is surely oversimple: in this case the tool is also coextensive with the product, and shares some identity with it. Language is both tool and product simultaneously. It is not simply the means of conceptualization and analysis.

Medicine is of particular importance, since it is an area in which the whole society is the potential clientele and where knowledge is quickly and frequently transformed into practice. It is perhaps the most obvious point of contact between science and society, and one at which attempts to popularize are inevitable. Medical practice is also a point of synthesis: 'Diseases, societies, and ideas may change independently of one another or concurrently; at their conjuncture lies medical practice' (Cook 1981: 88–90).

It is also the case that scholarship has focused its attentions on those aspects of Renaissance medicine which have been progressive and evolutionary to the neglect of the whole range of beliefs, attitudes, and practices which formed the basis of contemporary medicine, and in the context of which the singular steps forward were made. It is a salutary exercise to look at the words which were used for such progressive and evolutionary processes and their discoverers, such as **experiment** and **invent**, since it is immediately apparent that the language itself did not contain those concepts for which we now lionize the great medical figures of the Renaissance.[5] As it has been put elsewhere:

> modern writers tend to focus on the openly experimental literature and neglect the vast amount of humanist science, as general philosophy, Aristotelian physics and Galenic medicine, which not only formed the minds of nearly all the experimental scientists who had a university education, but still represents—for those with the knowledge and philological expertise needed to make use of it—a virtually untapped source of information about Renaissance intellectual attitudes. (Vickers 1984: 11)

The primary interest of this book is to examine the emerging specialist terminology of the medical profession in England in the sixteenth century as it appears in the opinions and practices of those publishing in English, and through a study of the way in which dictionaries, especially the *OED*, have dealt with words found in contemporary medical texts, particularly those medical terms from Greek, Latin, and Arabic not yet naturalized in form. From the beginning there has been no attempt, however, to survey the word-lists and glossaries in medical works available from this period, since Jürgen Schäfer was already hard at work on them in Augsburg as part of a larger project before his death. This important work, which adds significantly to our knowledge of the lexicon and lexicography of the period, has since been published (Schäfer 1989).

The data for this study has been built on the methods adopted by Schäfer and the many others who have from time to time collected extra data for the *OED*, often in the course of pursuing some other aim such as an edition. This is hardly new in itself, but this study shares with Schäfer's work that fact that the material has been deliberately sought for its own sake, and its excerption has been as thorough as circumstances and resources have permitted. It is different in having been concentrated on one semantic domain only. The book deals with the resultant word-lists and their relation to the *OED*'s own, but it does not attempt to use this material to analyse the structure of its main lemmas except in peripheral areas such as the field-marking of medical terms, even though the material available has now and then been sufficient to shed some light on it and comment is made on individual lemmas where it has seemed appropriate. Thus, for example, the overall conceptual subdivision of senses and their consequent sequencing within *OED* lemmas is not considered, but such things as the lack of a tagged or untagged medical sublemma, or the omission of a then frequently used, but subsequently obsolete, medical term are. The present study is limited mainly to issues of inclusion and exclusion, first citation and its implication, and the editorial problems raised by what the *OED* itself calls 'denizens'. Such studies as that by Ladislav Zgusta have therefore not been used as a theoretical basis, and the data now available has not been used to test the claims which he puts forward; indeed, given the inherently specialist character of the data collected here, it would be an inappropriate vehicle to employ (Zgusta 1988).

It is also important to consider the context of the works which form the core of this study, particularly those from which the additions have been excerpted, and to examine as far as possible what the relevant interests of their authors were and what they had to say on the subject of their own language. Many of them are unfortunately so little known that even reconstructing a minimal biography is impossible. The book will discuss the attitudes to the use of the vernacular expressed by those authors, and examine aspects of their actual linguistic practice. The core of the study, which explores the extent to which the specialist words (and therefore concepts) of English Renaissance medicine have subsequently been recognised, is 3,985 items of new data for the *OED*. The categories of new data included in this figure are antedatings, new senses, unrecorded words, and postdatings. The works from which this data has been drawn are:

1. Anon. [Plutarch], *The gouernaunce of good helth*, 1549
2. Bailey, W., *A treatise of the medicine called mithridatium*, 1585
3. Baker, G., *The composition ... of the moste excellent and prestigious oil called oleum magistrale*, 1574
4. Banister, J., *The historie of man*, 1578
5. Barrough, P., *The methode of phisicke, conteyning the cavses, signes, and cvres of the inward diseases in mans bodie from the head to the foote*, 1583
6. B[ostocke], R., *The difference betweene the auncient phisicke ... and the latter phisicke*, 1585
7. Clever, W., *The flower of physicke*, 1590
8. Cotta, J., *A short discouerie of the vnobserued dangers of seueral sorts of ignorant practisers of phisicke in England*, 1612
9. Hester, J. [Fioravanti], *A short discourse ... vppon chirurgerie*, 1580
10. Hill, T. [Fioravanti], *A ioyfull iewel. Contayning ... excellent orders, preseruatiues and precious practises for the plague*, 1579
11. Langton, C., *A uery brefe treatise, ordrely declaring the principal partes of phisick*, 1547 [cited as *VBT*]
12. Langton, C., *An introduction into physyke, with an vniuersal dyet*, *c.*1550 [cited as *IP*]
13. More, P. *The hope of helth*, 1564

A third area of consideration is the ways in which the early lexicographers, both monolingual and bi- or multilingual, dealt with the medical language of the time in the context of their lexicographic practices, whether stated or unstated, and a chapter is therefore devoted specifically to the earlier Latin/English lexicographers Elyot, Cooper, Thomas, and Rider, and to the earliest monolingual lexicographers Cawdrey and Bullokar.

There is at present no glossary of sixteenth-century English medical terms as such, although recent work has gone some way to identifying part of the corpus (Norri 1992). The terminology which is examined here may give some general indication of the size and extent of the potential corpus, but it is not claimed that the words which form the basis of this study are in any sense a complete corpus of sixteenth-century medical terms.[6] Clearly there will be a bias resulting from the nature of the terms likely to be discovered to be new data for the *OED* towards the more obscure and dubiously naturalized words rather than to those of more common currency; nevertheless many now familiar words do appear, both as antedatings and as new senses. Some of the words listed as unrecorded in the *OED* were in fact quite familiar at least to the practitioners of the age if not to the public at large, and appeared frequently in the medical writings. Thus the corpus presented here, while probably skewed as a sample, is at least partially illustrative of the kind of specialist medical language in use in the sixteenth century.

It was at this period that the medical writers themselves were just beginning to publish in the vernacular and, in the first half of the sixteenth century especially, exhibited a good deal of nervousness about this enterprise, apparently meeting persistent opposition to it. Attitudes changed, however, in the course of the century as will be shown in Chapters 2 and 3. It was not opposition to medical books as such, as is sometimes thought, but to books which stepped outside the bounds of acceptability by being too debased, or by being written in the wrong language. It was, however, also the time when the possibilities for the dissemination and popularization of knowledge through the printing presses were being enthusiastically recognized, ensuring a growing demand for medical works in English. The second chapter will survey the attitudes of the medical and other writers to their own language and to the business of translating medical texts, either from the classical languages or from other vernaculars, and Chapter 3 looks at the concept of authority and at details of the lexical practice of selected authors.

The fourth chapter briefly surveys the bilingual and monolingual lexicographers of this period from Elyot to Bullokar. It considers the differences between the two groups in terms of their significance as lexicographers, and looks somewhat more closely at their attitudes to and treatment of the medical lexicon. The question of which of these lexicographers the *OED* relied on is also examined.

The works from which information for Chapters 5 and 6 has been compiled form a modest percentage of the total published during the course of the sixteenth century. An estimate suggests that over 150 titles were seen through the press during this period (Slack 1979).[7] This, of course, does not represent the number of original titles, which is rather difficult to estimate, since many were reprinted and re-edited, or underwent major or minor rewriting. Old titles were changed without alteration to the text, and new texts were bound with old ones. The total number should also be considered in the context of the production in Western Europe during roughly the same period of some 600 editions of Galen, very few of which were produced in England. Other ancient texts were similarly published and republished. These were produced for use, not curiosity or artistic value, and the number of vernacular texts, especially those containing new material, was indeed paltry by comparison in sheer volume with standard editions of the medical classics. This reflects not merely an attitude towards classical sources but a real need for information and for certainty in the reception of texts. The interest in antiquity and the hunger for better and more scholarly editions was vital to the advancement of knowledge, and was not simply an antiquarian curiosity. History has subsequently shown that this perception was correct, if perhaps for other reasons than would now be advanced, since coming to recognize and understand the real shortcomings in the writings of the ancients was an essential stage in the process.

Chapter 7 is concerned with the genesis of the *OED* and the way in which the medical terminology of the sixteenth century was ultimately handled in the most comprehensive English dictionary. How was it compiled, on what assumptions, and how did these matters affect the final outcome? Is there any point in amassing details of the lexicon purporting to improve what has been done, as many have done ever since the appearance of the *OED*? Is the sixteenth-century medical lexicon adequately represented in the *OED* or not?

The mass of new data on which this book has been based has been set out in full detail in Appendix 1, which records each word excerpted from the thirteen works in the study under the various categories of new data for the *OED*, and provides the textual context of each excerpt. It is hoped that these quotes are for the most part sufficient to illustrate the sense of the items included, though this is not possible in all cases. I have hardly had to search for works which would yield fruitful evidence for this study, since virtually every work as it was taken up immediately began to prove its productiveness. No work of any size had to be rejected as barren of information.

To scant the medical terminology of the sixteenth century would be to preclude an objective view of the preservation of many long-established terms in an intellectual climate where a conservative tradition of scholarly rigour was felt to be creative and productive. It also simultaneously distorts the understanding of many commonplace modern words which began their lexical career in this specialist area, for example, **deflation** and **indication**.

It is often mistakenly assumed that the conceptual structure of Renaissance science must be the same as for modern science; a continual progress towards better and more complete knowledge sustained by a self-analysing procedure of hypothesis and testing. But is it realistic to make such a generalization about a science whose innovators, however praised, were very few, and whose assumptions were rooted in a backward-looking tradition of classical learning? Thus Juhani Norri, for example, introduces a discussion of fifteenth-century scientific terminology with the generalization that 'In science, facts earlier unknown are being discovered and new theories are being presented' (Norri 1989: 147).[8] But this is surely a modern view, and hardly seems to be a perspicuous description of the medical science whose language he discusses. Indeed, the terminology itself is the best evidence of the innate conservatism of the discipline. What is required is a new model for the science of these times, based on a thoroughgoing analysis of its conceptual basis. Only minute attention to its language can provide this, and what happens can be best understood in the light of contemporary preconceptions, not modern ones. In this task the language of the non-innovators is quite as important as that of the originators of new ideas and concepts.

Other preconceptions cloud our view of this period. There is, for example, the tendency to regard it as a coherent and consistent block of time about which one may safely theorize from any piece of evidence irrespective of its origin, its author, or the circumstances in which it occurred.[9] The tendency to consider the lexicon as an artefact whose creation was largely in the hands of literary authors appears in N. F. Blake's recent survey of research into the early modern period, in which discussion of the lexis immediately becomes a discussion of Chaucer and Shakespeare (Blake 1991: 31–3). I hope to provide some notion of the extent to which the *OED* has led scholarship astray in this respect in the course of this book. Blake's salutary account does, however, point out the still current deficiencies in our knowledge of the language at this period, and the need to redefine our fundamental assumptions. Görlach's 1992 survey of the situation in the lexical field, in which he alluded to the lack of follow-up to Schäfer's work and the failure to exploit the computerized lexicographic resources then to hand, was somewhat dispiriting (Görlach 1992: 25–7). Amid the notable advances being made in the wake of development of historical corpora such as the Helsinki Corpus (Kytö et al. 1994), the study of lexis still lags behind.[10]

Another assumption is that translators were hampered in their endeavours by the inadequacies of the language. What exactly this might mean deserves closer examination, though this study goes no further than to canvass some of their stated views. How does the scholar distinguish between a translator who struggles with his or her chosen text and one who struggles with the language itself? Since so many of the medical texts of the Renaissance are either translations or compilations deriving from them, the matter is crucial to our understanding of the development of the language and of the transmission of scientific knowledge.

Periodization is often non-existent in studies of the language of this period, claims about attitudes and practices being applied to periods sometimes extending to centuries as if they can be assumed to be reliable, consistent, and indeed unalterable from one period, author, discipline, genre or text-type to another. The most usual reason for this appears to be the transmission of assumptions from one scholar to another until they acquire the status of unquestioned academic folklore (see Schmitt 1983: 233).

Finally, the historiography of medicine itself has been a confounding factor in the long haul, having been rather regressively attached to notions of progress, of great and revolutionary advances, and to those figures who have determined the parameters of our historical concepts.[11] To understand the ordinary apothecary, surgeon, or physician of this time, we need to know who they were, what records they left behind, and above all what they wrote and what they meant by it.

We must look again at the original texts, since both as sources for medical history and for linguistic history they have been by and large neglected and discounted. The fact that almost none of these authors has been edited in modern times, Clowes being one of the few exceptions, is indicative of the neglect they have suffered. What was not progressive or revolutionary in medicine has not been of interest. Neither Banister, Gale, nor Baker discovered the circulation of the blood, or anything else which substantially changed the course of medical history; thus they are considered to be of no significance and it is not thought necessary to read them. Only two medical writers of this period, Elyot and Burton, have been credited with literary distinction. It is, however, the large trends, the subtle but ultimately pervasive shifts of attitude expressed in these writings as a whole, the incremental creep of language and thought in tandem, which ought to be researched in depth. It is here that the preconditions for the discoveries and the revolutionary changes are to be found, as well as the broader picture of society as it then was. These works are also surprisingly revealing of the state of the lexicon at the time. In particular we must attend to Jürgen Schäfer's plea concerning the revisions to be made to our view of the English lexicon in the sixteenth century:

> *OED*'s documentation, the richest presently available, is inadequate in the light of modern scholarship; the combination of the older EMED project, and present day computer technology offers a unique opportunity to remedy this situation and to arrive at solutions that might prove as indispensable and lasting for scholars as the *OED* has been for more than a century. (Schäfer 1989: 67)

Notes

1. Mats Rydén has shown the dangers of ascribing creative neologizing too readily to this or indeed any author. Of twenty-five antedatings listed by him discovered in an early herbal, nine are from Turner. The probability is that more will be found in time, and that the number of his neologisms have, on the evidence available from the *OED*, been overstated (Rydén 1985: 12–14). Although Rydén does not identify the nine, they are **bean [of Egypt]**, **dogberry**, **[great] rape**, **herb-grace**, **lunary**, **sindaw**, **[white] beet**, **clary**, and **[wild] saffron**.
2. For a cautious but enlightening discussion of the problems of definition and periodization involved, see Eisenstein 1979, vol. i, Ch. 3).
3. See Christianson (1989), however, for an assessment of manuscript production in London into the sixteenth century. Despite the decline in numbers working in this craft up to 1519 (Christianson, 89), medical

manuscripts no doubt continued to be used for various purposes throughout the sixteenth century.

4. The illustration of printed medical texts is, however, a different problem. The introduction of printing left publishers reliant on the woodcut, crude by the sometimes highly sophisticated standards of manuscript illustration, and my impression is that illustrations slowly disappear from medical texts. Braunschweig's *The noble experyence of . . . surgeri* of 1525 is relatively profusely illustrated, as is Turner's 1551 herbal, but the Vesalian illustrations reproduced in Banister's *The historie of man* of 1578 are both poor in quality and scant.
5. The present sense of **invent** (*OED* 3) was current in the sixteenth century, but was paralleled by the frequently used and perhaps earlier meaning 'find out', or 'discover'. The latter was often used in medical texts, the crucial difference being that in the latter sense a fact, object, or state of things could be repeatedly invented, not just once. Thus Banister can say: 'Wherfore *Vesalius* protesteth but onely once to haue inuented the same' on the subject of 'the wayes deducyng choler . . . vnto the bottome of the ventricle.' (Uii[v]). **Experiment** might mean a means of effecting a cure (*OED* 1b), or a test or trial (*OED* 1a), while also having a modern sense (*OED* 3). It is perhaps also worth noting that the quotation from Lanfranc (*c.*1400) clearly belongs to sense 1a, not 3a 'now /Æ/†/Æ/ese chapitles of /Æ/†/Æ/is book ben y-ordeyned, I wole fulfille my purpos pursuynge ech chapitle bi ordre, & confermynge my wordis aftir /Æ/†/Æ/e auctorite of myn auctouris and wi/Æ/†/Æ/ /Æ/†/Æ/e experiment /Æ/†/Æ/at I haue longe tyme vsed', thus compromising somewhat the early date given for this sense. The quotation from *Piers Plowman* is probably no clearer in implication: 3/Æ/Ó/Æ/et arn /Æ/†/Æ/ere febicches of Forellis of many manis wittes, /Experimentis of alkenemye of albertis makyng,/Nigromancie & per[i]mansie /Æ/†/Æ/e pouke to reisen' (Langland, ed. Kane, 1988, xi, 159–61).
6. The term 'sixteenth century' is used a little loosely—the actual range of dates of publication is 1547–1612. Earlier editions of *STC* had dated the anonymous translation of Plutarch *c.*1530.
7. Slack suggests that between 1486 and 1605, 153 medical works were published. See esp. 238–9.
8. Dr Norri has since produced a most valuable account of fifteenth-century disease names, a task which clearly takes as an assumption the need to survey the workaday terminology thoroughly (Norri 1992). For a perspicuous survey of trends in the historiography of medieval and Renaissance science generally, see Schmitt (1983).
9. Maurizio Gotti's examination of the development of scientific language in the seventeenth century freely appropriates the views of Thomas Elyot, Francis Bacon, Thomas Hobbes, and Robert Boyle, among

others, as if they were simply contemporaneously employed in the service of his thesis (Gotti 1991). Gotti surprisingly makes no mention of the extensive scholarly efforts of Vivian Salmon and others to elucidate the development of a real character and a universal language either, a subject beyond the scope of this book.

10. A most recent encouraging development is the appearance on the World Wide Web of the early modern English Renaissance dictionaries corpus, which provides convenient access for scholars to eleven dictionaries of the period. See Lancashire (1994*a*; 1994*b*) for information on the corpus itself.
11. For a summary account of this area at the beginning of the 1980s which is still useful, see Webster (1983).

2
The Inadequacy of English

I. SOME ASSUMPTIONS

It is an easy assumption to make that languages progress, that their progress is steadily evolutionary, and that there are always increases in sophistication, flexibility, and subtlety. What is less readily grasped is that this evolution reflects the requirements of their nurturant societies. A changing society will have a changing language, but a static one would have a static language. Progress is, however, not always steady and predictable; thus it is not necessarily the case that this development may be detected equally at all stages of a language's history.

It is not possible to speak with confidence about the English medical lexicon during the Renaissance. The documentation of the English language is not as complete as might be wished for the sixteenth century. Furthermore, what there is by way of material is relatively poorly understood, and much is infrequently, if ever, consulted. Not even the printed resources are fully utilized, let alone the manuscript ones. The picture we have of early modern English is therefore necessarily incomplete, and we are enjoined to discover the extent to which this is so. To generalize in this area at present is to skate on thin ice.

An assumption that the English language had stagnated while the English-speaking community had progressed does, however, lie behind some of the arguments about the state of English in the sixteenth century. Consider the following:

> In both translations and original works one is struck with the seeming unawareness of any obstacle other than language standing in the way of the education of the people, and also with the general assumption of the adequacy of the English language to express the thought contained in other languages ... this assumption, which represented wishful thinking rather than experience, was contradicted on every hand, but in most of the translations of this period, no hint is given of any inability to render the meaning

of an original in English, though much is said of the inadequacy of the vernacular to reproduce the eloquence of other languages. (Jones 1953: 39)

To summarize this argument: the only bar to understanding was the inadequacy of the language; almost no one among translators and authors of the time commented upon this bar, therefore almost all translators and authors were mistaken in being unaware of this obstacle; that is, that their presumed refusal to comment represented wishful thinking about the adequacy of English. Furthermore, it is contended that evidence exists 'on every hand' to demonstrate the truth of this conclusion. An examination of this curious proposition, based as it is upon the notion of a steady progression from inadequacy to adequacy in the English language, will show that first, it begs the question and second, it accepts as trustworthy some kinds of evidence, but rejects that which tends to confute the original premiss. In the medical field in particular the evidence simply does not point all one way, as is suggested.

There have been too many scholarly works on the history of early modern English which have assumed rather too easily that all matters of fact have long since been resolved. There has also been a tendency to disregard the writings of contemporaries not otherwise well regarded, usually for the lack of some literary or quasi-literary merit. C. L. Barber, for example, in considering attitudes to the English language at that time, argues that the medical profession was, of all disciplines, more likely than most to take exception to its use, suggesting that where it was a matter of professional status, changes would be most hotly contested.

People brought up in this tradition of Latin scholarship ... resisted attempts to popularize knowledge, and put forward arguments to show that the English language was unsuitable for works of scholarship. The hostility to de-Latinization was fiercest in groups whose professional status rested on their learning, like physicians. (Barber 1976: 67)

But he accepts this view too glibly, and cites only the well-known preface by Elyot to the 1541 edition of *The castell of helth* as representative evidence. It has been noted that 'It was not until after 1700 or thereabouts that Latin ceased to be usual for medical works written by, and meant for, experts in medicine' (Norri 1987: 336). But it was not that simple: the incautious reader might assume that the number of vernacular works prior to 1700 was negligible. It is, as will be seen, an assumption which does not hold good for England. In a summary chapter on the language in the Renaissance, Manfred Görlach puts the familiar view that the language was felt to be 'deficient and unsuited to the expression of complex arguments in such fields as medicine and science', but as evidence cites only the familiar counter-arguments of Hoby and Mulcaster, and the humanist views of Elyot, Ascham, and Wilson, rather than considering what the men of medicine or science at large had to say for themselves (Greenbaum 1985: 31–2).[1]

This view of the inadequacy of English, largely taken from work on non-scientific writings, is still current, and still unsubstantiated by evidence broad enough to support it convincingly.[2] I will suggest that the evidence needs a far more careful and thorough assessment, both for professional views on the use of English and also to establish who among the professionals was actually writing and in what language. The views of medical writers have also been disregarded, probably because their interest in language has been underrated. To take an earlier instance, J. L. Moore's compilation of opinions of the English language in Tudor and Stuart England lists Burton and briefly alludes to Borde, alone among medical writers (Moore 1910: 16).

Indeed, so far from there being little or no vernacular background to the early sixteenth-century medical book, there was a well-established and by then rich tradition of producing works in English in medical as well as other sciences, as has been pointed out by Linda Ehrsam Voigts (1996; 1989*b*). It now seems safe to say that English was well established and perhaps felt to be comparable with Latin by this time, having been in use for over a century for such purposes. Voigts has recently claimed that

> after 1475 we can find a full range of sophisticated university treatises—mostly on medicine and astronomy—in English-language manuscripts where Latin plays little or no role ... we find the earliest significant use of English in scientific and medical writing in the last quarter of the fourteenth century ... and that a century later the language had achieved a status equivalent to that of Latin for exclusive use in such texts. (1996: 814)

This fact provides a rational foundation for the findings in the present study, which takes up the story in medicine where Voigts and others concerned with the compilation of fifteenth-century texts have left it for the time being. The actual linguistic practices employed in these texts, such as Jones has examined for the translators of John of Arderne (Jones 1989), ought to reveal a good deal about the underlying attitudes of authors, translators, and compilers, which remain to be examined in full detail.

There is in fact quite a lot of evidence to suggest that the medical practitioners of the sixteenth century took a very lively interest in all kinds of linguistic matters. A summary survey will show that Thomas Elyot had a professed interest in medicine, and also wrote a dictionary. Andrew Borde claims to have at least a smattering of a considerable number of languages in his *Introduction to knowledge*; John Jones, who wrote a number of medical works, discusses artificial language in *The benefit of the auncient bathes of Buckstones*; Humfrey Lloyd's medical translation *The treasuri of helth* of 1558 contains a word-list at the end. William Turner, the physician and botanist, discussed the terminology of his profession at length in his works. The lexicographer Thomas Cooper was a trained physician, while John Baret and Peter Levins, also physicians, both produced dictionaries. Timothy Bright, sometime resident physician to St Bartholomew's and author of the first English work on melancholy, and William Folkington, who published on the medicinal properties of ale, both wrote works on stenography. Mark Ridley, who served for a time as physician to the Tsar of Russia left a manuscript Russian–English dictionary entitled *A dictionarie of the vulgar Russe tongue* and *A dictionarie of the Englishe before the vulgar Russe tongue* (MS Laud 47a, b; Stone 1987) and Thomas D'Oyly, whose work was the basis for Percyvall's *Bibliotheca Hispanica* of 1591, was also a physician, as was William Bullokar, the second English monolingual lexicographer.

Claims about the inadequacy of the English language have also to be considered in a somewhat wider historical view. The broad claim that the sixteenth century regarded the language as deficient seems to assume that the same would apply at an earlier period, but this now seems unsupportable. Janel M. Mueller has pointed out that in the fourteenth and fifteenth centuries many saw English as a fit vehicle for Scripture and that, while the impetus for this movement, which he dubs 'scripturalism', broadly coincided with the florescence of Lollardy, it did not die with Lollardy. A language fit for the word of God clearly might be fit for other purposes. The desire to have the fundamental Christian texts in the vernacular was, he suggests, 'a product of early modern English confidence in the capacities of the native tongue and its users to deal requisitely with the supreme instance of a text, the very Word of God' (Mueller 1984:

9–10). Mueller's work, taken together with that of Voigts, has restored balance to the picture.

2. THE NOTION OF INADEQUACY AND SIXTEENTH-CENTURY PRINTED MEDICAL WRITINGS

It will be proposed here that the evidence of at least one special category of sixteenth-century works, medical texts, does not support Jones's hypothesis, nor indeed his perception of the facts. The evidence examined in this chapter tends to modify and undermine such a hypothesis. The central practical problem is why the suggested bar is so infrequently noticed by contemporary authors.[3] I want to argue in this chapter that it is a sleight of hand to suggest that in these circumstances lack of notice implies a mistaken view, and that more credit ought to be given to these commentators for knowing the current situation.

Another assumption in Jones's position which needs to be questioned is that books addressed to the 'unlearned' are to be taken as suggesting an apology for writing in English. Jones rightly hints at a distinction between learned and unlearned; that is, between those literate in Latin and those literate in English only:

> The cleavage between the learned and the unlearned, in the minds of those employing the vernacular, was pronounced, and the latter make it plain that their efforts were directed to the unlatined. The consistency with which they designated the unlearned as the object of their writing suggests that such announcements were an apology for writing in English and also a precaution against a possible reprimand from the learned. (Jones 1953: 36)[4]

This is not, however, a sufficient ground in itself to argue that authors felt apologetic about the use of the vernacular. Jones himself has stressed that to write for the uninstructed (not the uninstructable) was itself a perfectly worthy motive and was widely espoused. Once again it is a question of looking closely at the evidence in medical works.

Neither will a chronological assessment wholly support this thesis. In fact, defences against the criticisms of the learned first appear only in the 1540s (e.g. Elyot 1541) and cannot therefore be taken to characterize the whole century. Several writers attack the learned early in the century for their indolence and unwillingness to publish. Further, it cannot be assumed that the unlearned were the unlettered—they could not have been except such as were read to. The term therefore generally means the unlatined, or those not educated in the classical tongues, a specific sense not firmly identified by the *OED*. Such remarks about the unlearned were probably no worse than patronizing to the readership, and cannot without further corroboration be assumed to have denigrated English by implication. We will see that defensive remarks were not always especially concerned with language and were more frequent than actual attacks; presumably these attacks were much more often personal than published, or the rejoinders to the sons of Zoilus were frequently merely conventional. Up to the 1550s it is more usual to hear authors and translators such as Turner and Andrewe criticizing scholars for being too indolent to do a service to their countrymen by committing themselves to print. Such reprimands have been ignored by historians of early modern English. Attacks on translators may have been a defensive response in the first place.

Not only has some evidence been left out of account, but some has not always been rightly understood. For example, Jones cites Walter Hilton (d. 1396) as explaining inadequacies or omissions in his treatise on the grounds of 'lackynge of englysshe' (Jones 1953: 70). There is no justification at all for this reading of the text. The passage in question is 'Also /Æ/†/Æ/ese wordis /Æ/†/Æ/at I write take hem not to streitli but /Æ/†/Æ/er[e] as yee thenkith bi good avisement /Æ/†/Æ/[at] I speke to schortli ei/Æ/†/Æ/er for lackynge of ynglisch or wantinge of resou[n]' (Hilton, MS Bodl. 592). Hilton's point is that he wishes to ascribe to God whatever is good in what he writes and the rest to his own shortcomings. He may also feel that he can express himself better in Latin, but in either case, the 'lackynge' is his, not the language's. About the end of the fourteenth century the use of English was defended by Wyclif's collaborator Nicholas Purvey in the prologue to the Wyclifite Bible of *c.*1395. He shared with the medical writers of the sixteenth century the view that English was sufficient to the task in hand, as well as the assumption that the utility of the language in itself justified the enterprise.[5] Making the Scriptures accessible to all was a religious duty; making medical practice comprehensible was seen as a social duty.

It is often said that English, like all major European vernaculars in the latter part of the sixteenth century, found itself having to cope with a rapidly expanding need for new technical and scientific vocabulary. Whereas at the beginning of the century it had been able to render most of the concepts inherited from the late Middle Ages, the race to find new terms intensified greatly as the century wore on. But this is not a convincing account of the state of things in medical science. A body of terms was already available to cover many of these exigencies, embedded in the universal language of medieval science, as well as in Greek and Arabic. The change can be seen to some extent as a shift from the use of a universal language for medical science to the use of a body of terms, insulated from common usage by their history and non-naturalization, embedded within the vernacular.[6] But more was required than merely the rediscovery of ancient concepts and phenomena, however. As will be seen in the case of botany, new phenomena required new words, and the terms were not always available from classical languages, though there was much ingenious adaption. Greek and Latin became a resource from which to supply the genius of the vernacular, not only with terminology, but with the means of word formation as well. The extent to which this adaption took place can be gauged by the lists of antedatings and neologisms to be found in Appendix 1 of this work, and discussed at length in Chapters 5 and 6, or by comparing in a more general way the richness of the technical vocabulary of the early sixteenth- to that of later sixteenth-century medical texts. The process is examined in more detail in Chapter 3, where the practices of some individual authors are considered. A close look at the medical texts will show that it was not, as Jones seems to imply, that the language's hitherto unconsidered but inherent inadequacies were suddenly brought to notice. It is possible that inadequacies in the lexicon had appeared by the end of the sixteenth century, and were inevitably discussed. But to notice inadequacies is to remedy them, so that it is more likely that the processes of change and addition to the lexicon had themselves come to be noticed, and, taken along with the rise in interest in linguistics in the second half of the sixteenth century, this is perhaps a more likely explanation for criticism of the language's perceived deficiencies. Indeed, it might be more perspicuous to say that the adjustments of the language to the new environment themselves were what caused the comment, rather than the need for those adjustments.

Another factor might be involved as well: that the formative role of translators in the development of the language has not really been fully understood either (Blake 1992). It is easy to assume that an author who obviously writes to fill a niche in the book market must simply be a hack, with no motivation other than making a living. But of course authors did not generally make a living at all from their work in the sixteenth century, not even the hacks, as the career of Thomas Churchyard amply demonstrates. The role of the translator is not always, as is generally assumed, that of the literary hack but, to an extent not fully realized, that of literary and linguistic innovator and pioneer. They set standards, even though these may not always meet with professional approval, and provide in some instances an ideal of language and rhetoric at which to aim, and indeed aimed at it themselves—at least the literary translators did. While the translators of staple, technical, and other non-literary texts were less obviously motivated by ideals, they still provided much raw lexical material for expansion and advance in the language, which they were obliged to assimilate and use in their own texts, a process which set many difficult tasks of selection of appropriate terminology and phrasing. For example, what Latin, Arabic, or Greek medical terminology was to be left in the original, or altered according to the demands of the potential market? The outcome of the myriad decisions of this kind which go to form a text are then disseminated willy-nilly, not so much by earnest literary emulation as by the sharing of common terms and scraps of translated, compiled, and partially plagiarized text through the various reworkings of the material, and the familiarization with terms of both practitioner and client through daily spoken usage. The distinctions between these processes are very blurred, and the commerce between the various workers was easy, being relatively unconfined by appeal to taste and refinement, let alone to copyright. Aesthetic considerations might actually have impeded the process.

Evidence for the views of authors, translators, and compilers of relevant works can normally be expected to appear in prefaces addressed to readers and other prefatory material, or in epilogues. Little appears in the texts themselves, though exceptions do occur. Early medical works, at least up to the 1530s and in many cases later than that, show no interest whatever in linguistic questions. Silence on a subject is of course difficult to interpret, but it is surely reasonable to suppose that writers or indeed publishers who felt a need to apologize for the use of English would at least in some cases actually have done so. One of the earliest printed medical books, the *Governayle of helthe* of 1490(?) (*STC* 12138) has no preliminary matter and nothing to say on the use of English. Neither does the popular and often reprinted *Treasure of pore men* of 1526 (*STC* 24199) a compilation of various remedies. Prefaces are also missing from the *Antidotarius* of 1542 (*STC* 675a) and the translation by J. Drummond (?) of Arnold de Villa Nova entitled *The defence of age and the recovery of youth*, c.1540, (*STC* 777). Two books on the speculation of urine, *The iudycyall of all vryns*, 1525 (*STC* 14836) and *Here begynneth the seynge of uryns*, 1540 (*STC* 22153), are similarly unconcerned about the position of English.[7] Laurence Andrewe's early translation of Hieronymus von Braunschweig's book on distillation likewise has no comment to make on the use of English, let alone suggesting that it is inferior.

It is counter to common sense to suppose that silence means that one and all have made a false assumption about the language when that assumption rests on the evidence from a later period and is unsupported by contemporary views. In any case, early publishers had as keen an eye as any to the whims of the market-place, and would have made whatever cap-doffings were thought necessary. The earliest printed medical works generally have no prefatory material at all, and it is particularly noticeable that this applies to the earliest herbals, the *Grete herball* published in 1526 and in three subsequent editions, as well as to the frequently reprinted herbal published by Banckes in 1525 (*STC* 13175.1, formerly 4720) and to works like the little treatise on the plague of *c*.1485 by Canutus, *Here begynneth a litil boke the whiche traytied many gode thinges for the pestilence* (*STC* 4589).

The problems of finding suitable nomenclature was crucial to the compilers of herbals, and the *Grete herball* of 1526 (*STC* 13176) does assist the reader with a list of 'wordes obscure and euyll knowen' at the end, consisting of eighty-five words, some still in Greek and Latin form, which comprise a little less than one quarter of the total. The rest are anglicized. Thus we find **condilomata**, **serpio**, and **benedicta** alongside **tutie**, **dysentere**, and **appoplexie**. It is characteristic of the function of a herbal at this time that the great majority of these terms are the names of diseases, medicines, or morbid processes. Unfortunately no further explanation for the presence of this list is offered, but it is notable that most of these supposedly ill-known terms are already naturalized, suggesting that the motive might be a perceived lack of erudition in practitioners rather than an inadequate wordstock.[8] What the *Grete herball* does not do is to suggest that new words are still required; the implication presumably is that English has sufficient words, if only they were better understood.

The antecedents of these two herbals are medieval,[9] and it is not until Turner that a genuinely enquiring concern with terminology in herbals appears. Turner is, by contrast with earlier works, forward-looking; he has debts to English nomenclature and the original efforts of sixteenth-century Continental botanists while looking to the development of an adequate vocabulary in the future. In charting the course of the language in this period, a distinction must be made between the legacy of the Middle Ages and the contribution of the Renaissance. The medical lexicon does not undergo a slow awakening from a rustic or medieval slumber. Certainly, deep demands were made upon the native ingenuity of the language in the course of the century to augment its vocabulary, but the view expressed later in the century that the language's resources were inadequate and its position was deteriorating is more likely to have been erroneous. This is not so surprising, since there have always been people only too willing to point out what they suppose to be deficiencies of their own language, whether real or not.

Thus the evidence of the modest early medical works does not on the whole support the conventional modern views on the status and use of English. We must now look in some detail at the more important individuals who actually did comment on the use of English. Often their evidence has not been read sufficiently carefully, and has on occasions been taken to support the accepted hypotheses when it actually does not. They will be dealt with in approximate chronological order of publication of the first work of each author discussed where this is practicable. Neither dates of birth of individual authors nor exact dates of publication of their works are known in a number of cases.

3. THE EVIDENCE FOR INADEQUACY IN PRINTED MEDICAL WRITINGS[10]

Thomas Paynell[11] *(fl. 1528–1567)*

Thomas Paynell's translation of the *Regimen sanitatis Salerni* of 1528 (*STC* 19496) argues that a book is pointless if it is not understood, as well as suggesting that it is to benefit the unlearned that the labour has been undertaken: 'Wherfore I consydryng the frute [tha]t myght come of this boke if it were translated in to the englishe tonge (for why euery ma[n] vnderstandeth nat the latine) I thought hit very expedient at some tymes for the welthe of vnlearned p[er]sones to busy my selfe ther in' (Aiii^r^). But he offers no criticism of English itself, and speaks of the skill not merely of the learned in physic but of those who have come by their knowledge in perhaps less formal ways: 'For lerned p[er]sones and suche as haue great experie[n]ce nede no instructions to diete them selfe nor to conserue theyr helthe' (Aiii^r^). Similarly his translation of Braunschweig's surgery adds no prefatory material except that provided by Braunschweig's original, in which it is argued that the book will help to overcome the prevalence of ignorant practice. The labour has been undertaken 'for the helpe of mankynde' (Aii^r^). The colophon reiterates that the work has been translated 'afterwarde in to our moders tonge of Englysshe moche necessary & profytable for surgyans as wel for the[m] that haue conynge as for the[m] that be lerners' (Tvi^v^).

Paynell's translation of Ulrich von Hutten's work on guaiacum identified two areas which made him pause before accepting the task, since they were likely to be difficult. 'It is in ernest a matter straunge inough to translate, not onely for the names of herbes and other dyuers thynges therin conteyned, but also for the phrase and eloquente style' (Paynell 1533: preface). It is the former which concerns us here, and his difficulty may be partially the result of the then relatively advanced state of herbal and botanical publication and research in Germany. English publishing had not yet felt the influence of the Renaissance in this area. Paynell, already an experienced translator, went on to explain that 'somme wordes haue I lefte barely englyshed, and somme not at al, but they be suche, as are by those names in latine vsually knowen to phisitions'. His text actually reveals only a modicum of such words; e.g. **absinthio** (8^{v}), **mentagrum** (26^{v}), **cassia** (58^{r}), or **Rhenus** (Rhine, 51^{r}), and the general impression is that a great majority found English equivalents or English form in the event. In this, the general sense is that he could have largely agreed about the state of English with the author of the *Grete herball*.

Thomas Moulton

Thomas Moulton's work *This is the myrour or glasse of helthe*, 1539 (*STC* 18214a), for which *STC* suggests a date before 1531, makes the distinction between the learned and the unlearned, but suggests that both may benefit from his translation, this being his only remark on language. He has decided 'to set it in printe so in Englysh that euery man both lerned, and lewde ryche and pore may the better vnderstande it, and do thereafter' (Avi^{r}). This may be authorial arrogance and aggressive marketing, but at least it is not a defensive cringe. He shows no apparent reluctance to include the learned among his intended readership, though how literally such a formulaic phrase may be taken is open to question.

Sir Thomas Elyot (1490?–1546)

In the edition of his well-known work *The castell of helthe*, of 1541 (*STC* 7644), Elyot takes issue with those physicians and others who he claims are upset that he should have written the work. The reasons are, in order, that he is a knight and that to do such a thing is beneath his station, that he has not undergone the full professional training of a doctor, and that he has written the work in English. To this he replies that the ancients wrote in their own tongues and that had they been so jealous of their art as his contemporaries, they would have taken steps to conceal it. This preface is one of the few in which one senses that there really has been criticism: 'Sayth one, syr Thomas Elyot is become a Physition, and wrytethe in phisick, which beseemeth not a knight' (Aii^{r}); but that does not necessarily apply to the defence of using English, which he expresses conditionally: 'But if phisitions be angry, that I haue wryten phisicke in englyshe, let theym remembre, that the grekes wrate in greke, the Romanes in latyne, Auicena, and the other in Arabicke, whiche were their own propre and maternal tonges' (Aii^{r}). Thus the actual criticism concerned his rank and what was a fit occupation for it, while his comment on the ire of physicians is anticipatory.

Andrew Borde (1490?–1549)

Borde's first work is probably *The boke for to lerne a man to be wyse in buyldyng of his howse for the helth of body* of 1550(?) (*STC* 3373), which was succeeded by the *Dyetary of helth* in 1542 (*STC* 3378.5), an expansion of the earlier text. Neither has any comments on language. In his *The fyrst boke of the introduction to knowledge* of 1555(?) (*STC* 3383), not a medical work as such, he shows a considerable and wide-ranging interest in languages, citing smatterings of Cornish, Welsh, Irish, Scots English, 'base Doche', High German, Italian,

Spanish, Latin, Moorish, Turkish, Egyptian, and Hebrew. He cites in addition some verses in the form of a dialogue between an Englishman and a 'Latyn man' which includes these lines from the Englishman:

I am an englyshman latyn welcome to me
In thy tounge I am wel sped & neuer was in thy cou[n]tre
For thou arte indyfferent here and euery place
If a man wyll study and lerne the bokes apace.
Wherfore bitwixt thee & me we wyl haue some alteracio[n]
That vnlerned men may know parte of our intention.

Exactly what he means is not clear. There is no help from *OED* with the obscure sense of **alteration** in this context. Surely the intended meaning is some sense of 'exchange'. Thus it is possible that this is a typographic error for **altercation** which would at least improve the sense a little. The *MED* provides **altercacioun**—'an argument . . . advanced in a disputation', and this seems to be the most likely sense, even though it is a rare one. Possibly the sense of the passage is that a formal disputation between Borde and the 'Latyn man' would, presumably with Borde as the translating intermediary, be of help to the unlearned. In spite of the difficulties, it is at least clear that the passage gives no sense of being unable to achieve this aim with the resources of English; indeed, the implication must be that the outcome of the exchange makes satisfactory sense to all concerned.

The breuiary of helthe of 1552 (*STC* 3374) undertakes to explain to the reader the obscure terms of medical practice, as the title indicates. This promise is expanded upon in the aureate preface: 'olde auncyent, and autentyke auctours, or doctours of Physicke in theyr bokes doth wryte many obscure terms, geuyng also to many and dyuerse infirmyties, darke and harde names, dyffycyle to vnderstande, some and mooste of all beynge Greeke wordes, some and fewe beynge Araby wordes, some beynge Latyn wordes, and some beyng Barbarus wordes. Therfore I haue translated all suche obscure wordes and names into Englysh, that euery man openlye and apartly maye vnderstande them' (Av^{r}). Borde also explains that these terms will be set forth in full alphabetical order. In spite of the obscurity and difficulty of the words to which he refers, he does not suggest that there has been any difficulty in finding translations, that the terms were not available in English, or that the translations would be anything but clear. This method was not new—such a glossary had appeared in Turner (q.v.) and earlier herbals. In this list, cognates and synonyms are given under their respective entry-heads and cross-referenced.

Thomas Phaer (1510?-1560) [Goeurot][12]

In a lengthy preface to *A new booke entyteled the regiment of lyfe*, 1543? (*STC* 11966.5), Thomas Phaer offers us some early and useful comments on translation. First he remarks that he wishes others of his calling to make an effort to spread knowledge, a sentiment which first appeared in Laurence Andrewe. A second occurrence of this view in the first part of the sixteenth century adds some weight to the idea that criticism by the learned might have been to some extent a reaction against such public rebukes. Second, Phaer wishes for a time when matters such as the nature of simples will be clarified. 'I hope to see the time, whan the nature of Simples (whiche haue been hitherto incredibly corrupted) shall be reade in Englishe, as in other languages: that is to saie, the perfect declaration of the qualities of herbes, sedes, rootes, trees, and of all commodities that are here amongest vs, shall bee earnestlie and truely declared, in our owne natiue speche . . . To the whiche I truste all lerned men (hauinge a zeale to the common wealth) will apply their diligent industries' (Aiiii^{r}). There is here a tone of confident assurance, and no suggestion that this 'perfect declaration' is not attainable. The botanical works of Fuchs and Brunfels had already shown the inadequacy of the neoclassical terminology derived from Dioscorides. Phaer is thus a strong advocate of publishing in English.

An addition to the preface appearing in the 1553 edition suggests that Phaer had been under attack since the work was first published. The grounds for this criticism seem, however, to have been his references to ingredients for remedies which could not easily be procured rather than for linguistic impropriety:

> And where [i]n the regiment of lyfe, whiche I translated out of the frenche tonge, hath appeered to some, more curious than needeth, by reasone of the straunge ingredience, wherof it often [tr]eateth: Ye shall know that I haue in many places amplifyed the same, with suche common thynges as may be easyly gotten, to satisfie the myndes of them that were offended. (Av^{r-v})

Richard Jonas [Roesslin]

The care and diligence of translators is stressed in the 1540 translation *The byrth of mankynde* (*STC* 21153) by Richard Jonas, who also calls attention to the enrichment of the language consequent upon their activity. The work by 'Eutharius'[13] which he translated had already been rendered into Latin from the original German, and into some other vernaculars as well (preface, ABii^{v}). He commends his work to common use and especially to the assistance of women in England. The treatises to which he refers are twice called 'proper', and it is certainly not suggested that a vernacular version renders them any less so. Jonas does have something to add concerning the names of diseases using particular terms from Latin and Greek, advising the reader that the apothecary will know them. He refers to these as 'there owne proper names of Greke or laten'. Does he mean that there are no English equivalents or that if there are, that they are not 'proper'? Or is it merely that these names are those which are 'proper' in the tongues and that laymen cannot be expected to be familiar with them? It is certainly the case that apothecaries sometimes used terms not regarded as the correct ones in Latin and Greek.[14] He appears, however, to slide to names for ingredients: 'and they are ... to be had onely at the Apothecaries, beyng of them ryght wel knowen wherfore when ye shal nede any such thyng yf ye sende the same names in your byll to the apothecaries they wyll soone spede your purpose' (Ciii^{r}). Jonas's labours were soon to be revised by Thomas Raynalde.

Thomas Raynalde [Roesslin]

Little is known of Thomas Raynalde, who describes himself as a physician, and who published two works in mid-century, *The byrth of mankynde* 1545 (*STC* 21154), and *A compendious declaration of the excellent vertues of a certaine lateli inventid oile* 1551 (*STC* 20779). He seems to have secured for Merton College, of which he was Warden from 1545 to 1549, the two lectureships in physic bequeathed to the University by Linacre in 1524 (Rolleston 1932: 6), Merton being the college most frequented by medical students. His first book, a treatise on the diseases of women and midwifery, is prefaced by a lengthy self-justification in which he suggests that some will reproach him for writing in English. His reason for this is that the disclosure of these matters might lead to a disrespect or even loathing for women, or perhaps to odious jokes at their expense 'sume alledging that it is shame, and other sume that it is not mete, ne fyttyng such matters to be entreatyd of, soo playnely in our mother and vulgare langage: to the dishonour ... of womanhed, and the derision of their wount secreates' (Ci^v^).

The work is a revision and augmentation of Richard Jonas's translation. The preface, in which Raynalde urges a proper attitude to the subject matter and the essential value of such a work, contains no linguistic arguments, except that he sees good reason why 'this lytell treatyse [should be] made to speake Englysshe, as it hath ben long sith tought to speke dutche, frenche, spanissh, and diuers other langages' (Cviii^r^); neither does he manifest any awareness here of the use of English as an issue—there is simply a job to be done.

The notoriety attendant upon publishing did not seem to affect Raynalde's attitudes in any negative way. His second work exhibits an ebullient confidence in the progress of science generally and of medicine in particular, speaking of 'suche an increase, yea perfection engendred & upsprung' (Aiii^r^). He is very positive about the benefits of publication to all concerned with medicine, looking to a spirit of cooperation and enquiry. There is nothing added here to the question of the use of English, although whether he understood 'one [physician] descanting oppon a nother, to inuestigate and right oute enithing mistaken or mistought by there predicessors: to explicate and cleare thi[n]gs obscureli & darkli bi onother eather throu breuite, orels rudenes, entreatid of before' (Biii^v^) as a virtue of the maintenance of communications in Latin or as a benefit of the influence of the press upon the use of vernaculars remains unclear.

William Turner (15?–1568)

William Turner, who probably took a medical degree at Ferrara and was at one time physician to Protector Somerset, is a crucial figure in the history of the acceptance of English in medical writing in the sixteenth century. His remarks on English need to be understood in the light of his contemporary reputation, and of the significance of his contribution to the botanical lexicon.[15] Apart from anything else, he is the English writer most often alluded to by his contemporaries, and his contribution was acknowledged by them to have been considerable. Though he published works which are rather natural history than medicine, at least to the modern mind, Harrison was moved to describe him as 'the father of English physic' (Harrison 1577/1968: 289).

The preface to his *A new herball* of 1551 (*STC* 24366) anticipates adverse criticism. 'Other will thinke it vnwysely done, and agaynst the honor of my art that I professe, and agaynst the comon profit, to set out so muche knowledge of Physick in English' (Aiii^{r-v}). But this is not intended as a slur on English itself. His reason is that incompetent practitioners might be encouraged by the easy availability of information, and his reply to the accusation is purely practical: that since physicians do not oversee either the apothecaries or the grossers in the collection of simples and preparation of recipes, and since the latter have little or no knowledge of Latin, it is essential that they have guidance to ensure that prescriptions are correctly filled. Opinions of the competence of apothecaries in Latin vary widely. He notes in addition that 'the Physicians of England (sauing very few) committ not [th]e knowledge of herbes vnto the potecary', and names some who he thinks might have made a useful contribution.

In the preface to the 1568 edition, a good deal more is added. It does not agree, however, in all points with the earlier account, seeming also to be wrong in certain matters of fact. Turner claims that he was while still a Fellow at Pembroke [Hall in Cambridge] unable to learn anything at all of the nomenclature of herbs, and also that there was 'no Englishe herbal but one'—but there were in fact two, even though one would not necessarily wish to dispute his claim that they were 'al full of vnlearned cacographies and falselye naminge of herbes' (*ii^{v}). There are some fascinating remarks on his methods and he recounts that he was able to 'learne neuer one Greke, neyther Latin, nor English name, euen amongest the Physiciones of anye herbe or tre' (*ii^{v}). The preface to the earlier edition makes the claim that he was unable to learn anything at all seem extravagant. This amended preface does not contain any further discussion of the status of English.

Turner's abiding concern with terminology emerges, perhaps unexpectedly, in his small, late work on the nature of wines, *A new boke of the natures and properties of all wines commonlye vsed in England* 1568 (*STC* 24360). At one point he takes rather a crude and dismissive swipe at those who prefer to read Galen in the original: 'These wordes peraduenture some learned Gentleman or other learned men, had leuer reade in Greke than in the Latine or rather Englishe alone, for whose sakes I will rehearse *Galens* owne wordes in his owne tongue, that men maye iudge the better of the nature of the wordes, and thereby of Galens meaning' (Ci^{v}). But it is English with which he is mainly concerned. In discussing the nature of wine by taste, he gives a long disquisition on the subject, examining at length the English terms and their Latin equivalents, the nature of dictionary entries, and even calling for the reform of a contemporary dictionary, namely Thomas Cooper's *Thesaurus linguae romanæ & britannicæ* of 1565. His difficulty is that he is unable to find suitable English words: 'What shall we call *acre, austerum* and *acerbum* in common vsed English: surely I cannot tell, for I cannot giue to euery one of these wordes one seuerall used English word, without circumlocution' (Diiii[r]), although not all the examples he cites support this claim. A long explanation and an attempt to construct a suitable dictionary definition follows. Turner obviously spent much time in the classification of plants and in the field identifying them, and it seems likely that the hunt for the correct, or at least commonly used, word also occupied much of his time. It is clear that his efforts were often practical, not merely theoretical.[16] He also claims to have been urged to produce a vernacular work, as Leonhard Fuchs had done, and this advice led to the publication of *The names of herbes in Greke, Latin, Englishe, Duche & Frenche* in 1548 (*STC* 24359), a work which is clearly an interim production. What he does in these works is not to classify in the modern sense, but to fix the names; as he puts it, to finalize his 'iugeme[n]t of the names of so many herbes as I knew' (Aii[v]). A further medical work on 'the great Triacle made by *Andromachus*' is appended to his book on wines, since this little work had apparently been pirated and corruptly printed some years before (Turner 1551: Evi[v]; 1568: *ii[v]). In it he claims to undertake the task since no other Englishman seems willing to do it, in spite of the accounts produced by Italians, Spaniards and Germans (Ev[v]).

Christopher Langton (c.1521–1578)

Christopher Langton is clearly one who would prefer the vernacular to be used. Nevertheless, he does claim that there are deficiencies in the specialist vocabulary and cites a particular instance, the word **cerebellum**, to show that there were cases in which English possessed no appropriate word for a particular medical concept, which he found to be a lamentable want. It seems that he feels the lack of an authoritative precedent for the use of the word. In his *An introduction into phisyke, with an vniuersal dyet* of *c.*1545? (*STC* 15205) he lays the blame for this lack at the feet of his unproductive fellow physicians:

a greate parte of the brayne, whiche the Grecians call /S/παϱεγκεφαλισ/S/ [*sic*], in latyne it is called *Cerebellum*; in oure tungue we haue no propre name for it, whiche I can do no lesse then count the negligence of our Phisitions to be the cause of: for yf they had wrytten of theyr arte in theyr mother tunge, as they do in other places, why shulde we lacke englysh names, more then we lacke eyther Latyn names or Greke names? and yet to saye the truthe, it is better for vs English men to haue English names, then eyther Latyn or Greke. (Diii^{r})

The lack in this case is probably more apparent than real. The *OED* cites 1565 as the earliest instance of the word, but the *MED* provides **cerebellar** from Chauliac, *c.*1425. Thus **cerebellum** probably had been in the language for some considerable time. Langton therefore can be assumed with some confidence to have failed or refused to recognize this term as having 'proper' acceptability in the English lexicon, a phenomenon which it will be suggested was widespread and may lie behind much of the treatment of medical language in the sixteenth century. Similar considerations appear to underlie his remark on the concept of the **master vein**, occasioned by his discussion of the **vena cava**: 'th[e] veyne which is called *Porta*, & also of th[at], that is called *Caua vena*, we haue no names in our tung whych be propre or peculier to them onely, but muste be fayne to call them master veynes, and in dede so that we vnderstande the thynge, it shall make but lytle matter for names' (*IP*, Eiiii^{v}).

OED records **master vein** as early as *c.*1400. Another interesting suggestion is that apart from the terms **chorion** and **secundine**, midwives may have yet another term of their own for this concept. He describes it as 'a crust, not unlike the vtter cote of an egge, whiche the Grekes call /S/χοριον/S/, & in latin is called *secu[n]dine*, or *secu[n]dina*: what oure mydwyues call it I can not tell: howbeit, it may well be called a skin wherein is wrapped th[at] that is co[n]ceiued' (*IP*, Ciiii^{r}). It would have been good to know whether there was another term in use in the jargon of midwives, and to know what it was. More generally, we hardly know whether there was such a jargon at all, since comments about this matter are rare.

Robert Recorde (1512?–1558)

Recorde defends the use of the vernacular at length in the preface to his book on the speculation of urine, *The vrinal of physick* 1548 (*STC* 20817). He distinguishes far more clearly than his contemporaries some of the problems involved in translation, realizing that technical terminology, the syntactic units ('phrase'), and the idioms ('the kindes of speaking') are all distinct, if interrelated, difficulties for the translator:

it is more harder to translate into suche a tonge, wherein the arte hath not ben written before, then to write in those tonges that ar accustomed, and ... acquainted with the termes of the science.
Nother is it so easy a thing ... to translate well. For unles that a man be able to perceyue not onely the wordes, but also the phrase and kyndes of speking of the tong, out of which he doth translate ... he shall not be well able to translate. (Biii[r])

He advances two reasons for writing in English himself. The first is that he is English, and finds it easiest in his own tongue, but this he claims is too easy an excuse, given that to translate from a tongue in which the subject matter is familiar into one where it is not is a difficult matter—the problem is that the language should be 'acquainted with the termes of the science'. This notion requires some further examination. It might mean that the target language ought to have its own set of such terms, or that the set of terms belonging to the tongues should be familiar to the target language and acceptable in it for this purpose. It seems in the context that he means the latter, and there is an assumption therefore that the terms of science are a given for any target language. To put it a little differently: Recorde's use of the article could suggest a set of terms appropriate to the language, or a particular set of terms which any target language would have to find acceptable. The quote below suggests the latter. Thus Recorde appears to imply that the English language is not well acquainted with this set of terms; unlike most of his contemporaries, the difficulty of finding the right medical term in English is a matter of concern to him. He expands on this problem:

I am sure that the true iudiciall of vrines ... is very harde ... partely by cause that sundrie wordes vsed in the same [as in the rest of physicke] ar obscure to them that haue not ben exercysed ... in all kindes of lernynge, and that with the knowledge of both the Greke and Late[n] tonges. (Bv[r])

On the other hand, he seems also to suggest that such Greek and Latin terms are in proper use in English, a point not often acknowledged in the sixteenth century, but one which relates crucially to the way in which non-naturalized terms are used, especially later in the century.

His other reason is that it is desirable to disseminate knowledge as widely as possible. 'What is learnyng vnlearned, or knowledge vnknowne?' He puts forward many examples of other 'learned men' on the Continent who have written in the vernacular, and praises Elyot for his efforts in this direction, for which England must be grateful. But he has little respect for the paltry efforts of the learned physicians of England: 'vnto this day do not lerned wyttes sleepe ... England may reioyce of soch a knyght: yea, England hath to few that foloweth soch example' (Bvi^{r-v}).

He is therefore a strong advocate of writing in the vernacular, while at the same time admitting the superiority of Latin in the medical area when he mentions writing a book 'of the same tytle, but in the Latyn tonge, as more meete for learned eares, & for them that neede more precise iudgment' (Liii^{r}). In this he clearly concedes a greater precision to Latin in specialist terminology.[17]

John Caius (1510–1573)

One of the few writers who did not write primarily in English was John Caius, who was one of the leading physicians of his day, being a court physician, President of the College of Physicians, and a distinguished lecturer to the Barber-Surgeons' company. He preferred using either Greek or Latin to avoid charges of publishing irresponsibly, and to reach a wider audience than was available in English. In his *A boke, or counseill against the disease commonly called the SWEATE* 1552 (*STC* 4343), he exhorts compatriots to follow his example; 'to leaue the simplicite of the same, and to procede further in many and diuerse knowleges bothe in tongues and sciences at home and in vniuersities' (4^{v}) for their own and their country's greater glory. Thus we find an exception to the general trend in the writers we have so far surveyed who use much the same arguments to advance the opposing cause. The present work was written to meet a present need, and to be available immediately and generally to those 'to whom it ... most behoueth to haue spedy remedie' (7^{v}). His view of the usefulness of English is therefore actually much the same as that of many who advocated it against the claims of Latin. Mueller proposes him as an exception for another reason: his Catholicism runs against 'the Protestant tenor of vernacular medical handbooks at mid-century', but, while accepting the continuity of the paradigm of prose composition which leads Mueller to this conclusion, it is not immediately obvious that in his science being a Catholic was of greater weight than being a classically trained professional physician (Mueller 1984: 285).

Nicholas Udall [Geminus] (1505–1556)

In penning the dedication to the surgeons of England which prefaces his translation of Geminus, the *Compendiosa totius anatomie delineato* of 1553 (*STC* 11715.5), Udall makes the claim that the work in hand will benefit the unlatined through the provision of illustrations, and will at the same time improve knowledge of the basis of the art, written as it is by one of 'high learnyng and profound science of naturall thynges' (ded.). Udall suffers no qualms, it seems, like those of Securis (q.v.) and does not fear a falling-off in the process of translation. The preface to the 1559 edition, in Geminus' own voice, claims only to 'make common and familiar to al Englysshe people, that which in the Latine hath byn founde profitable amonge so many foren nations'.

Humfrey Llwyd [Pope John XXI] (1527–1568)

In about 1550 in *The treasuri of helth* (*STC* 14651.5), Humfrey Llwyd drew attention to the problem which had concerned Turner, and also appended a list of words to the end of his work. He distinguished a difficulty in deciding which Latin term is appropriate as the nomenclature for particular plants, attempting to follow the best available precedents. At the same time, he echoed Turner's complaint that English lacked botanical names, and paid his learned predecessor the kind of compliment which physicians would not normally have contemplated bestowing. He wished:

> to set the same furth as truly & as nye the authores mynd as I could, not thynckynge but that there do some faultes remayne therin both because the barbarous and arabicke termes whych the author dothe chyefly vse, and of the dyuerse and sundry opynyons of moyst notable and well lerned Phisicions alswell in the names as in the natures of herbes and symples, and especially that we be eyther ignora[n]t or destytute of Englyshe names for a great sorte of them, yet I dyd as nigh as I could folow Dioscorides and in such thynges as I could not fynd in hym, I dyd confer Fuchsius, Ruellius and Dorstenius together, and folowed [th]e judgement wherein they dyd al or the most part of them agre, and in the Englyshing therof I & al other whych intend any such worke are muche beholden to Mayster Wyllyam Turner, who wyth no small dylygence hath in both hys herballes most truly and syncerly set furth the names and natures of dyuerse herbes, vnto whose iudgement and correccio[n] and all other lerned in the most necessary scye[n]ce of Physycke, do I submyt thys lytle worke (Aii^{v})

The problems are here set out with more than usual clear-sightedness. The use of the word *sincerely* in its contemporaneous sense of properly and without falsification is useful, though it would be nice to know if he had the English and other vernacular names in mind as well. If it is only the Latin ones to which he refers, it is still an advance in nomenclature on his classical and medieval predecessors. Debts to contemporaries are duly noted, and there is in these modest disclaimers a perceptible quickening of critical enquiry.

William Warde (1534–1604?)

In the same year as Llwyd's work appeared, William Warde, the translator of the remedies and formulas of Alessio of Piedmont under the title *The secretes of the reverende Maister Alexis of Piemovnt* (*STC* 293) also argued in favour of rendering foreign works in the vernacular, though his readership is certainly not understood to be a professional one.

> *Scientia non habet inimicum præter ignorantem.* Whiche saiynge (I feare me) is verified more in some of vs Englishe men, than in anye other nation ... And yet I thincke there is no man so bestiall, so rude, or so blunt of wit, but that he is ... desirous to know things not before knowen, to heare newes not before heard, and to vnderstand bokes in his maternall tonge, written first in a forein langage, to thende not to seme altogether ignoraunte in matters both of the liberall sciences ... and specially in Phisick. (+iii^{v})

He proceeds then to inform the reader that this work had already been translated from the original Italian into both French and German ('Dutche'); texts were increasingly being translated from one vernacular to another by this time.

William Bullein (15?–1576)

While William Bullein has no direct addition to make to the question of the use of English, he does provide a snippet or two of circumstantial interest. On one occasion in the work entitled *Bulleins bulwarke of defe[n]ce againste all sicknes, sornes, and woundes* published in 1562 (*STC* 4033) he refers to the difficulty of rendering technical terms into English, mentioning four terms, two of which have been thoroughly naturalized since, **sanies**, **pus**, **virus**, and **sordities**: 'For our Doctors and chief Phisicians saie, there bee fower kindes of matter or *sanies*, whiche the Latines thus terme, and cannot well bee Englished *sanies*, *pus*, *virus*, *sordities* whereof, thei surname them, with like diriued termes', and on another the folly of relying on apothecaries to know the correct Latin and Greek terms for simples;

that is, medicines consisting of one ingredient only, or the individual ingredients of compound medicines (Eeiii$^{r–v}$).

On a third occasion he draws attention to the fact that

Even so be riche also for sicknes, as we doe daiely see, doe not perticulerlie dwell in poore men, but rather generally in al although the kindes of sicknes be variable, and the complexions diuers, and the causes many, and euery sicknes, and sorenes, haue his proper name, although men, either through ignoraunce, shame of crafte doe abuse their names, although the effect doe stille remaine as in clenlie termes by your lisence, thei will call it nothing els, but a sausie flemed face, redde or high coloured, whan many times in deede, it is not onely so, but the verie Leprosie with all. It is nothing saie thei, but breaking out, or paines of the body, weakenesse of limmes, or a grene sicknes, through the obstruccion of the liuer. &c, with soche nicke names, whose very sure name is, the buttens of Napelles, *Gallicus morbus* commonlie called the Frenche poxe. (Bbiii^{v})

In the margin he has, 'Men doe vse pretie termes for foule sores and call them by one name, when thei are an other', but whether he means that they have another name or that they really are some other phenomenon and are misnamed is not clear. The text itself would seem to suggest that incorrect diagnosis is what is at issue.[18] But the context is problematical. The use of the word 'cleanly' suggests that it is the elegance of the word which commends it to those who abuse such terms, and that Bullein is being ironic at their expense. He seems to be objecting to a wrong diagnosis rather than an unsatisfactory term for the same disease. Both **leprosy** and **sawcefleme** are historically equally technical in application, and both are naturalized terms.

Thomas Gale (1507–1587)

Gale was one of the first English surgeons to go into print on his own account, and probably the first to attempt a complete method for the discipline in English. His large, four-part textbook appeared in 1563 under the general title *Certaine workes of chirurgerie* 1563 (*STC* 11529). The lack of learned Englishmen willing to publish is noted in a dedicatory letter by the physician William Cunningham, who takes up the cudgels against the reproaches of those who 'be … arrogant & loiter in idlenes' (Aiiii^{r}). He is at pains to note his friend's assiduity in reading his surgical sources, and concludes that 'I dare bouldlye affyrme, that neuer in Englishe was so perfite workes in Chirurgerie set out' (Av^{v}). He goes to some length to point up the particular merits of Gale's work. But his complaint is essentially Laurence Andrewe's: the English language community simply lacks people like Gale to set about the work.

Gale also puts the practical argument that the language is actually not relevant, serving simply to facilitate learning the skills. It does not matter, therefore, whether the text is in Latin or English. This argument is taken up by Clowes as well (q.v.). Gale also argues that experience is essential to making a competent surgeon, not merely book learning. 'It doth manifestly apeare by Galen, that the tongues maketh not an Artist, but reasonable knowledge being ioyned with experience, maketh the Artist.' At the same time, he wants surgeons to understand the tongues, because in the past those who did have been more industrious '& careful to further their common welthes in those countries, then they be in ours, by meanes whereof they haue brought many noble Artes into their owne tongues, which we haue not so largely set forth in our English tongue.' (Aiiii^{v}, 1586 ed.)

In the second part of the work, the *Enchiridion*, Gale pauses to explain the fact that while the text is in English, the recipes are in Latin. This is possibly the lengthiest explanation of this practice from the period, advancing two reasons. His first, the deficiency in the language most discussed by medical writers in the mid-sixteenth century, recalls the difficulty faced by the botanists: 'we cannot aptly giue all these simples Englyshe names ... for as much as herbes and other symples are called by dyuers names, accordyng to the use of the countrye in oure Englyshe tounge that they growe in' (Hv^{v}). It is important to note the distinction between the generalized critiques that were frequently offered and the very particular difficulty which is discussed here, stemming from dialectal diversity. The latter we can discuss with much more confidence than the former, for which convincing evidence is hard to come by. The regional variation in terminology had also been noted by Turner.

Gale's second reason is again a pragmatic one: it will force students to learn sufficient Latin; 'it shall cause you to vnderstande your recepts or medicines in the Latyne tounge, not onely by the vse of compositions but the symples also' (Hv^{v}). He takes it for granted that apothecaries will assist in this teaching in the process of filling orders, a confidence not universally shared, as we have seen. Gale also pays considerable attention to the uncertain nomenclature, not only of simples, inherited from his sources. The question recurs in dedicatory poems prefacing three of the four parts of the work. He took the matter of simples very seriously, declaring his intention, ultimately unfulfilled, to produce a herbal 'with manye other simples appertaynynge to the arte of chirugerie' (Hv^{v}), and to give names both in English and 'all other tounges.' We will presumably never know how substantial his progress towards this goal had been.

John Securis

Securis, in his attack on the contemporary abuses in medicine, *A detection and querimonie of the daily enormities co[m]mitted in physick* 1566 (*STC* 22143), asks of those who abuse the profession, 'Where is their great and manifold knowlege of the tounges' (Avii^{r}), putting the answer into their own mouths: 'Syr although we haue not this exquisite knowledge that you require in vs, yet we haue had experience of many thinges, we haue Englishe bokes enough to teach vs diuers medicins for diuerse purposes' (Avii^{v}). His answer to this is that 'the englishe bookes teacheth nothinge of the trewe foundation of Phisicke. For if there be any that doo it, howe can it be well vnderstanded without logike and naturall philosophie' (Bi^{r}). His complaint appears to be that English books are not supported by the theoretical superstructure required to understand medicine. 'I doo not denye but to haue some bokes of phisicke in englyshe specially of the Simples, well and cunnyngly set foorthe for Surgeons, Apothecaries, yea and for sober and wyse men, that delite to reade in suche thynges, and know not the Latine tongue, is not vnmete nor hurtefull' (Bi^{v}).

There are limits, however, to the amount and kind of learning available through this medium. 'Doo you thynke to haue in youre Englyshe Bookes, all the perfecte knoweledge that is required in Physicke? ... We coulde neuer have it yet in Greke and Latine perfectly (not wythstandynge we haue it nowe better then euer we hadde afore) howe thenne should you haue it?' (Bii^{r}). Thus his view is that medical knowledge itself is imperfect, and the state of understanding of the classical texts is imperfect. The fitness of English itself is not mentioned.

*John Jones (*fl. c.*1565–1580)*

John Jones was an engaging figure, about whom very little is known. It is recorded that he studied at both universities, and seems to have practised in Bath, Nottingham, and near Derby.[19] Widely read, and of a catholic interest in contemporary affairs, he stands apart from most of his colleagues in writing two works on spas, Buxton and Bath—he shared an interest with Turner in these, as well as having a high regard for him. He also wrote a treatise on fevers, and a curious last work which is a kind of physical and spiritual *regimen sanitatis* for the rearing of children. His work on the waters at Bath, *The bathes of bathes ayde* 1572 (*STC* 14724a.3), had nothing on the use of English in the prefatory matter. He was nevertheless aware of the deficiency in published works in English in this particular area and remarks that 'there is not one that hath written of ours in England, Brytayn, sauing Doctor Turner' (Ai^{r}), who had in Jones's view provided only a superficial account.

His treatment of recipes does add a little to what we have previously seen. He does not share Gale's confidence in the linguistic abilities of apothecaries, and makes a point of putting recipes in both languages 'for the Apotecaries, in English, for your better vndersta[n]ding.' (Hii^{v}). He sets out the two side by side in the text. Names of specifics in the text are frequently in English.

The preface to the book on Buxton, *The benefit of the auncient bathes of Buckstones* 1572 (*STC* 14724a.7), comments that there are those who 'suppose knowledge nothinge worthe vttered in their own language' (*iii^{v}). Jones replies that a thing presented plainly and without obscurity is a far better means of instruction, and uses the argument employed by Elyot that the ancients wrote in their own native tongues and that had they desired obfuscation they would have invented a secret code or language (McConchie 1987: 7–8). 'I would haue them to reme[m]ber . . . whether their own familiar spech . . . or the Romains be better, & easyer, too Judge of' (*iiii^{v}). Jones revives the kind of argument met much earlier in Norton's *Ordinal of Alchemy* (Norton, *c.*1477, 6).[20] It is best that the matter should be put as plainly and succinctly as possible. This is far from claiming that English ought to be more elegant, and the anxiety that the language may lack terminology seems to be far from Jones's mind:

> If the phrase be best that is most playn, the[n] this is not worst. If the style or endyting be best which co[n]tinueth the matter: then this is not vtterly to bee disallowed. In fyne, if the mother tongue be most meete for hir own children, and easyest to be vnderstanded, then this in our own, you will affirme, is not to bee abandoned. (*iiii^{v})

His first work, *A dial for all agues* 1566 (*STC* 14726), contains the observation that the world is already overstocked with books in all languages: 'the worlde is pestered not onely with a superfluous plenty of ... treatises'; he is also sure that many 'perceaue and inwardly bewaile this insaciable gredines of writing and printing' (Aviii^{r}). Much of it he sees as unworthy trash, and he trusts that the worthwhile will eventually supplant the trivial. Throughout his preface he consistently offers glosses of foreign quotes and words, including triple glosses, which anticipates the methods used by Phillip Barrough.[21] He is also one of the first to record that many people had already written in English to the credit of their country. Galen and the rest wrote for the common good, and so should Englishmen. 'Why shall we so imbase the laude of our language,' he asks (Ci^{r}). The argument of Mulcaster concerning the nature of language is also anticipated. Knowing Greek and Latin does not in itself assure skill in physic: 'the perfectnes in Artes is the cause of cunning as maye appeare very well by infinite number that can speake Hebrue, Greke, Latine, &c. yet no Poetes, Deuines, Lawiers, nor Phisitions' (Ci^{v}). It is the particular body of knowledge which is crucial, not the language. It might also be added that Jones is among a very few physicians who obviously read copious amounts of the medical writings in his own tongue. His advocacy of what we would now agree to call professional training is also apparent throughout.[22] Further evidence of his linguistic concerns appears in his allusion to a 'compe[n]diu[m] of myne Anotamy which sheweth [th]e greke termes, Arabick, Latine and Englysh, of al the whole body' (Hviii^{v}–Ii^{r}). Jones's *Anatomy* is presumably a fine idea like Gale's *Herbal*, but either was never completed or has been lost. The Peroration touches our subject briefly, to encourage those who can to read further in the tongues, since the present work is compendious and the matter available elsewhere so vast.

That Jones's interest in these matters was more than merely professional is demonstrated in the preface to his final work, *The arte and science of preseruing bodie and soule in healthe, wisdome and catholique religion* 1579 (*STC* 14724). It also suggests his awareness of a native tradition both in utilitarian prose as well as literature. At this late stage of his career, he seems to have veered into the camp of those wholly opposed to borrowing and neologizing. He upbraids:

> some other that seeme to write as they knowe in their proper tong Englishe, and yet their termes must be altogether forsooth in Latin and Greeke, or in some other forraine speach, as though our la[n]guage could not comprehend so muche as their fresh wittes can discourse, or that truth cannot be

deliuered but in vnknowen words and terms far fet, clean contrarie not onlye to the iudgemente of our Elders, but also to the beste of oure dayes, as in the skilfull workes of oure countreymenne, *Chaucer*, *Gowre*, *Surrey*, *Cheeke*, *Chaloner*, *Recorde*, *Phaire*, *Wilson*, *Iewel*, *Dee*, *Digs*, *Fox*, *Holenshead*, &c. . . . is apparent. (Bi^{r})

He makes no particular complaint about specialist medical terminology, nor alludes to the special role of the tongues in providing such terminology. There seems to be a presumption that English terminology is quite sufficient for his purpose. Phaer and Recorde, the two medical writers mentioned, are apparently praised for the relative purity of their diction. The particularly eclectic collocation of literary figures, historians, scientists, and grammarians which he cites seems to suggest a view of staple English prose as competent in various fields.

John Banister (1533–1610)

Banister was a significant contributor to the medical literature of the last quarter of the sixteenth century, publishing works in 1575, 1578, and 1589. His first work, *A needefull, new, and necessarie treatise of Chyrurgerie* 1575 (*STC* 1360), has little to say on the subject of English, although a lengthy dedicatory epistle deals with detractors, especially those who practise physic. In the epistle to the Company of Surgeons his complaint is rather that it is pointless to reveal the mysteries of the art when the activities of quacks are so damaging to its reputation.[23] He does contribute a list of simples appended to the work, in which they are listed first under a Latin name and then, in the majority of cases, under an English cognate or translation, **ambra–amber**, **cherifolium–cheruell**, etc., along with some explanation of the nature of the ingredient. The qualities of each are listed in a separate appendix, a typical entry being '*Acorus*, Gladin, hot and drie in the third degree, resolutiue'. These lists are only loosely alphabetical, by first letter only, and the latter does not list English equivalents. There are some in the first list which do not have them either; e.g. **camepitheos**, **filipendula**, **nux indica**. Unfortunately, he offers no explanation for the appearance of these lists, and we must deduce what we can from their character.

His second work, the substantial *The historie of man*, 1578 (*STC* 1359), which is an anatomy, is declared to be 'sucked from the sappe of the most approued Anathomistes, in this present age' (title-page), and his announced reason for undertaking this work on surgery is that 'no English Author, which hitherto hath written, hath sufficiently applyed his tyme to the amendement therof' (Aiiii^{r}). In the dedication, he launches into an extraordinary attack on his critics in a passage replete with biblical allusion and hence fulsome self-righteousness. His foes, the 'Impes of Hell . . . [who] . . . deuoure the sheepe of Gods pasture', have apparently forced him to compromise:

> If therefore I haue any where frequented a phrase aboue the common vse of our Englishe language, or vsed woordes litle different from the Latin, esteeme the same to be done onely for your cause, since ... I haue endeuoured euery where, to shade the kernell with a harder shell then you shalbe able to cracke (Bi^{r})

and it seems that this is at worst a reluctant concession and at best an instance of *litotes*. There is also some praise in a dedicatory poem from his friend William Clowes for writing in English and not bothering to address the learned. There is, however, no more than this on the subject of the English language in the prefatory material. In the text itself there is a suggestion that he regards some of his fellow English surgical authors as particularly lacking in the tongues, and hence in appropriate knowledge, this accusation probably being well-founded. He speaks of Englishmen who might object to his omitting certain information on the grounds that 'our meaner sort of Chirurgians, who are not able to dispence with the Latine Author, haue learned to many such phantasticall imaginations of sundry Englishe workes, which heretofore haue bene Imprinted', and he recommends that they should have 'sweat more in the workes of *Gal.*' (Oiii^{v}), even if he was not always correct. Banister also shows, as others had done, that the attitudes expressed to neoclassical terms were not always approving. He notes that the names for the articulation of bones are confused and disordered: 'you shall commit vnto your memory, a word or two of the maner how mans body is construed, and combinated, as touchyng the frame and *articulation* of bones: as also of the straunge, and diffused names, wherewith their kindes of knittynges, in eche respect are nominated' (Ciii^{r}). Ignorance is obviously objectionable in whatever language. His objection is not, however, to English works as such, but to those which are ill-informed and misleading.

The last work, his *An antidotarie chyryrgicall, containing great varietie and choice of all sortes of medicines* (*STC* 1358), adds nothing new, at least not in Banister's own voice. There is a good deal of attention paid to the carpers, especially once again in the dedicatory epistle by Clowes, who suggests 'impropernesse of the phrase . . . inckhorne termes, or some imperfection for want of knowledge in tongues' (A3^{v}) as reasons for adverse criticism. This is one of the rare references by medical writers to inkhornisms, indeed to matters of style generally, but since inkhornisms are hardly the besetting sin of the medical literature of the time, one wonders whether this has been picked up in an unconsidered way from more obviously literary circles. Another dedicator, the surgeon William Goodrus, also takes up the well-worn theme of detraction, but offers nothing on linguistic matters. Clowes suggests with characteristic acerbity that 'too much frequenting the hot-house, hath sweat out all their wittes' (A3^{v}). He also hints that they did sometimes commit themselves to print in his reference to their 'rotten and confused pamphlets' (Ai^{v}).

There is in none of this any substantial evidence for the argument that English is by nature inadequate as a medium of use in medicine, although the carpers themselves may have said as much. The views expressed both pro and con are extraneous: a want of style, lack of argument, the dangers of half-baked practitioners, and so forth do not bear materially on the linguistic question. Banister's attack on his detractors may actually arise from such criticism, but the welter of argument *ad hominem* hardly permits us to draw such a conclusion confidently. The appendix of the names of simples in the *Treatise* might seem to suggest a lack, but in the absence of comment by the compiler, it may equally well be for the convenience of apothecaries who needed to interpret Latin terms, rather than as a conscious attempt to make up deficiencies in the vernacular. As it is set out, it is a translation table, not an encoding device.

Henry Lyte (1529?–1607)

Henry Lyte, translating Rembert Dodoens' herbal from French (the original was written in Dutch) as *A nieuue herball, or historie of plantes* 1578 (*STC* 6984), remarks that some may reprehend its being in English, suggesting that personal gain or a sense of superiority may cause such dislike: 'neither thinke I, that any will mislike or repine thereat, except such, as either envie the Weale of others whom they accompt simpler then them selves, and therfore recken vnworthy to be in their language made partakers thereof: or els are so studious of their owne priuate gaine, that they feare, least by this meanes some parte therof may be lessened' (*iii^{r}). The tacit assumption seems to be that one's own language is perfectly adequate, since otherwise the medical knowledge it contains could not be acquired, or become the object of envy; the sense that the learned practitioner who thus repines is superior is presumably largely social and economic rather than linguistic in this case.

William Clowes (1544–1604)

Clowes published a treatise on syphilis (**morbus gallicus**) in 1579, *A short and profitable treatise touching the cure of the disease called (Morbus Gallicus) by unctions* (*STC* 5447), though he appears to have completed, and perhaps published, an earlier version of this tract about 1576.[24] In the prefatory remarks, Clowes offers us no views at all on the propriety of writing in English, which is taken for granted. Whereas in 1579 he had felt the need to enlist George Baker in justifying his use of quicksilver to the world, in the 1585 edition he now appends not only his defence of the use of English,[25] but also an epilogue by another surgeon, William Pickering, who takes up this theme as well. Clowes had earlier roundly attacked a foreign quack, Valentine Rasworm, who 'in most shameful sorte abused [th]e Queenes Maiesties good subiects' (Cii^{r}). In the 1585 version, *A briefe and necessarie treatise*, Clowes upbraids those who took offence at 'so simple a treatise, & so obscure a writer' (Liii^{v}), and who 'myslike, not onely that this Pamphlet, but any other worke of Phisicke or Surgery should be penned in the English tongue' (Liiii^{r}). Perhaps these were the friends of the reviled Rasworm. Certainly Clowes was attacked on purely medical grounds, probably by those who opposed the use of quicksilver and who also 'laboured to deface this maner of cure, as dangerous & vnsufficient' (Liii^{v}), but it is now impossible to know whether those who did so found the dispute over English merely a convenient additional stick with which to beat him. The concerted defence seems to suggest a serious attack, but it is worth noting that this and the prefaces by Elyot and Phaer are the only instances so far identified where a specific attack on the author can with any confidence be assumed to have taken place. What form these might have taken remains unknown.

Thus stung, Clowes lists those medical writers of his acquaintance who have furthered learning in English with whose work he was presumably familiar. The list is a compendium of sixteenth-century medical authors, those 'many notable men [who] haue written sundrie kindes of learned workes in English, their naturall language'.

He cites Gale as having argued that knowledge may be communicated in any language: 'And therefore was it wiselie sayd of our Maister *Gale*: In what tongue so euer a man may get knowledge, the tongue serueth no further, but to the learning of the art.' He names Phaer, Turner, Langton, Borde, Bright, Gale, Hawle,[26] Baker, Banister, Eliot, Treheron, Lyte, Barrough, and Bullein, and suggests that these are but a selection (Liiii^{v}). He finds it reprehensible that such authors should only receive 'churlish vpbraiding' for having published in English.

This represents a considerable list of supporters. It is also an unprecedented acknowledgement of intellectual debt in this time and on this subject, as well as suggesting that those who do not write in their own language are, in the face of so extensive a list, simply out of touch with their times. A similar spirit of learned enquiry prompts his declaration in 1588 that should anyone undertake to better what he has done he 'will ... be thankefull to God that it hath pleased him to make my simple Booke the cause of the publishing of any learned worke' (Clowes 1588; Epistle to the Reader);[27] moreover, a rare glimpse of a more sceptical and progressive scientism intrudes into an attack on those who had recently denigrated traditional methods: 'truth is truth from whome so euer it come, be it from *Hipocrates*, *Galen*, *Paracelsus*.' He suggests that the detractors examine the works produced by 'our late London English writers', claiming that they will find them competently professional (Ai^{r}).[28] In confirmation of Clowes's generally progressive outlook, his friend John Banister, in his Epistle to the Reader, points out that, against the traditional garnering of secrets he is able to 'testify that you haue concealed nothing from the reader' (Biii^{r}).

It is also plain that Clowes had in fact read Gale (q.v.) with approval. Gale's comment in his *Certaine workes of Galens* (*STC* 11531) that language, no matter which one, will serve the scholar no further than what is actually read—'it serueth him no more but for the further vnderstanding of that thing which he doth read' (Aiii^{v}–iiii^{r})—is obviously echoed by Clowes in his *A briefe and necessarie treatise* of 1585 (*STC* 5448). Knowledge of the tongues in itself does not make a man a physician, or in Gale's words 'the tongues maketh not an Artist (Aiiii^{v}, 1586 edn.).

Timothy Bright (1551–1615)

The particular interest in linguistic matters evidenced in Bright's

Characterie. An arte of shorte, swifte, and secrete writing by character of 1588 (*STC* 3743) is not obvious in his English medical works. In his second English treatise, on melancholy, as much is revealed by the confident tone of his address to the dedicatee as by what he actually says. There is no hint of self-defence, only a modicum of self-deprecation and the choice of language seems a matter of convenience; that is, a decision not made in spite of a sense of compromised standards. Indeed to do anything else seems to him pretentious:

> I write it in our mother tongue that the benefit (how small soeuer it be) might be more com[m]on, & as the practise of all ancient philosophers hath bin to write in their own language their precepts, whether concerning nature, or touching maners of life, to the end their country me[n] might reape the benefit with more ease, and seeke rather for sound judgement of vnderstanding, the[n] for vaine ostentatio[n] of strange tongues. (*iii^r)

In embracing English, Securis and Phaer had been rather shrill by comparison with Bright's almost bland assurance. One is made to feel comforted that the arguments have already been won. Bright then adds the revealing suggestion that the 'vaine ostentatio[n] of strange tongues' has appeared elsewhere; it is a manner which 'is also after a sort followed in translations'. Even more tantalizingly, this was one of the few passages altered in the second edition of the work where it reads 'also allowed in translations'.[29] The change to a more confident assertion looks deliberate. Although it not now possible to know to what stylistic excesses he refers, the reasonable assumption is that translators, as in the known cases of Llwyd and Paynell, borrowed terms directly from their originals; but whether this was to impress the readership or to make up deficiencies in the language is not wholly clear. On the whole the lack of comment on stylistic matters in our authors would suggest the latter. It does seem less likely that Bright could have been referring to the words already well known to physicians which Paynell mentions. Thus it seems that he had recent coinages or borrowings in mind. His other works, *A treatise: wherein is declared the sufficiencie of English medicines* 1580 (*STC* 3750) and *A treatise of melancholie* 1586 (*STC* 3747), add nothing of interest, apart from the general suggestion that Bright's outlook was decidedly patriotic.

Other authors and works

There were many other writers on medicine in the latter half of the century who had nothing or very little to contribute. These include

Thomas Cogan, author of the *Hauen of health* of 1584 (*STC* 5478), a dietary; Walter Cary's *A briefe treatise called Caries farewell to physicke* 1583 (*STC* 4370), the anonymous translator of Fuchs in *A worthy practise of the moste learned phisition L. Fuchsius* 1563 (*STC* 11408), John Partridge in *The widowes treasure* 1582 (*STC* 19433.2), A. Hunton, the translator of Guillemeau's treatise on the eyes, *A worthy treatise of the eyes* 1587(?) (*STC* 12499), R. Surflet, who translated another French work on the same subject, *A discourse of the preseruation of the sight* 1599 (*STC* 7304), and the anonymous discourse on scurvy, *A profitable treatise of the scorbie* 1587(?). Among authors with nothing of significance to say on our subject and generally very little else in any case is Henry Wingfield. Neither is much added by Mosan's translation of Christopher Wirzung, but the preface acknowledges that much has already been done by various translators, and that their labours thus imitate the efforts of the ancients in providing for the common weal. There is a little added by Phillip Barrough in *The methode of physicke* 1583 (*STC* 1508), to the effect that he anticipates criticism from colleagues who will castigate him for the use of 'so base a tongue' as English, but he goes on to claim that many write in English as well as other vernaculars, and that some works have been translated from vernaculars (he mentions French and Italian) into Latin to ensure wider dissemination (*v[v]). A number of other works by the authors already individually dealt with in the above have been read, but they also yielded nothing of interest.

The translator of Gabelkhover's *The boock of physicke* 1599 (*STC* 11513) and Guillemeau's *The french chirurgerye* 1597 (*STC* 12489), known to us only by his initials, A.M., is especially apologetic in his prefaces, apparently because he was not English himself. All the deprecatory remarks about rude style and other infelicities are personal. In fact, although there are some awkwardnesses in his work, the most obvious characteristic of his English is the command of a considerable vocabulary of a somewhat pedantic kind. Examples are **perpolite**, **ebulliated**, **cenation**, **floscles**, and **supranominated**. He does at least indicate that Guillemeau had written with students of surgery in mind rather than the learned, but the overwhelming impression is of the translator's own anxiety (ep. ded.). Thus he contributes nothing to our debate.

John Cotta makes it clear that his book on medical abuses, *A short discoverie of the unobserved dangers of severall sortes of ignorant practisers of physicke* 1612 (*STC* 5833), is intended for the general reader, and, without adversely reflecting upon English, indicates the kind of register which he has employed:

For the meanest readers sake (whom in this whole worke I labour equally to obserue) I haue suited the plainnes and simplicitie of a familiar style: and for facilitie of common reading haue also smoothed and cleared the streame and current of this little volume, from the stops and interrruptions of vnusuall sounds and language (as farre as the subiect will permit) refreshing onely the learned in the margine. (To the Reader, A3^{v})

While the great majority of his marginalia are in Greek and Latin, placed there, as he says, for the purpose of 'refreshing onely the learned', there are a few in English as well, e.g. 58–9. He is clearly aware that there are limits to the simplification of medical language. He also was concerned at the profusion of books on the subject, and their effect in promoting abuse of professional practices:

And hereby may be iudged and discouered the indiscreete thoughts of light braines and vnderstandings in these dayes, of men, that so preposterously diuulge in all places so many bookes and paper-Apothecary-shoppes of secretes and medicines, better iudgement and learned soath teaching the wise and discreete, that things without reason in themselues are by reason and wisedome to be guided and ordered; lest in ignorant handling and vnwotting abuse their faire promising seemings proue gilded poysons. (23–4)

4. DISCUSSION

A preliminary difficulty in understanding the foregoing survey is to free one's view from the many preconceptions imposed by literary scholarship and by the many contemporaneous comments on the language by its literary authors. The first thing to notice is that the criteria which were applied in that field do not necessarily apply to medicine. Our assumptions incline to over- or misinterpret remarks found in medical texts. What our survey actually indicates is that there is little general criticism of English and its status or fitness in the first half of the century, even though the majority of these commentators were translators and compilers who would naturally have had a vested interest in the promulgation of the vernacular. But this interest did not apparently move them to offer much by way of self-justification, and there are, especially early, many translators who did not choose to comment on the rationale for their work; not that they had no precedents for such comment, since Caxton (to take an instance) had added lengthy prefaces to his early translations, and one might have expected a specialist area such as medicine to have provoked interest in the problem. Some of them, while taking up the subject, have nothing pejorative to say about the language. There is very little to suggest that these early sixteenth-century authors felt the inadequacies of the language; indeed, there is some evidence that they felt comfortable with it.

Changes in attitude begin to appear in the 1530s, and the matter of nomenclature begins to assume importance. Such criticism as there is from this time concerns the specialist vocabulary available to the language rather than the language more generally. By now it is the specialist lexicon of medical science which commands the attention of authors such as Moulton, Paynell, Turner, Recorde, and Llwyd, especially the language of botany as we have seen. Those who consistently identify a problem are compilers of herbals and the few who prepared word-lists. They point out particular deficiencies in the naming of medical phenomena, especially herbs, but there is really not much more worth comment up to the completion of the first three-quarters of the century.

At that point, another shift in attitudes emerges. This time general complaints about the status of English, not restricted to lexical matters but concerning the unworthiness of the language in comparison with the tongues, its inability to convey scientific knowledge, and the inappropriateness of its use, begin to be widely voiced.

There is a perceptible drift in the complaints of the translators. Early on they are concerned with obscure words for the most part naturalized in English. By the mid-century they are more interested in the problems of translating specialist medical terms, specifically for diseases and for herbs. Complaints are not directed to other parts of the lexicon. There is no reference to the idea of borrowing words. Was this because these words were already felt to be a part, if not a 'proper' one, of the language's lexicon, or was it that learned physicians maintained knowledge of a lexicon which could never be thought to be 'proper' in English? As the century proceeded, complaints became more generalized and more frequent. Failure to contemplate borrowing or neologism is interesting, given their long recognition in other areas of the language. This does suggest that practical recognition was given to encysts, those words used in the language but not fully incorporated into it,[30] but that very status led to public denials of the legitimacy of these words.

Thus the voices raised against the English language are for the most part those of the mid- and late century, but once again scholars have failed sufficiently to appreciate the evidence before them. Thus Barber is able to write that 'by the end of the sixteenth century, uncomplimentary comparisons of English with other languages have largely disappeared', when this patently did not apply to the medical professions, in which such protestations had greatly increased (Barber 1976: 76). It seems that the changes to the lexicon actually preceded the perception of the need for them, and the criticism of its inadequacies. This phenomenon is not, I suspect, confined to the late sixteenth century.

It also seems perverse, therefore, to maintain with Jones that translators were almost to a one deluding themselves about the serviceability of English in the first three-quarters of the century. The evidence of those who published must be supposed to mean that English was genuinely felt not to present a problem to the translator. If it is assumed that early in the century English was correctly thought by its users to be an adequate vehicle for use in science, many obstructive difficulties are resolved.

Some perceived that certain words might be difficult to understand or to translate, but this was not always seen to be due to the shortcomings of English. The difficulties were also those presented by the terms in the source languages themselves, and in the opacity of the specialist lexicon in whichever language it was to be found. It seems better to suggest that the earlier sixteenth century had not made fallacious assumptions about the capabilities of the language, and that those who fell upon its perceived shortcomings after 1575 were discussing their own English as they understood it, not that of their predecessors. They do not advert (and why should they?) to the English of previous generations. They were not interested in a historical view of the recent development of the English lexicon.

The bar to the transmission and comprehension of texts might have been either of two extralinguistic phenomena: the lack of translations, or the inability of readers to comprehend those which were provided. Neither of these is in the strict sense a linguistic problem. If there really was a bar which probably did not consist in the nature of the language itself, what then was the real problem? A simpler explanation of the apparent contradictions is to hand, as has been shown in the case of the medical texts.

Three possible solutions are suggested here which need not be mutually exclusive. First, that the bar was not, as already suggested, as obviously a linguistic one as has been thought, being at least partially an educational and social one. Second, that insufficient allowance has been made for shifts in the views of those actually doing the translation and compilation in the course of the sixteenth century, some of which have been discussed here. It can now be seen that most adverse criticism of English was a late sixteenth-century phenomenon, and that its occurrence was by no means uniform throughout the century. The third suggestion is that English found itself in a very different position in the last quarter of the sixteenth century to that which it had occupied at the beginning. The extra-linguistic environment had not remained static, and there is other evidence than writing and publishing to suggest the magnitude of the change. The academic environment was also beginning to feel the temper of the age.

The shift in the course of the century to the use of the vernacular emerges not only in the appearance of many texts in English but also strikingly in the proposals put forward by Sir Thomas Gresham and by the adventurer Humphrey Gilbert for the establishment of academies (Gilbert 1898). Gresham's college did, of course, actually come to fruition. He endowed lectures in physic and surgery in both English and Latin. Gilbert's unfulfilled proposals are rather more radical. He suggests that the Orator of his Academy should conduct his exercises in English, citing Cheke in support of this proposal. It is argued that 'in what language soeuer learninge is attayned . . . by such exercizes learning shall haue brought vnto yt the Choyse of wordes, the building of sentences, the garnishmente of figures, and other beautyes of *Oratorie*' (2). He also suggests that the lecturer in physic and surgery should likewise teach in the vernacular. There is no suggestion that these lectures should be paralleled by a set in Latin as in Gresham's establishment. But it is to be noted that by the time of Gresham and Gilbert the vernacular was well on the way to predominance in scientific writing.

Further advances in the scientific thinking of the day are indicated by Gilbert's demand that no reader in medicine should recommend a remedy without accounting for the '*reason philosophicall* of euery *particuler ingredience*' (5), as well as his injunction to experiment and to report the findings of this research annually. More appositely to our own investigations, he insists that this should be done 'without *Equiuocac[i]ons* or *Enigmaticall phrases*' (6). Although he does not mention it specifically, there is no reason to suppose that such a report should not be made in English and, this being so, what he points out as a flaw is the tendency to high-sounding circumlocution and verbal obfuscation certainly noticeable in the texts of the day.

We should also look at the role played by the three main branches of the medical profession in the formation of attitudes to the use of the vernacular, and to their actual practices. It has previously been noted that there was a difference between physicians and surgeons in these respects, but the evidence from the presses has not always been rightly assessed. We need to look again at the view that physicians were generally unproductive, first of all to see what they actually did do, and also to compare what they did in Latin with what they achieved in the vernacular. Comments such as Antonia McLean's 'Although most physicians wrote in Latin if they wrote at all, there were one or two conspicuous exceptions in the Tudor period' turn out to be rather misleading (McLean 1972: 192). In fact her exceptions are more than one or two, since Borde, Recorde, Turner, and Caius are all discussed, and Phaer is mentioned as well, but this fact seems to show an unwillingness to admit in the face of the evidence that a majority, even in the first half of the century, published in English, and a minority in Latin.[31]

One would certainly expect many physicians, given the nature of their training, to have had a career as an author somewhat like that of Linacre, who wrote in Latin, or Caius, who wrote one of his works in English, or perhaps John Case, an Aristotelian scholar and commentator who was admitted MD in 1589 (*Ath. Ox.* 259), none of whose works was published in English. But our evidence suggests otherwise, in that the average physician in England was loath to publish at all, and most of those who did saw the need for vernacular writing. But the fact is that what they were conspicuously failing to do was to write even in Latin—Linacre, Caius, Bright, and Wootton being the most distinguished exceptions. There were others of less note, for example, David Edwards (d. *c.*1542), who wrote two Latin treatises, (Edwards 1532*a*; 1532*b*),[32] and John Frere, or Fryer, who translated the aphorisms of Hippocrates (Frere 1567). Later in the century and in the early seventeenth century Moffett added his name to the list, but it is neither long nor impressive, and it is really only Linacre among these who made a major contribution. Not only are Latin works by Englishmen hard to find, but the indolence of English physicians is mentioned on a number of occasions, as we have seen, by different authors including Andrewe, Cuningham (in Gale), Recorde, and Langton, and must therefore be taken into account as a previously overlooked motive for writing in English. Many obviously felt that if their betters would not publish in Latin, then they themselves had better do so in English.

A list of early printed medical works in English[33] shows that a significant number of them were by physicians. In the following list it has been possible to determine the profession of their authors in some cases, and these are marked with an asterisk where they are known to be physicians, and with ¶ for surgeons: there are others whose calling it is now impossible to identify:

Andrewe, L. [Hieronymus], *The vertuose boke of distiylacyon*, 1527 (*STC* 13435)
[Anon.] *The antidotharius*, 1535? (*STC* 675.3)
[Anon.] *The boke of knowledge: whether a sycke person . . . shall lyue, or dye*, 1548? (*STC* 3319.5)
[Anon.] *Here begynneth a newe mater the whiche is called an herball*, 152? (*STC* 13175.1)[34]
[Anon.] *The judgment of all vrynes*, c.1540 (*STC* 22153)
[Anon.] *The judycyall of vrines*, 1527? (*STC* 14836)
[Anon.] *A lytell boke of the xxiiii stones pryncipalles that profiteth most to a mans body*, 1535? (*STC* 3361)
[Anon.] *The ordre of the hospital of .S. Bartholomewes*, 1552 (*STC* 21558)
[Anon.] *The practyse of cyrurgyons of Mountpyller*, 1540? (*STC* 18052)
[Anon.] *The seynge of vryns*, 1525 (*STC* 22153)
[Anon.] *The treasure of pore men*, 1526? (*STC* 24199)
[Bacon, R.] *The beste waters artyfycialles*, 1530? (*STC* 1179.5)
Borde, A., *The boke for to lerne a man ... for the helth of body*, 1550? (*STC* 3373)*
—— *The breviary of helthe*, 1547 (*STC* 3380)*
—— *A dyetary of helth*, 1542 (*STC* 3378.5)*
Caius, J., *A boke . . . against . . . the SWEATE*, 1552 (*STC* 4343)*
[Canutus] *A litil boke . . . for the pestilence*, c.1485 (*STC* 4589)
Caxton, W., *Gouernayle of helthe*, 1490? (*STC* 12138)
[Chauliac, Guy de] *The questyonary of cyrurgyens*, 1542 (*STC* 12468)
Drummond, J. [Arnaldus de villa nova], *The defence of age and recouery of youth*, 1540? (*STC* 777)
Elyot, Sir T., *The castell of helth*, 1539[35] (*STC* 7642.5)
Hales, J., *The preceptes of Plutarch*, 1543 (*STC* 20062)

[Hieronymus] *The noble experyence of the vertuous handywarke of surgeri*, 1525 (*STC* 13433)
[Hippocrates] *Prognosticacion drawen out of ... Ipocras, Auicen and other notable authours ...*, 1545 (*STC* 13521.7)
Jonas, R., [Roesslin], *The byrth of mankynde*, 1540 (*STC* 21153)
Langton, C., *An introduction into phisycke*, *c*.1545? (*STC* 15205)*
——*A uery brefe treatise, ordrely declaring the pri[n]cipal partes of phisick*, 1547 (*STC* 15204)*
Llwyd, H., [Pope John XXI], *The treasuri of healthe*, *c*.1550 (*STC* 14653)*
Moulton, T., *The myrrour or glasse of helth*, 1539? (*STC* 18214a)
Paynell, T. [Mediolano], *Regimen sanitatis salerni*, 1528 (*STC* 19496)
—— [Ulrich von Hutten], *De morbo gallico*, 1533 (*STC* 14024)
——*A moche profitable treatise against the pestilence*, 1534? (*STC* 19492)
Phaer, T. [Goeurot], *The regiment of lyfe, whereunto is added a treatise of the pestilence with the boke of children*, 1544? (*STC* 11966.5)*
[Plutarch] *The gouernau[n]ce of good helthe*, 1549 (*STC* 20060.5)
Raynalde, T. [Roesslin], *The byrth of mankinde*, 1545 (*STC* 21154)*
——*A compendious declaration of the excellent vertues of a certaine lateli inventid oile*, 1551 (*STC* 20779)*
Recorde, R., *The vrinal of physick*, 1548 (*STC* 20817)*
Turner, W. *The names of herbes in Greke, Latin, English, Duch, & Frenche*, 1548 (*STC* 24359)*
——*A new herball*, 1551 (*STC* 24366)*
Udall, Nicholas, *A Compendyouse Rehearsall of all Anatomie*, 1553 (*STC* 11715.5)
Vicary, T., *Anatomie*, 1548 (see *STC* 11715.5)¶
[Vigo, J. de] *Lytell practyse of J. de Vigo in medycyne*, 1550? (*STC* 24725)
—— *The most excellent workes of chirurgerye*, 1543 (*STC* 24720)
Wingfield, H., *A compendious or shorte treatise ... of healthe*, 1551 (*STC* 25852)

Where it is possible to distinguish the author's profession, most of the early vernacular works were by physicians rather than by barber-surgeons. The evidence of this chapter shows clearly that it was physicians such as Turner, Recorde, Phaer, Raynalde, Langton, Askham, and Borde who were the first generation of medical professionals to make their influence felt in print, being for the most part busily engaged in publication in English well before the earliest surgeons. Thus the view that the physicians were less active than the surgeons or that they were all but supine needs revision, since slightly less than one third of vernacular works are by physicians. It was in Latin that they failed to produce work. This list shows that it was in fact the physicians rather than the surgeons who led the initial assault on the academic and professional prerogatives of those learned in Latin and Greek. The first and only work on this list known to be by a surgeon is Vicary's derivative anatomy.

It has hitherto been assumed that in English it was the barber-surgeons who took the lead. Margaret Pelling comments on barber-surgeons who showed initiative; e.g. in 'their prompt adoption of new remedies and in their creation of a body of medical literature, much of it in the vernacular; the academically qualified physicians of the London College lagged behind in both respects, and were not very productive even in Latin' (Pelling 1986: 83). But this view is not supportable either, only one appearing in our list. It is also generally assumed that the translators, compilers and popularizers were not always fully learned and were not the professionals of their discipline, but the involvement of physicians shows that this was not necessarily the case. We will see in the next chapter to what extent the achievements of these authors were recognized in their own tongue.

The rise in the status and articulateness of the barber-surgeons, whose professional need was for works in English, stems from the mid- and late sixteenth century rather than from the earlier period, emerging first with Hall, who translated Plutarch, and seems to have been a surgeon, Vicary, and then Gale in the 1560s, followed by Banister, Clowes, and Baker a little later, by which time the surgeons are almost the dominant force in medical publishing.[36]

Thus the university-trained physicians commit themselves to print sporadically throughout the century after the first three decades, while the views of the barber-surgeons are infrequently voiced up to the 1560s, but are heard frequently thereafter. Authors with no demonstrable professional affiliation contributed consistently from the 1520s on, and perhaps Paynell and Moulton are best thought of as professional translators. The apothecaries are rarely heard; their most notable voices are those of the distillers, such as John Hester, who in the late 1560s come under the influence of Paracelsus. They were not professionally trained like the physicians and later the surgeons, and presumably were never a very articulate force.

The belief that physicians were as one opposed to the use of the vernacular is partly created by the almost universal disclaimers of the latter half of the century. The problem of the detractors is usually addressed in the prefatory material, and is so widely mentioned as to give the impression that there were hordes of acerbic critics awaiting the appearance of a book to do their worst, but these disclaimers are so universal and so formulaic that it becomes difficult in the end to see them as very much more than a topos. Two possible early exceptions are Elyot, who actually refers to a critic in the present tense, rather than as normal, in the future or the conditional, and Phaer. Actual instances of such attacks on authors are rather hard to find. The proponents of the use of English, in their anxiety to deflect attacks on their work, may have helped create the sense of an overwhelming opposition mainly from physicians which we have consequently overestimated, while underestimating the considerable fruits of their labours. The fact is that most of the information about critics of those writing in English comes from the often strident disclaimers in these authors' own prefaces.

Against such attempts to deflect real or imagined attacks are the arguments for the use of English and the dissemination of knowledge which are also somewhat formulaic and owe their form to some extent to the long-established parallel arguments put for the translations of Scripture into the vernacular.[37]

In the next chapter I will examine some of the lexical problems faced by medical authors, the solutions to which were not merely a matter of coining new words to fill gaps. It was often one of reworking the older vocabulary of the tongues, and of grappling with well-established views as to their authority. Hard evidence for coinage is rather difficult to come by for individual authors and particular words, as the next chapter will show. The more general evidence of antedatings to *OED*, especially in Chapter 6, will on the other hand reveal general trends in word creation, and demonstrate that a revision of our notions of the scope of the medical terminology in this period, as well as its time of and means of introduction where it really was new, is in need of revision.

Notes

1. Misinformation continues to thrive, it seems. As recently as 1994, Mattei writes that medical concepts were 'couched in Latin terminology, not in English' (251), overlooking the fact that they were variously in Greek, Arabic, and English as well.
2. Most recently in Koivisto-Alanko (1996), who simply reiterates the views of Vickers (1987) and Gotti (1992).
3. The question of the inelegance of English may be dismissed from this discussion as having no especial relevance to the compilation of medical texts. The unimportance of this aspect of the debate to medical work will emerge in the course of examining the evidence presented in this chapter, but I do not propose to deal with it directly. It is considered at some

length by historians of early modern English (Jones 1953; Barber 1976: 76–8, etc.)

4. Such a disclaimer appears on the title page of Walter Bailey's *Mithridatium*, but the distinction is not quite as Jones would have it—'Compiled rather for those which are to vse it, then for the learned.' The learned physician only attended upon the patient in exceptional cases, so that apothecaries and other medical attendants and the patients themselves are the intended audience.
5. For a fuller discussion of Purvey's remarkable prologue, see Mueller (1984: 111–15).
6. Voigts 1996 shows both that my view here is rather ingenuous, and that a good deal of research must be done on the details of code-switching and other relationships between the various languages in use in late medieval and renaissance medical writings. See also Voigts (1990: 30–3).
7. I have been unable to consult the 1525 edn. of the latter, which is in the Huntingdon Library.
8. A number of these words which appear in non-naturalized forms elsewhere, e.g. **narcotyke**, **tutie**, **asma**, and **erysiple**, appear in Barrough 60 years on.
9. The *Grete herball* derives its text from the *Ortus Sanitatis* (1491) and *Gart der Gesundheit* (1485); its illustrations have a lengthy ancestry (see Greene 1983: i: 235). Turner's herbal, on the other hand, derives from Leonhard Fuchs.
10. Dates for the authors listed are given only where available, usually from *DNB*.
11. I have found no evidence to suggest that Paynell was a trained physician. Thomas Gale, in his *Certaine workes of chirurgerie* 1563 (*STC* 11529) (Aaiiii^{r}), calls him 'Master', but not 'Doctor', as with the other physicians in his list. *The noble experience of … surgeri*, 1525 (*STC* 13434) has been previously ascribed to Paynell, but not in the edn. of *STC* used here.
12. The first name is that of the translator and that in square brackets the author of the text translated.
13. Eucharius Roesslin, who published a German work in 1532.
14. Turner's work consistently identifies 'apothecaries Latin'.
15. The place of sixteenth- and seventeenth-century botany in establishing a taxonomic model has been discussed by Slaughter (1982: 48–82). What was true of scientific taxonomy was also by necessity true of the lexicon itself: exact terminology and exact description and classification were ultimately indistinguishable. Thus the attempt to define reality became an attempt to refine the lexicon. As Slaughter puts it, 'To the extent that the taxonomic structure includes definitions, and definitions constitute names, Aristotelian taxonomic naming reflects taxonomic structure in the most transparent manner possible. The taxonomy is an encyclopaedia, nomenclature and dictionary all at the same time' (66).

16. The advice he received from physicians concerning his earlier work was that 'I shoulde cease from settynge out of this boke in latin tyll I had sene those places of Englande, wherein is moste plentie of herbes' (Turner 1548: Aii^{v}).
17. There is no record of this proposed work in *STC*.
18. *OED* gives for **cleanly** in reference to language, etc., 'neat', 'elegant'. **Sawcefleme** 'a swelling of the face accompanied by inflammation, supposed to be due to salt humours' (*OED*) had a well-established place in the lexicon at least from the end of the fourteenth century; see both *OED* and *MED*. See also Norri (1992: 367), etc.
19. *Ath. Ox.* 1858–1913, i: 419 claims that there is 'no record therof', but this is amended, iii: 98, in a record of 1563–4 stating that 'Conceditur Jo. Jones vt studium viii annum in medicina sufficiat . . . Presentatus eodem per doctorem Walker.' A handwritten note to the *STC* microfilm of his *The bathes of bathes ayde* records that Jones practised at Bath 'with great reputation' as well as at Nottingham and King's Mead, near Derby.
20. 'The subtile science of holi Alchymye; Of which science here I entende to write, How be it I may not curyously endite, For he that shuld al commyn peple teche, He most for theym vse playne & comon speche.' (ll. 54–8).
21. An example is '/S/*εη*[?]*αϱτικα*/S/ in Latine, meatus repurgantia, or driving forth' (Bviii^{r}).
22. For instance, in *The bathes of bathes ayde* he discusses the registration of physicians on Ii^{r}.
23. On the activities of empirics, quacks, and charlatans, and the attempts to establish and defend professional privileges, see Lingo (1986: 583–603).
24. No trace of this work is found in *STC*. In the work discussed here, *A short and profitable treatise* . . . 1579, he reports 'I was bolde about three years since . . . to offer vnto you a very small, and vnperfect Treatise of mine touching . . . Morbus Gallicus' (Aii^{r}).
25. Entitled 'An admonition to the frendly Reader, for the defence of publishing this worke in English' (Liii^{v}).
26. Probably the Hales, Hawle, or Hall, apparently a surgeon of Maidstone, who translated Plutarch under the title *The preceptes of Plutarch* 1543 (*STC* 20062). He is mentioned in William Clowes's *A short and profitable treatise touching the cure of the disease called (Morbus Gallicus) by unctions* in the 1585 edn. as the 'Chirurgion Maister Iohn Hawle of Maydestone in Kent, a brother of our Companie' (Iii^{r}).
27. Clowes was also up to date in his English reading—Lyte's Dodoens was published in 1578, Timothy Bright's first work in 1580, and Barrough's as late as 1583.
28. Possibly the denigrators referred to are Bostocke and I.W. The old foe, Rasworm, 'whome heeretofore I haue deciphered in my Booke *De Morbo*

gallico', is abused as having more recently 'spurned against incarnatives' (Ai[r]). There is also according to Clowes 'a new adopted chick of this old Cocke' (Ai[v]) who may be Bostocke, since he is accused of having refused to 'follow the method and wayes of curing after Hipocrates and Galen, because they were heathen men'. The evidence suggests that the Paracelsian opposition was not all that potent, English medicine having received him only very cautiously. The sense which Clowes and others sometimes convey of being embattled is hardly justified by his actual circumstances as a leading member of an increasingly respectable profession.

29. Published by Windet in 1586. Always assuming, of course, that it was Bright and not someone else, perhaps even Windet himself, who made the change.
30. What the *OED* introduction calls 'denizens.' 'DENIZENS are words fully naturalized as to use, but not as to *form*, *inflexion*, or *pronunciation*' (*OED*, p. xxix).
31. Of course, one or two who published in Latin published a great deal. Although the history of science is not our primary concern here, in considering the weight of publications by, say, Linacre, it should also be noted that their influence was ultimately conservative by comparison with, say, Turner's *Herball*, which in the longer view was probably a more significant contribution to scientific progress.
32. For details of his life, see Talbot and Hammond (1965: 33). The same work indicates that there was some writing in the late fifteenth century, suggesting (386) that William Bokynham of Norwich may have written two short treatises on urines (Wellcome MS 408), and the same MS contains another work on urines attributed to William Kylinghale (Talbot and Hammond 1965: 405). Another late fifteenth-century treatise, this time on fistula, is by William Seyton (Talbot and Hammond 1965: 414).
33. They are listed, as far as it is possible, complete up to 1552, with dates of publication where possible. Short titles only are employed, but reference to *STC* numbers is included. Names of the original authors are in square brackets where they have been translated into English. Note that the *STC*'s practice is to list them under the original authors, not the translators, who are cross-referenced.
34. Subsequently known in its various editions as either Banckes's, Macer's, or Ascham's herbal.
35. Elyot shows an abiding interest in and wide knowledge of medicine, but there is no evidence that he was formally qualified. See Elyot (1541, Aiiii[r]).
36. It is impossible to ascribe *The noble experience of . . . surgeri* of 1525 positively to a surgeon.
37. Janel M. Mueller's exhaustive stylistic and discourse analysis of Scripturalism in English prose of the period approaches medical writings from a very different standpoint, preferring to treat them as a manifestation of

'the Scripturalist cast of mind' of the time, and thus of 'the genial standing assumption that vernacular works would benefit a popular readership' (Mueller 1984: 280). He associates the appearance of a number of texts during the years 1537–40 with the ascendancy of Thomas Cromwell (282–3).

3
Language and Authority

This chapter will discuss two aspects of authority in medical writings. The term 'authority' may refer either to those linguistic standards upheld and appealed to in medical practice or terminology, or to a person or work whose status is regarded as for the most part beyond question. The two are obviously interlinked inasmuch as the authority of the ancients is also the authority of Latin, Greek, and, though to a decreasing extent in the postmedieval period, Arabic. The extent to which the authority of these languages held firm during the course of the century is crucial to this enquiry. The first form of authority requires us particularly to examine the language used by the medical literature, to try and determine the extent to which it is naturalized in English, the extent of borrowing and neologism, the means (if any) of rendering difficult terms comprehensible, and the extent of re-alienation of terms. Changes in the terminology might reveal changes in attitudes rather more subtly than direct statements of principle, and are more likely to anticipate such statements. Convention continued to dominate publicly stated principles for most of the century, but actual terminological practice does not always accord with these principles, as we shall see.

It is now clear that there was an established tradition in the fifteenth century of writing medical texts in both English, Latin and Anglo-Norman, and indeed of using all these languages in a particular text (Voigts 1989*a*: 95–6). English had been established as a language in which serious scientific texts could be written. Voigts and Jones have also made it clear that the simple divide between learned, Latin knowledge and writing in English was far less marked than has been supposed, at least in England (Jones 1989: 62; Voigts 1989*b*). The present inquiry is therefore more concerned with the specific issue of medical terminology, whether Latin, Greek, or English, and its status and use in English texts in comparison to English terminology than with the more general question of whether English should be used or not. As we have already seen, it was raised by some of the medical writers themselves, but may have been less urgent in fact than their own exculpations suggest.

Completely uncritical veneration for figures of authority is normally assumed to be the background to sixteenth-century medical science, and by and large this is so, but there is a consequent tendency to ignore deviations from this attitude, or to notice them only when they appear in the works of recognized pioneers such as Vesalius. It is therefore a salutary exercise to look at some attitudes and linguistic practices as they actually appear in the texts of that time.

A complete survey of the usage of particular authors is not practicable within the limited scope of the present study, but the practices of the two largest contributors, Barrough and Banister, will be examined in the first part of this chapter, which deals with terminology in some detail,[1] and the views of some others who also contribute useful material are added in the second section on authority figures. Sufficient material is to hand to indicate the kinds of problem with which the medical professions had to deal in putting its corpus of knowledge both to practitioners and to the public. What is of especial interest is to detail the ways in which the lexicon itself was a problem to authors, and how these difficulties were managed.

In the second part reference to authority figures will be canvassed, though here the intention is to find deviation from already well-known practices. Reference to the ancients can be taken for granted, since it is frequent, uncritical, and for the most part reverentially stereotyped. It is departures from these conventions which are noteworthy rather than the numberless standard occurrences of them. The extent to which Englishmen, especially contemporaries, are acknowledged is the special concern of this section, since it can be supposed that extensive reading of contemporaries in the vernacular will have helped to spread, standardize, and consolidate the usage of vernacular terminology, and especially to have determined the limits to the incorporation of neoclassical terms into the vocabulary, as well as the extent to which full anglicization might occur.

The kinds of misconception the scholar of this subject must deal with seem to arise from a failure to make proper and full use of the available primary resources. To take an example, John Banister interrupts his anatomical treatise *The historie of man* to sum up the forward-looking attitude of the time, both in respect to style and to authority:

But since in a later Writer is expected a newer stile, and that I not onely professe more appertinent prolixitie then the rest of our Nation, that before haue trauailed herein, but also to haue for my guides the most princely *Anathomistes* of latter yeares: If I thus forsooke, or breake of my descriptio[n] of the head, in professyng to open I should but shut, and in meanyng to discouer I should but hyde the light. (Fii^r)

Banister is unfortunately almost always quoted for his conservatism than for his obviously clear perception of the way forward, but misconceptions based on flimsy evidence die hard in medical history. Copeman (1960: 87) and subsequently McLean (1972: 196) cite Banister as someone who, faced with the appearance of something unexpected in the course of a dissection, would rather argue that the human body had altered since Galen's time than admit that the master was wrong, as he certainly does in his preface. But this familiar argument hardly originated with Banister,[2] and such anecdotes completely overlook other evidence from *The historie of man*. In the body of the text he points out Galenic errors quite frequently. He suggests for example that 'noble *Galen* ... was not a little deceiued' about synarthrosis (Di^r) and elsewhere claims that 'agayne it is manifest, that *Galen* (for all his industrious search) fayled to finde the truth, in affirmyng these *Appendances* to be added to the bones for the conseruation of the marey' (Cii^r). He also argues that the truth is to be preferred to the magisterial assertion of it:

I shalbe perhaps misliked agayne for swaruing so much from the auncient Authors: yet vnto the wise I meane to giue no such occasion. For in expressing of both, I leaue vnto euery one that readeth the best to be chosen. The circumsta[n]ce therfore equally wayed, yeld auncientie vnto the truth whether the Author therof was first or last. (Oii^v)

Such a comment is surely more illuminating of Banister's attitudes than one which simply repeats conventional and long-held beliefs, if only because it runs against expectations.

At many other places he is prepared bluntly to reject Galen, and also to acknowledge the superiority of recent anatomical work. The master is roundly reproved elsewhere for believing something contrary to the experience of the working surgeon:

This is that *Muscle* that *Galen* sayth he commaunded to be cut in a certaine currour, who neuerthelesse could runne more swiftly: which thyng is most vnworthy, for such a prince of Phisicke to imagine, or say. For this muscle being taken away: direct flexion can in no wise be brought to passe ...

> although the wound be not very great, yet when they are healed, it shalbe a labour vnto them to bowe the same legge. (Rii^{r})

Banister's index contains references to eighteen Galenic errors (Ii i^{v}), and other omissions are also mentioned. To cite examples, the second muscle of the shoulder blade 'is nothing seruiceable to the shoulder, what soeuer Galen thought therin' (Pii^{v}), and elsewhere he claims that Collumbus 'triumpheth ouer all before his time' in his description of the upper jawbones, and he continues by asserting the primacy of truth: 'the truth is to be embraced, and the inuentor accordyngly reuerenced' (Eiiii^{v}). Similarly, John Hester begins the preamble to his *Short discourse* with the claim that 'There is no doubt, but that our newe Physicke and Ch[y]rurgerie, is better then that, [th]e which the Auncients haue used' (¶iii^{v}). It is simply essential to return to the texts themselves and to study them.

I. LINGUISTIC AUTHORITY

The orismology of a typical *OED* entry for the specialist words of this period in the development of the English lexicon is often less revealing than might at first appear. Senses of words, especially some pertaining to medicine, were sometimes missed, and those entered were sometimes given a weighting which might need revision. There are occasions when restructuring the entry might be appropriate in the light of further information. The existence of technical terms and senses is only patchily acknowledged in the field markers, and sub-technical words, an important class since they provide the contextual matrix for the use of technical terms, are not identified at all. Thus the *OED* is not always a reliable guide to assessing the lexical status of medical words, making it necessary to reconstruct actual practice from the extant texts. While the collection of entry material was extensive, there was no thoroughgoing attempt to find either trends or processes in the naturalization of words at this period, let alone to compare it with those of other periods, and this area of research is still deficient. The corpus of terms discussed here is probably too slight to make any confident generalizations, but may at least be sufficient to show the possibilities for further work. It is also the case that what is available in *OED* is under-utilized and needs to be much more fully analysed.

The phenomenon of denizens, as the *OED* describes them, is also a problem. These are words retained in the lexicon without full naturalization. The term does not now seem entirely appropriate, so that I propose to call them encysts and the process encystation. It also seems appropriate to refer to this as a process, rather than merely a state of affairs; though the effects are long-standing and on the whole stable, the conscious application of linguistic assumptions about the status of competing lexicons is nevertheless involved, and practices do vary somewhat from author to author, as we shall see. It seems that in the sixteenth century the status of encysted words was less legitimate than now, inasmuch as there are frequent parenthetical observations that these were the words used by the Greeks or the Latins, and that this explains comments that no English word for such and such a phenomenon was known when clearly there was a fully available and well-known denizen; indeed, in many instances there was an oversupply of vocabulary. It is of course the familiarity of those writing on the subject with the languages from which the encysted words originally come which maintained this assumption.

A related process not taken into account at all is the tendency among medical writers in the sixteenth century to remake words in their original forms even though they have been naturalized morphologically, and many instances of this process appear in the works discussed below.[3] Bostocke provides an example on Hiiii^{r} 'For this *Aeschrion* was *Empiricus* and *Galens* master' where the familiar **empiric**, dated by *OED* in this sense to Copland, 1541 is re-formed. This process I shall call for convenience re-alienation. In other words, some earlier naturalizations are subjected to a process of alienation from the lexicon at this period by being given Greek or Latin form anew, and the assumption that all new words are consistently assimilated, though possibly at different rates, is not always reliable. English words are in some cases given a neoclassical form, even though they have not originated from such sources.

The reasons for this process, an aspect of the terminology of the discipline not often considered, are obvious enough, though not always easy to demonstrate. Since many of the terms borrowed from the classical sources[4] are etymologically parallel to the English term where one exists, one must assume that the classical terms were no more accurately descriptive than the native in many cases. Thus the reasons for using them are not primarily etymological. The terminology borrowed is not obviously capable of finer medical distinctions. There is no obvious gain in explanatory or discriminatory power in using *patella* or *rotule* rather than the **eye of the knee**, or in *gladiform* for **shieldlike**, *linea alba* for **white line**, *deltoid* for **three-square**, or **triangular**, *ginglymos* for **hinge-joint** or **bone-joint**, or in *skirrhos* (or *scirrhus*)for **hard coat**.[5] Instead of **pylorus**, from late Latin, Clever (7) uses **pylon**, going back to Greek, but makes no obvious gain in clarity. The usage is unrecorded in *OED* and is perhaps a case of his 'neologizing'. He also uses both **tympany** and **timpana** (7). Indeed, the linguistic practice of both Barrough and Banister tends to imply that in many instances the terminology is less than satisfactory at this level. Bostocke's *Difference* supplies the rather subtle example of **actor**, cited in apparently full naturalization: 'there must be an Actor before there be action' (Aii^{v}); however, on Ivi^{v} we get 'there must be *Actor* before ther be *Actio*, for *Agens* begetteth *Actionem*', where the context, the grammar, and the capitalization and italicization all suggest that it is non-naturalized. The same work offers **occult**, also an antedating: 'eche thing hath two natures, that is *occultum* and *manifestum*' (Dvii^{r}). Both are recorded earlier in the *OED*, **manifest** in 1374 and **occult** in 1533.

Two factors seem relevant to the adoption of this terminology: first and most apparently, the terms used carry the accumulated prestige of classical learning and authority with them. Second and less obviously, the fact that they are borrowings allows these terms some immunity from the tendency to polysemy and to the 'corruption' of popular use. Monosemy and semantic integrity is more easily preserved by the encystation of terms within the disciplinary context. The process is of course not wholly successful and terms will 'escape', as in the more modern instances of **neurosis**, **hysteria**, the very recently escaped **virus**, and others.

Since Phillip Barrough and John Banister are the authors most frequently cited in this study, they are an obvious and appropriate subject for lexical analysis. Both make much use of borrowed words and neologisms. It is not necessarily that they are typical of their age in these matters of terminology—such a generalization would have to await further research—but their usages may put into perspective the kinds of lexicographic difficulty which such terms present, both to them and to the compilers of later dictionaries. The two next most productive texts, those by Cotta and Bostocke, are less medical textbooks than books about certain medical subjects, and are relatively rather less revealing.

Barrough is more obviously concerned with the selection of the right term than Banister, and shows a particular preference in his use of specialized terms for the exotic as against the anglicized form. Not that it is an exclusive preference by any means; but it is not clear that he would have regarded such terms in all cases as aliens. There are many instances in which having declared that such and such is the Greek or Latin term, he proceeds to use it as his own preferred form.[6] Nevertheless words which are established in anglicized forms, some of long standing, are often eschewed. For example, **betony** is generally referred to as **betonica** (e.g. 194), in spite of the fact that naturalized forms are recorded at least as far back as the OE *Leechdoms*, *c.*1000.[7] **Achor** he refers to as **achora** (276); **apozem** as **apozema** (285); the fevers called **diaries** he calls **diaria** (168), and so forth. *OED* lists **lentisk** (1398, Trevisa), but Barrough uses **lentiscus** (134); *OED* records Chaucer's **narkotykes** while Barrough employs **narcotia** (225). **Oxymell of squills** also occurs in the *Leechdoms*, but Barrough uses **oxymel scillicitum** (8). He can hardly have been in doubt as to the meaning of the English term. He obviously does show some concern to disambiguate terms, but whether that is the only reason for his preferences is another matter. The evidence collected here suggests that it was only one motive among several, but the question must await further sustained research, which is beyond the scope of the present work. In many such, it can hardly have been the case that the English term was ambiguously polysemous, though instances of this problems can assuredly be found.

It is not that the naturalized forms do not appear; there are many instances of both being used, often in close association. **Bolus** and **bole** (66) are both used, though when the preparation of these medicaments as a type is being discussed (288) the exotic form is used. It is presumably regarded as more formal and perhaps a more impressive usage.[8] Other pairs include **embrocha** (4)–**embrocation** (4); **nasales** (9)–**nasalia** (9); **narde** (11)–**nardinum** (11); **tutty** (41)–**tuthia** (276); **cerusa** (238)–**ceruse** (238). There is no suggestion on Barrough's part that the English was ambiguous or imprecise: indeed, his own tendency to slip from one term to another suggests full interchangeability, so that in many cases his reason for preferring one usage to another was probably extralinguistic. In other texts there seems to be a tendency to use the latinized form when introducing a term, but the anglicized equivalent in subsequent entries in running text, one example being John Hester's initial reference to

quintaessencia solutiua (*Short discourse*, ¶4^{r}) but his subsequent use of **quintaessence solutiue** on ¶4^{v}—'giue ... halfe an ounce of our Quintaessence solutiue with broth.' The same does not, however, apply to **balsamo** on the same pages. Such pairings of course frequently occur elsewhere; for example, Langton in *IP*, 'properlye that is named *nutrimentum* and in our tonge, nouryshment' (Gvii^{v}).

Sometimes there are literal translations, not merely anglicized forms, the pair **sanguinea pustulae–blood pushes** occurring on 226. **Coniunctæ** and **continentes** he also calls **ioined causes** (207). He is frequently at pains to point out equivalences, as in the explanatory rubric 'Of Tumours aboue nature, which the Latines call inflationes, but they are commonly called windie Apostemes, *apostemata ventosa*' (250). Thus glosses may expand into explanations in English and into definitions in a more obviously dictionary sense. As in the example given, the provision of an explanation does not necessarily depend on the availability or otherwise of a native term, and the choice is not always a simple one between the neoclassical (proper) and the English (improper).[9] Presumably Barrough regards *apostemata ventosa* as a legitimate Latin gloss for the English term, but **inflationes** as the only proper Latin term of the two available choices in that language.

The putative linguistic status of some terms used can become quite complex, since ascription to a particular language does not obviate the possibility of the term having an established history in English. On 201 he employs the term **carbunculus** for the already well-established **carbuncle**. For the same complaint he also introduces **anthrax**—'*Carbunculus* also called of the Greeks *Anthrax*'. **Anthrax** is, however, well attested from the late fourteenth century,[10] so that the ascription to the Greeks cannot be understood as introducing an unfamiliar term to the readers. Another curious instance is **canker–cancer**. The *OED* notes the reformation of **cancer** from the Latin original to make a finer diagnostic distinction than was possible with the fully anglicized **canker** 'about 1600'. Phillip Barrough not only makes this distinction—**cancer** is an antedating in this study—but also distinguishes **carcinoma** from both. The latter is an antedating from 1721. If, however, Barrough intended a similar distinction with **carbunculus** it failed to supersede **carbuncle**, and the *OED* does not record it at all. A somewhat more subversive explanation of the kind of situation exemplified by **anthrax** is that Barrough was unfamiliar with earlier medical works in

English, a circumstance which would hardly surprise the modern commentator, but only substantial research into the reading habits of physicians at this time would inspire real confidence in this assumption.

At the same time it is by no means the case that all latinisms indicate finer distinctions or a better usage. On page 210 he pairs the latinate adjective **complicate** with 'greatly folded', but on 171 the same word is given the gloss 'ioyned', suggesting that both senses were present in this neologism for Barrough and that the finer distinctions were made in the native periphrases. **Complicate** is once again an antedating. Another useful example occurs on 171, where Barrough links the terms **confusion** and **complication**. 'Complicatio[n] (as Galen witnesseth) is when the feauers inuade the patient at diuerse houres. And confusion is, when they begine at one time.' The term **confusion** goes back to the twelfth century at least according to *OED*, but **complication** is an absolute first citation from Barrough. Thus an old term and what appears to be a new one, **complicate**, being a sixteenth century introduction,[11] are used to form a pair expressing a fine diagnostic distinction. The use of both these terms might ultimately be new senses for *OED* if further examples were forthcoming, but it is not in this case Barrough's own distinctive usage—it occurs in Jones's *A dial for all agues* of 1566 and no doubt elsewhere.[12]

It is possible that Barrough uses terms in new ways, or in ways suggested by the logic of the etymology, but not employed in English as such. The term **inclination** appears to be a case of a previously unrecognized sense which shows Barrough employing a characteristically strict etymological logic. He appears to use it (174, 183) in apposition to **declination**; the obvious sense in reference to the rise and fall of fits in fevers. He also speaks of the **remission** of the fit (174). *OED* gives a sense which seems the same as **declination**,[13] but here Barrough surely intends a juxtaposition, so that this becomes a new sense.

The predominant concern with the minutiae of terminology is evident throughout *The methode of physicke*, and he is constantly giving multiple forms of words, or alternate names—often Galen's and those of 'the Greeks' as against those of Avicenna or Celsus. Less frequently an English word is supplied, but it is often a more familiar loanword rather than a common native name. This concern is nowhere more apparent than in the ten pages at the opening of Book V which he devotes to the classification of what he calls 'tumours'. At this period, this involved diseases as diverse as carcinoma and erysipelas, scabies and psoriasis. Barrough employs a multitude of terms in English, Latin, Greek, and Arabic in this painstaking exposition; one which is much more concerned with the niceties and proprieties of nomenclature and of classification than with the diseases themselves. He pauses at one point to state his intentions—with undue self-effacement, in the circumstances—'I haue thought it expedient, and a thing worthy the labour, to set downe in this place the names of them, bothe in Greeke and in Lataine, and also their barbarous title, with a certaine rude discription thereof' (203). It was a matter which concerned him deeply, and reflects a long-established humanist approach to such problems.

After a protracted discussion of scabies, impetigo, ringworm, and their various synonyms and pseudonyms, he concludes that there is much still to be explained in such matters, and that the ancient and therefore the contemporary nomenclature may be unsatisfactory, 'Whereby we may coniecture that little credite is to be attributed to wordes or names, vnlesse the matter be throughly discouered' (204). The matter to which he refers must be presumed to be primarily lexical rather than pathological. As Barrough complains 'one and the selfe same worde by varietie of authors hath [*sic*] enforced to vphold many diuerse & different significations, as in their commentaries doth euerie where appeare' (204). He obviously feels a need for the lexicon to reflect these finer discriminations, as well as for some standardization of nomenclature in the medical literature. At the same time, it is not necessarily a lack of words which troubles him; rather, it is a plethora, a fact which is generally ignored by those who claim that the language at this time lacked terms. What concerned him was the proprieties of choice, not the lack of choice.

It is evident that Barrough's writing is a kind of battleground which is being contested by the conflicting claims of various recognized authorities from different medical and, more significantly, linguistic traditions. However, there was no English authority with permission to enter the lists and to whom Barrough could have recourse in solving particular problems of nomenclature.[14] It seems that Barrough, although writing in the vernacular himself, recognized no contemporaneous English authority. No English medical writers or treatises are mentioned in his work, although there were many he might have alluded to. There was nothing unusual in this, since references by English authors to their contemporaries or immediate predecessors were infrequent as we have seen—the matter will be discussed more fully below. The weighty eminence of a Linacre, Caius, or Vicary, or the popularity of Gale or Borde, by no means entitled them to this sort of notice or to the status of an authority, whether they wrote in Latin or English, and in this Barrough is decidedly conservative. Although many of these authors contributed to the emergence of English as a language for scientific use, the correlative judgement that English itself was also authoritative simply did not emerge and was not acknowledged until very much later. That it was at least functional was, on the other hand, taken for granted for the better part of the century.

Thus Barrough nearer the end of the century, writing extensively and painstakingly in English, consistently denies by implication that his own language has authority, in spite of his disquiet over the insufficiencies of terms from languages which for him do possess that quality. The majority if not all of his fellow physicians would have acquiesced in this assumption, while surgeons would have been increasingly likely to question it. A medical work in a contemporary language, or indeed by a contemporary in Latin, was seen as doing no more than explicating and supplementing the ancients.

John Banister

The surgeon John Banister also has much to offer on this subject. His *The historie of man* is largely unillustrated, and what illustrations there are do not support and supplement the text.[15] Banister therefore depends entirely upon verbal descriptions of the body. It is perhaps odd that an anatomical work published at least a generation after Vesalius should rely so little on illustration. His work contains only five—two of the skeleton, two of the musculature of the whole body, and one of surgical instruments. The work is thus necessarily rich in anatomical terms, its author spending some time in explanation of terms as well as of his methods of explication. There are also occasions on which he lists terms without explanation, e.g. 'Membranes of the eyes . . . The first . . . hath many names, as all these, *Adnata, alba, adhærens, and coniunctiua* (Ffiii^r). He must also painstakingly explain structures which may be obvious and self-explanatory in an illustration, but for which there is no particular term.[16]

Banister emphasizes as might be expected from a surgeon the obscurity of anatomical terms in Latin and Greek:

> Now forasmuch as in this our narratio[n] of bones, diuers straunge names, & such as to the simpler sorte are altogether vnknowen, be here & there scattered: It shalbe very conuenient before hand, briefly to table out an expositio[n] of them: That therby the reading of such in their places (being now first cracked and shaled from their obscure *Huskes*) may be more perspicuous, and pleasaunt to your contemplation; which otherwise would be loadsom, and tedious. (Ci^{v})

He exhorts the reader to 'haue in mynde ... those fewe decyffered names, which the au[n]cient *Anathomistes* haue giuen accordyng as it seemed best to their learned opinions' (Ciii^{r}). The sense of 'deciphered' here is unclear—it could just conceivably mean 'enciphered' (see *OED*), but if 'decipher' is really the intended meaning, then does he imply that the ancients enciphered them, and we have now deciphered them? or that the ancients deciphered them? Neither does 'fewe' seem an apt assessment of the number of words from ancient sources in this work. But perhaps he refers here only to **appendance** and **process**, the two terms which he does immediately explain at some length. A little later, he explains that one must understand not only how bones are joined, but also 'the straunge, and diffused names, wherewith their kindes of knittynges, in eche respect are nominated' (Ciii^{r}). The fact that 'diffused' almost certainly has here its older sense of disordered or obscure seems to suggest that some of the terms of the ancients will be so at least for his readership, and that he is able to clarify them.

But of the two examples he undertakes to 'table out', **appendance** and **process**, early in the work, only the second had a clearly established medical sense in Latin. These are mentioned specifically presumably because they themselves are often part of definitions or descriptions, being generic or sub-technical terms rather than fully technical ones. Certainly **process** is used very frequently throughout the book; **appendance** rather less so.

Appendance is a word which he feels a need to explain at some length, although his explication, apart from giving the Greek equivalent, is anatomical, not linguistic (Ci^{v}–Cii^{r}). This word is first cited in the *OED* for 1523; the first medical use is listed as 1615 (Crooke's *Microcosmographia*).[17] Senses 1 and 2 are marked obsolete, sense 3 is marked legal; thus there is no evidence in the *OED* of a current medical sense in Banister's time. Neither is there any obvious medical sense in Latin.[18] This might therefore be a case of Banister (or of the surgical profession) reworking a word for a particular purpose. It is obviously of importance to know whether this state of affairs reflects a deficiency in the *OED* or an original lexical discrimination by Banister, and therefore a gap in contemporary English medical terminology. The scrupulousness of his discussion suggests that it might be the latter, but it is notoriously difficult to be certain, given the current state of research into the sixteenth-century lexicon. Somewhat similar considerations apply to **process**,[19] which he is also at pains to explain as if it is an unfamiliar term, but in this case the first citation of this sense (12) in *OED* is from Banister himself. Furthermore, the medical sense was available from Latin.[20] Thus Banister's sense once again might originate with Banister or be a transfer of the Latin sense.

On another occasion Banister discusses the types of flesh in the body, concluding with Vesalius that these are two, proper and improper. The meaning of **proper** here is covered only in the *OED* by a reference under sense 1 to an archaic use of the word. Medicine itself is not mentioned, only that it is 'chiefly scientific'. He means to distinguish those kinds that are, according to the theory of the time, engendered from blood, and those which are not, proposing therefore to call them *sanguinea* and *exsanguis* respectively. 'It shalbe sufficient inough with *Vesalius* to deuided [*sic*] them into two, and so (if it be lawfull) to call the propper *Sanguinea*, and the impropper *Exsanguis*' (Tii^{r}). The disclaimer suggests deliberate coinage in this case.

Acetabulum receives a much fuller linguistic discussion, being cited as a word for which Banister claims to have found no wholly satisfactory English equivalent. He offers a number of alternatives, some of which he makes use of himself later in the work; **acetabulum** is 'a deepe hole, or cauitie therfore, you shall call after the Latins *Acetabulum*, after the Greekes /S/χοτυλγυ/S/ or /S/χατυλ δωγα/S/, our English phrase offereth vs no proper terme for it, vnlesse we shall call it a caue, case, or cuppe' (Cii^{v}). The context suggests that there is nothing to choose between these three alternatives, but there is a sub-lemma for **cave** with this meaning in *OED*. The next recorded use of **cave** in this sense is in Bacon, and it might well be that Banister's suggestion is a genuine innovation. At the same time he uses **acetable** (Cii^{v} margin), a naturalized form which, though in a different sense, is first recorded in 1551 (Turner).

Another instance of his providing some English equivalents is the case of **larum** or **supercilium**, which are the upper edges of such cavities in bones. These he suggests might be called 'the lippes, or browes, or as we may terme them the brinkes to those caues' (Cii^{v}).

OED does not list such a sense of **brink**, limiting it to geographical features and figuratively to times and events. He seems to be searching for a new application of the term. Similarly, **brow** has no such sense in *OED*.

Banister also takes the trouble to point out 'barbarous' terms; for instance, the case of the bones of the arms, the ulna and the radius, which he claims are known as **focile minius** and **focile maius** respectively. Writers of this period are inclined to treat 'barbarous Latin' almost as a separate language, or at least to distance themselves from it; certainly to treat it as a distinct and non-authoritative lexicon, and Banister is no exception. On another occasion he mentions that the **casula cordis**, the involucre of the heart (pericardium), is referred to by 'the barbarous number' who 'by the addition of one letter pronounce it *Capsula*' (Cciii^{v}). But his comments on barbarous Latin are less frequent than, say, Turner's.

There always seems to be a concern to find the right, or practical term, rather than painstakingly to sift the options as does Barrough, and Banister certainly does not work on a principle of clear linguistic authority and decorum. One may find Latin or Greek terms in profusion, and even Latin phrases: 'the first bones of the fingers are ioyned aboue, with the *Postbrachiall* bones *per enarthrosm* [*sic*]' (Kiii^{r}). He generally shuns Arabic terms, which Barrough is at least prepared to discuss, except for a few towards the end of the work, but frequently offers alternatives, especially in Latin: 'the *Triangular Cartilage*, named *Mucronata*, because it is downewardes sharpe poynted, and edged like a sword: wherfore some also call it *Ensiformis* and *Gladialis*; other, for that it ha[n]geth like a shield, say *Clypealis*: some agayne, *Malum granatu[m]*: but the Greekes, *Xiphoides*' (Hiiii^{v}).[21]

There seems to be little consistency in usage. The **arteria aspera** is indifferently called the **rough arterie**; the **os sacrum** is always just that, and the **scapula** is always the **scapple bone**. The **sternum** is often also the **brest bone**. In at least one case, the **pericardium**, a rather lengthy discussion mentioning **pericardium**, **cordus involucrum**, **casula cordis**, **capsula cordis** ends with 'but we wil vse here to say the inuolucre of the hart' (Cciii^{v})—and he does thereafter, preferring the naturalized term. There are other occasions in Banister's work where, against expectations, no neoclassical terms occur at all; as in 'the aforesayd gutter of the shoulderbone' (Iiii^{v}).

Many instances of the appositive coupling of terms, one native and one latinate, occur, as is usual in medical texts.[22] These are superficially similar to the aureate appositions so much liked by some prose writers from the fifteenth century on, but unlike literary and religious writing, where their function depends on an assumed synonymy, even if the aureate synonym may not be well known, in medical texts their basis seems rather to be an assumption of potential unfamiliarity. Thus the function of those appearing in medical texts seems generally to be instructive, first in the light of the deficiencies in Latin of some of the readers of these works and, second, possibly because of a need to naturalize the large body of encysts in medical terminology and to establish vocabulary in the reader's not fully educated mind.[23] The former motivation seems obvious enough, but the latter is more difficult to establish. Clearly, however, the neoclassical member of the pair will often have been familiar to the learned from their Greek and Latin textbooks, and thus will have served a bridging function for those less thoroughly educated. In the absence of statements about motivation, it is not always clear either whether an author means to reinforce the neoclassical or the native term. Some of the couplings discovered in Banister's work may be instances of his searching for an English term, but it is hard to be certain, as the technique is so widespread and conventional.[24] For example, he speaks of the 'circumaction and round, or wheelyng motion of the shoulder' (Iii^{r}), and in discussing what he calls the sigmoid processes of the shoulder mentions that 'the same *Processes* might complect, and embrace the hollow or rounded gutter in the lower end of the shoulder bone' (Iiii^{v}). Both of these sound as if he is casting about for the best term among some obvious alternatives in English. Many variations on coupling are possible, which may involve short descriptions rather than single words, e.g. 'a more blunt bowyng, and *Semicircled* corner' (Gii^{r}), or explanation rather than literal translation, as in the 'stiliforme, or spurrelike processes' (Ei^{r}); 'no lesse than a stabiliment, stay, or ground' combines other than neoclassical words. There are also some which are expanded into similes; e.g. 'many other little perforated places & chinkes, as it were the small siftyng holes of a searse' (Fiii^{r}). In his discussion of the eye he says of the crystalline humour that it is 'almost the principall member of sight, pleasaunt to be marked, and worthy to be knowe[n], not iniuriously therfore called the idole, or Image of seeing' (Ffiiii^{r}). It is possibly a case of Banister wishing to establish an English usage for what is obviously an important phenomenon and being forced back upon inventing a metaphor, but it is hard to be certain. None of these seems simply to be straightforward synonymy for rhetorical purposes, but conscious attempts to clarify terminology. On at least one occasion he is obliged to comment, on the term **larynx**, that 'I know not properly what English terme to giue it' (Fiiii^v), and indeed the word **voicebox** appears in *OED* with a first citation for 1912! On this occasion he makes no attempt to find a satisfactory English term.

Coupling may not always be strictly technical; for example, Banister's 'as well by election or choise' (Qi^r) or 'to make the third process recited, better knowne, and more manifest to your intellection' (Ei^v), but on the whole instances of aureate periphrasis are not common. At least it is possible in dealing with couplings in medical texts largely to discount the suggestion which arises in discussing this device in other forms of prose that it often arises from literary pretension, and is at heart tautological.[25] Cotta (88) provides an example of a physician using a word whose use is probably medical coupled in a non-medical context: 'they exenterate and eate out the bowels of poore mens purses.' Some examples are quite difficult to interpret. Does Bostocke intend equivalence between the three items in the following example, or is some difference in meaning implied (that is, is it a genuine list): 'those qualities be onely signes, colours and *Symptomata of* diseases' (Ei^v)? Another motivation for coupling is the assertion of literary authority, and while this would be difficult to determine in particular cases, the impulse not being context-specific, the explanatory function of couplings in Banister is often, as we have seen, contextually transparent. In spite of being so frequently used in medical texts, coupling is hardly explained at all by the authors. Perhaps the device was so conventional that no need for explanation was felt. At least it is useful for the modern lexicographer in establishing synonyms.

The origins, or at least the impetus to employ coupling in these texts, is more likely, therefore, to be found in the multilingual glossing commonly practised in herbals and medical texts. Another practice which perhaps conduced to this device is the pretty well universal habit in medical works of placing Greek and or Latin marginalia, many of which are glossarial, alongside English running text.

The difficulties in adapting the vernacular which this raises are clear in the category confusions inherent in finding an equivalent for the term **postbrachial**: 'which is the middle of [the] hand, (wherto

I can giue no propper Englishe, except I shall call that part the backe of the hand, or after the Latins the *Postbrachiall* bones' (Iiiii^v). Definition often creates confusion; perhaps an understandable problem when one considers the awkwardness of having constantly to identify the thing in question either through a welter of competing terms from different languages, or a dearth of them, and in an age when dictionary or glossary definitions were inadequate, frequently not specific, and often only one-word glosses, many of which simply assigned a word to a class, rather than delineating the characteristics of that member of the class. Many contemporary dictionaries define any malady as 'a disease', or any herb as 'a herb', sometimes with equally unhelpful adjectival qualifications such as 'well known'.

On some other occasions the Latin is simply perceived by Banister to be the more elegant or appropriate term; for example, the muscle adjoining the shoulder blade, which 'accordyng to the raritie of his shape obtaineth a rare & peculiar name, that is a hoodlike *Muscle*, or more seemely in Latin *Cucullaris Musculus*' (Pii^v). Another occurs later in a triple coupling: 'The right veyne, and arterie ... beyng together, after a space, so contingent, and mutually growyng together, as that most elegantly this word of the *Grecians Anastomosis* may be to them applyed' (Bbii^r). But such comments are rare.

Banister is not always clear in matters of the definition of terms. He also has an extended discussion of the term **shoulder**, which he defines as 'the mouinge that is geuen to the upper bone of the arme'. There is no evidence in *OED* that the term ever had such a sense other than the power of motion or the action of moving given in *OED* 1c and d. But it is also clear that **shoulder** is intended to be a translation of **humerus**. He continues: 'that is the most propper terme for it, for the same bone in Latin is called *Humerus*, which in English is shoulder, although in our domesticall phrase, we say the shoulder, when we meane the highest part aboue the arme, which in deede is the *Processe* of the scaple bone called *Acromio[n]*, in like sort, as by the arme we meane both the shoulder bone, and cubite. Thus for thy better satisfaction' (Piii^v). Thus shoulder may mean the humerus and/or the process called the acromion, which is still the proper term (Dorland 1988). His contemporaries used shoulder for what he would call **acromion**, but he regards **humerus** as preferable, and the latter as 'domesticall'. The term 'mouinge' remains problematical, and must await further research to know if it is a genuine new sense. A fascinating instance of re-alienation occurs in the case of **kell** (Tiii^{r} ff.) which he uses a number of times. The word perhaps relates to Fr. *cale* (see *OED*), a small cap, but there is clearly no classical precedent for it. Nevertheless, both **kellum** and **kellum intestinum** are used. It is a clear example of investing a word with neoclassical robes. Perhaps not quite so obviously, he also uses **lasertus** (Niiii^{r}) where **lacert** was already extant by the fourteenth century. **Planta** (Liiii^{v}) may be another example of re-alienation since it is not recorded in this form by *OED*, and the earliest citation for **plant** *sb*^{2} is from the fourteenth century.

As with Barrough, the problems arise from a surplus of words rather than a dearth of them. Although lacks are sometimes commented upon, it is very often the case that Banister has to choose between options. It is his practice in many instances not to exercise this option and to use synonymous terms or equivalent forms indiscriminately. Choices are familiar to the compilers of herbals also, who were as concerned to find the right terms among competitors to name known plants as they were to find new names for new ones. Although a special reason for this particular set of terms is offered, it is interesting to note that according to Harvey, 'The membrum virile has various names as penis from "that which is pendent", yard; it has twenty names in Greek and sixteen in Latin according to Laurentius. Because it is the symbol of fertility in procreation it has got for itself so many names' (Harvey 1964: 209).'[26]

In general the frequent authorial claims of introducing a new term to the reader are illusory, in that the language often contained the term in question already. It cannot be assumed that authors reliably identify neologisms and recent borrowings; or to put it another way, educating the readership should not be confused with enriching the lexicon, despite authorial intimations of omniscience. The emphasis is frequently on giving a previously naturalized term a Greek or Latin form, as much as on enrichment and expansion, and the lexical processes involved are far more often conservative than progressive or innovative.

Thus the idea that English lacked words, at least for medical science, has been a response to an insufficiently flexible view of the English medical lexicon, and there may be an inadequately researched generic principle of lexicon recognition involved here; that is, encysts have been treated on the whole as not being part of the lexicon, when in practice they were and are. Not only does the process of encystation need to be taken into account, but also re-alienation of fully adapted or encysted words, examples of which we have seen, as it is a markedly conservative factor in lexicon formation in medical writings.

2. AUTHORIAL AND TEXTUAL AUTHORITY

It is possible to distinguish, though not always clearly, between the authority of an author and the authority of a text. Textual authority is partly that of *a* text, partly that of text itself, the latter being firmly established during the century as a consequence of the reliability and accessibility of the printed word:

> the overall effect of printing, especially in medicine, was to reinforce the authority of the ancient texts . . . The real benefit of the printed book was not in the spread of new thought, but in the raising of the general standard of learning of the medical profession by the provision of an increased number of accepted texts. (McLean 1972: 185)

The former is more a matter of the improvements brought about by humanist scholarship. But the situation was by no means simple: at the same time as a rejection of medieval 'barbarism' and more attention to textual purity as against exegetical sophistication enhanced the authority of a text or author, so the increasing revelation of the deficiencies of that source had the contrary effect.

While these scholarly humanist endeavours continued, an inexorable linguistic change which influenced the position of Latin in the sixteenth century in England was taking place—the great vowel shift affected the pronunciation of Latin, cutting it adrift from already divergent Continental practices; furthermore, spoken Latin declined as classical rather than medieval Latin became the preferred form. William Bullokar, the father of the lexicographer, was able to comment on the divergence in Latin pronunciation which had occurred by the end of the sixteenth century that 'some single letters in the Latine are diuersely sounded of any nation, and one nation differeth from another in pronouncing Latine' (Bullokar 1970: 2 (original pagination). A further factor in these processes in England was the dissolution of the monasteries. Latin increasingly became the restricted preserve of esoteric areas of knowledge, rather than familiar as the language of religion, thus increasing its inaccessibility to all but the intellectually privileged. By the early seventeenth century the decline in spoken Latin as an international language had become obvious (Salmon 1979: 3–4), and it was declining as the language of instruction in the grammar schools (Görlach 1985: 30). It has been suggested that the decline had already gone so far at the beginning of the seventeenth century that it 'was to be learnt as an international quasi-scientific language, desirable for the naming of objects in the real world and not primarily for the reading of ancient authors' (Salmon 1979: 13). Bailey in *Mithridatium* alludes to the increasingly perceived corruptions of older texts and the discovery of new and better information. Discussing the quality of imported cinnamon, he remarks that 'We may also vndersta[n]d, how in old time things were sophisticated by the monume[n]ts of old writers. And who doth not now perceaue and acknowledg many errors in *Dioscorides* bookes, in deliuering the descriptions of simples, not so well knowe[n] in his time, as now by these nauigatio[n]s made manifest' (C6[v]).

It is frequently remarked that the widespread publication of scientific texts made knowledge far more freely available after the development of printing than had previously been the case, especially to the literate, middle-class stratum of society. Undoubtedly this is largely true, even though it is a proposition about which circumstantial evidence—contents of libraries, sales of books, identity of purchasers, reading habits, and dissemination of books—is often conspicuously deficient. On the other hand, it does not follow from the emergence of such an apparently liberating phenomenon that vernacular writers influenced each other or acquired reputations like those of the ancients. Chrisman remarks that 'the discoveries of these trained scientists [Vesalius, Brunfels, etc.] were made available to the broad spectrum of burgher society through the medium of illustrated books' (Chrisman 1982: 191). What is less clear is that physicians would have read such works, and her view should be considered along with the claim of H. S. Bennett, who commented that in England in the first half of the sixteenth century, 'printers exploited the popular market and ignored to a large extent the professional one' (Bennett 1969: 109). It has been argued that it is perhaps unlikely that many of the books, especially the vernacular compilations of remedies, were taken very seriously, but that argument really comes to little more than a twentieth-century disgust at the kinds of remedies suggested:

> given the false remedies and impossible recipes contained in medical treatises, one hopes that they were studied more by poets than by physicians. Given the exotic ingredients described, one may assume that few apothecaries actually tried to concoct all the recipes contained in early printed

pharmacopeia, although they may have felt impelled to stock their shelves with bizarre items just in case the new publicity might bring such items into demand. (Eisenstein 1979: i. 65)

But this view is surely apologetic; apothecaries, surgeons, and other less official practitioners were probably the main readers of such works, since physicians were less concerned with the course of treatment, and there is no evidence to suggest that they did not take them seriously. Why indeed would anyone other than those with a particular concern for medicine read them, when what they purveyed were the orthodox procedures and standard recipes? Some exotic and bizarre items were substituted with locally obtainable ones, but of course many which seem outrageous to us, such as pigeon droppings and crushed centipedes, must have been regarded as perfectly normal and acceptable.[27] The existence of many manuscript compilations gathered by enthusiastic amateurs, by those who practised professionally but unlicensed, and by those who were in charge of the medical well-being of some institution, along with the fact of borrowing and reborrowing recipes repeatedly, is sufficient to indicate that such activities were entirely serious, and that printed works of this kind are not merely eye-catching sports.[28] Walter Bailey makes it clear on the title-page of his work on mithridatium that he intends it for use; it is 'Compiled rather for those which are to vse it, then for the learned'. This is no very accurate directive as to readership, but it seems likely that apothecaries are the intended market.

That physicians accumulated and maintained professional libraries and felt that they were worth bequeathing to the next generation is clear enough, as is shown by the bequest of William Turner's books to his physician son.[29] What the contents of these collections were less well known. Presumably physicians in England as in the rest of Europe read Galen, Hippocrates, and the rest (in editions mainly printed in Continental Europe), but it is their attitude to what was being read which is of particular interest. Did they read Vesalius or Linacre in the same way as they read the classics? And what was their view of vernacular works? The written evidence suggests that, with the partial exception of surgery, the wide dissemination of books did not mean necessarily a corresponding attention on the part of the professionals either to the writings or to the discoveries of their colleagues.[30] Thus it remained true that not even the maker of a conspicuous advance in technique or the discoverer of a new truth in medicine became as a consequence an authority in the full sense. Knowledge in the vernacular grew through an accumulating exegesis of the classical texts. The remarkable career of Paracelsus encapsulates the difficulties. In this respect, the failure of English medicine to notice the Paracelsian Bostocke in the 1580s was characteristic. It was not as if Paracelsus had not been noted before, at least by some, and attention to him grew for the most part through the adoption of some of his remedies rather than the acceptance of his theories. At least a couple of authors tried to wave him away with the mulish remark that they by no means pretended to understand him, Clowes being a good example,[31] while at the same time making use of some of his formulations.

Some firm evidence as to what medical practitioners read can be got from references to particular authors in their published works. In the case of English authors, such references normally indicate that the author in question had really been read, since there was no tradition of citation of English authorities which could be employed as a matter of course from the works of other compilers. Needless to say, not being cited cannot mean that an author was neither read nor used, but a citation should generally indicate a particular debt or token of appreciation, unless some particular reason for the citation which might indicate disapproval is stated.

Laudatory comments on the works of contemporaries do appear, however, in certain areas, although references to Continental authors are far more frequent than to English ones, and also appear earlier in the literature. Before 1600 they are most frequent in herbals, a fact which seems to underline the relative importance of this particular form of taxonomy. Leonhard Fuchs was translated into English quite early, although it was not his herbal but a tract on the plague which was chosen (Fuchs 1563). Turner had similarly paid his respects to recent work in his field, acknowledging among others Fuchs, Gesner, Bock (Tragus), and Brunfels. He had no debt to English authors, but scrupulously and, with a hint of regret that there were learned men in England who might have made as worthy a contribution but did not do so, remarked:

> There haue bene in England, and there are now also certain learned men: whych haue as muche knowledge in herbes, yea, and more then diuers Italianes and Germanes, whyche haue set furth in prynte Herballes and bokes of simples. I mean of Doctor Clement, Doctor Wendy, and Doctor Owen, Doctor Wotton, & maister Falconer.[32] Yet hath none of al these, set

furth any thyng, ether to the generall profit of hole Christendome in latin, & to the honor of thys realme, nether in Englysh to the proper profit of their naturall countre, wherfore some will laye vnnaturallnes and vnkindnes vnto their charges, whyche myght haue done these thynges and dyd them not, and could do the same and wold not. (Aii^v^)

Writing at the end of the century, Gerarde has a list of acknowledged debts in his herbal of 1597.

In a lengthy preface to *The regiment of lyfe*, Thomas Phaer offers us some early and useful comments both on translation and on authority, calling for Englishmen to do for medicine in England what contemporaries had already done on the continent in their own vernaculars, and specifically to make improvements in herbal description. He cites a number of contemporaries or near-contemporaries with approval, calling them the 'men of high learninge nowe of oure daies as Manardus, Fuchsius, Ruelius, Musa Campegius, Sebastia[n] of Austrik, Otho Brunfelsius, Leonelus, &c.' (Aiii^r^), and as such may be the first English physician to do so in print. He hopes 'to see the time, whan the nature of Simples (whiche haue been hitherto incredibly corrupted) shall be reade in Englishe, as in other languages: that is to saie, the perfect declaration of the qualities of herbes, sedes, rootes, trees, and of all commodities that are here amongest vs, shall bee earnestlie and truely declared, in our owne natiue speche . . . To the whiche I truste all lerned men (hauinge a zeale to the common wealth) will apply their diligent industries' (Aiiii^r^).

Reference to English contemporaries during this period is much more grudging than that accorded to Continental authorities. It should also be noted that authorities are not cited in the sixteenth century in order to acknowledge intellectual debts and, although the precise motivation for citation may vary a little from author to author and in different circumstances, it was generally done to demonstrate the respectability of a particular view or assertion. Some kind of verifiable assent was useful, and the more venerable the authority cited, the less assailable the claim. Citation was, however, not felt to be mandatory, and plagiarism was widespread. Thus citation represents a more genuine feeling for the authority of the source than would be the case today.

Citation of English authors in printed works begins with the very early notice of an English contemporary occurring in a herbal published by Banckes in 1525, which takes the opportunity of cashing in on the putative and by the time of publication posthumous reputation of the renowned Thomas Linacre. It purports to be a herbal 'practysed by Doctor Linacro'.[33] This physician seems to have been the only Englishman to have published in Latin during the century who received real credit, though later John Caius is very occasionally mentioned.[34] It is also another hint that the compilers of herbals were as interested in the practice and experience of the present as in the legacy of the ancient or medieval past.

There is, then, a gap of a quarter of a century until another citation of an English authority, namely the one in Turner's *Herbal* of 1551 already mentioned, which is hardly flattering. He was perhaps not to know that Wootton would venture into print the very next year, though not on the subject Turner hoped for.[35] He implies that others might very well have also made some effort without mentioning further names. Linacre's translation of Galen is cited in his treatise on wines of 1562 (Ci^{r}). In 1558 Humfrey Llwyd gratefully confesses that he is 'muche beholden to Mayster Wyllya[m] Turner, who wyth no small dylygence hath in both hys herballes moste truly and syncerly set furth the names and natures of dyuerse herbes' (Aii^{r}).

The Salisbury physician John Securis, who published *A detection and querimonie of the daily enormities and abuses co[m]mitted in phisick* in 1566, occupies an ambiguous place in this discussion, as if to demonstrate that no scheme is ever cut and dried. He was clearly a conservative in his attitudes, but on the other hand was acquainted with recent writings. He published two works, one now lost, which is referred to in his later book.[36] The latter attacked the abuses in medical practice of his day. It is possible that, as the title suggests, the subject of his earlier attack was the spate of then recent translations, but this must remain speculation.

Securis has criticism of all three branches of the profession, the most general being a lack of the appropriate education. He inveighs against those who 'so fondly and so wickedly do abuse the noble art & science of Phisicke. Where is their great and manifold knowlege of the toungues?' (Avii^{r}), but he reserves his especial condemnation for surgeons and apothecaries. Surgeons are in his view too frequently unlearned, not to say unlettered. He points out that surgery has a more profound and abstract aspect, which goes beyond practical experience. 'Surgerie although it be a manuell arte, yet it hath his speculation, whiche can not be had without readynge of diuers authors' (Evii^r), but his references are not only to the ancient and medieval canon, and he also directs practitioners to some of 'the latter writers, *Tagaultius*, *Hollerius*, *Bologuinus* and others'. He does in fact give reason to suppose that his own reading was well up to date for his time. He advises apothecaries to be more discriminating as to whose guidance they might follow, suggesting:

the chiefe guide & Instrument, that shold rule al the rost, I meane the boke of *Bernardus Dessennius Cronenburgius*, *de compositione medicame[n]torum* ... I would wish also, that [th]e poticarie mought not be without the dispensatories of *Valerius Cordus*, of *Fuchsius*, or *Nicolaus Mirepsius*, or the .ii. bokes of *Siluius* contening the chosinge, kepinge, and making of medicines commonlye vsed: or *Examen tam simplicium* [?] *compositorum*, *Antonij Muse*; and not to followe still their blinde *Nicolaus Præpositus*, which is full of errours. (Dv^v)

Thus Securis refers quite extensively to recent authorities, though it must be noted that none of them is English. He also praises Silvius, under whom he appears to have studied in Paris, as 'that man of high learning & famous memorie' (Avi^r). This is not unusual; in the end, language of whatever kind, as long as it was not one's own, remained that last great arcanum of the late sixteenth-century physician.

The next major series of allusions to English authorities comes in 1562 in the writing of William Bullein who, in his *Bulleins bulwarke of defe[n]ce againste all sicknes, sornes, and woundes* (Aaiiii^r–v), makes mention of no fewer than twenty-three, for the most part his own contemporaries. They include those who wrote in Latin, such as Caius, whom he describes as 'the seconde Linacar', and in English, including Turner, Recorde, Borde, Phaer, and Gale, and some who are not known to have published at all, including Porter, Ludford, Clemens, and Butts. He also mentions the translator Paynell. Some of these are mentors, others colleagues, or practitioners he has heard about. There is also a mixture of surgeons, namely Gale and Vicary, and physicians, although the latter predominate. Bullein was himself a physician, so that his willingness to recognize and to write about surgery is progressive, inspired perhaps by the example of Caius, whom he particularly praises for service to the craft in his lectures to the Barber-Surgeons' Company. He was also aware of the fact that Gesner had praised Turner 'whose learned actes, I leaue to the wittie commendacio[n]s and immortall praise of *Conradus Gesnerus*'. Neither are all the practitioners mentioned confined to

London—there is 'Porterus' of Norwich (Aav^r) and Mighell (or Michell) the Frenchman of Newcastle (Aii^v), among others. Bullein's work on pleurisy (*Pleurisi*, 1562), however, contains no mention of Englishmen.

The first part of Gale's *Certaine workes of chirurgerie* is in the form of a dialogue between himself and two contemporaries, Field and Yates, which gives the text a contemporaneous feel, and is certainly a departure from the more normal learned debate usually put in the mouths of known figures from antiquity, or of characters with Greek or Latin names. This dialogue, however, contains few other references to English writers or practitioners.

Another surgeon, John Banister, has one allusion to Linacre in *The historie of man* but hardly a flattering one. Discussing the misunderstanding of a passage in Galen, he ascribes it to the 'imbecillitie of his interpretour *Thos. Linacre*, not perfectly vnderstandinge the sense or meaning in that place' (Uiiii^v). There are no further references to Englishmen, though his reliance upon Vesalius, Collumbus, and others is heavy.

The little-known physician John Jones is also a copious source of contemporaneous references, and of praise for his countrymen. He offers the general remark in his treatise on the waters of Buxton that English physicians are comparable to any other, claiming that 'there were neuer better, nor greater store in our lande, euen of oure owne Nacion, than bee at this day: comparable (I dare saye) both for wysedom lerning, and experience, to any in all *Europe*' (Bi^v). Apart from allusions to such disparate authors as Chaucer, Savonarola, Tusser, and Erasmus, he also mentions specifically Chaloner (*Bathes*), Turner (*Arte* Fiii^r), Elyot (*Arte* Iiiii^r), Recorde and Phaer (*Arte* Bi^r), Banister (*Arte* Gi^r), Bullein, one Doctor Francis (*Dial* Av^r) and Caius (*Dial* Fvii^v), among others. A dedicatory note by Thomas Newton (*iiii^r) refers to 'Turnerus, Caius, Bullenus, Linacrus, Askham ... Phairus ... Hallus ... Argenterio Frerus & Hatcherides'. Several of these people are cited on more than one occasion throughout his works. His reading appears to have been up to date—he mentions Bullein four years after the appearance of his *Bulwarke*—as well as extensive.

William Clowes's work is characteristic of the publications of surgeons in showing a practical interest in contemporaneous writings and in innovation in the discipline. His earliest extant work, on *morbus gallicus*, immediately shows his concern to acknowledge real rather than fanciful or expedient obligations, being dedicated to his colleagues in the Barber-Surgeons' Company of London. In the preface he generously acknowledges those teachers past and present who have been his benefactors. His emphasis is on practical experience: not on his reading in his subject so much as on the 'lectures, anatomies, co[n]ferences, and practises of the notable and skilfull chirurgio[n]s that heretofore haue bene, and are at this present the worthy members of this house' to whom he feels indebted (Aiii^{r}).

By the time this work was refurbished and reissued in 1585, it appears that much had changed. The attribution of debts to teachers has been stripped of references to lectures, but the personages themselves are now 'the shining starres and light of our most excellent art and mysterie' (Aiii^{v}). An attack on a quacksalver called Valentine Rasworm, which had appeared in the 1579 edition, is now considerably enlarged and much more acerbic; a long list of the patients he is supposed to have killed by his bungling is added to the original accusation that Rasworm was a fraud—surely a savage indictment even in an age whose freewheeling personal attacks are best characterized by the vitriolic Harvey–Nashe controversy.

Perhaps more than any other in the sixteenth century, William Clowes both acknowledges debts to other Englishmen and praises the efforts of his contemporaries. In his work on the cure of *morbus gallicus* published in 1585, Clowes provides a long list of authors who, he argues, have benefited their country by their endeavours, speaking of the

> many notable men [who] haue written sundrie kindes of learned workes in English, their naturall language ... And therefore was it wiselie sayd of our Maister *Gale*: In what tongue so euer a man may get knowledge, the tongue serueth no further, but to the learning of the art. This hath made many of our Countrie men to publish many profitable works in English, both of Phisicke and Chyrurgerie. As maister Doctor *Record*, maister Doctor *Phare*, Maister Doctor *Turnar*, maister Doctor *Lancton*, maister Doctor *Bourd*, and maister Doctor *Bright*, with many other learned Physitions & Chyrurgions, as maister *Gale*, maister *Hawll*, maister *Baker*, master *Banester*, and many other Chyrurgions. What shall we thinke of [th]e worthie knight sir *Thomas Eliot*, of maister *Trehiron*, of maister *Lite*, maister *Barrow*, maister *Bullen*, & such other worthie Gentlemen. (Liiii^{v})

This list is very up to date, since Barrough, for example, had published his *The methode of physicke* only two years previously, and both

Lyte and Bright had published not very much earlier in the late 1570s.

Clowes's work is, apart from his earliest treatise, rich with mention of contemporaries, not only writers, but people from whom he had learned something, or had got useful remedies or methods, including Bailey, Yates, Trip, Foster, Crowe, Goodrus, and others. In *A prooued practice* he refers, for example, to the skills of 'Maister *Banester*' (Piiii1^{r}), 'Maister *Archenbole*, a very skilfull Chirurgeon' (Piiii^{v}), and to the learned lectures of 'Doctor *Foster* ' (Piiii3^{r}). In a rare allusion to a female practitioner he also mentions a Madam Donnell whom he records as having done many 'charitable deeds in the curing of a many [*sic*] wounded soldiers', and from whom he had got a useful wound-drink (113).[37]

In the course of his career, Clowes deferred at least once to the skill of a contemporary, and showed a knowledge of other work in progress in refusing to complete a larger work on *lues venerea*, knowing that another learned work 'writte[n] by that great doctor Theredehere of Fraunce, a man of a profound iudgeme[n]t, and very great experience ... is now translated out of French into English, by M. William Martin Surgeon of London' (148).[38] The combative Clowes returned to blast the carpers in 1597 in a dedication to the reader in Peter Lowes's book on surgery, attacking them not only for a destructive attitude but, as earlier in the century, for their own negligence in not publishing anything themselves. A considerable shift in attitudes to received wisdom has occurred, and Clowes is prepared to echo Banister in claiming that 'truth is truth from whome so euer it come, be it from *Hipocrates*, *Galen*, *Paracelsus*, (Clowes 1588 Ai^{r})'.[39] By the time of his last treatise, the controversies have apparently died away, aside from a reference to the strife which continued between the Galenists and the Paracelsians, but his career clearly shows his productive immersion in the day-to-day problems and developments in his profession.

The extent to which writers such as Clowes, to whom no major discovery and no pioneering research can be attributed, represented a progressive stance in their profession can perhaps be shown more objectively and effectively with the use of diachronic corpora. A recent study employing such techniques, albeit narrowly statistical and based on the single linguistic feature of first- and second-person pronouns, has been able to confirm the rather strikingly progressive attitude apparent in his texts (Taavitsainen 1994*a*; 1994*b*: 208).

William Clever published his *The flower of phisicke* in 1590 (*STC* 5412). It exhibits greater apparent conservatism, or perhaps simply discretion, than Clowes's work. The preface to *The flower of phisicke* conceals rather more than it reveals. He declares in pastoral imagery the virtues and authority of his compilation in which its author has 'presented ... all the whole counsels and high iudgements of Physicke, written by the monarch Phisitions of the world, Galen, Hypocrates, Auycen, and Dyoscorides'. Clever stresses the ancient authority from which 'you shall find most rich treasures, discouered from a fruitfull soile, A pure water running from a cleare fountaine, And most sweet flowers, from the pleasant garden of humaine and liberall arts' (ep. ded.). He disingenuously asserts that his task has been merely to have 'broke the yce, and smoothed the path from the greeke and Latine'. This suggests to the reader that such sources were not already plentifully tapped, but also conceals the fact that his text is actually liberally sprinkled with references to rather later and more sullied springs—there are, for example, numerous references to Paracelsus, with whose work he was obviously familiar, and whose arguments against Galen he is prepared to notice. There are frequent references to other sources, but of those which can be confidently recognized Leonhard Fuchs is probably the most recent. Others such as Jérémie de Dryvere, Giovanni Manardo, and Jean Ruel represent the early sixteenth century, but there is an absence of contemporaries, and in this Clever contrasts with the current reportage of Clowes. Established authorities, many of them medieval, are still of paramount importance in his text. By contrast, an approving reference to the work of the 'no lesse learned than worshipfull' (¶¶4^{r}) Thomas Elyot occurs in Cogan's *The hauen of helth* of 1585, from whom he freely admits to having borrowed verbatim (¶¶4^{v}).

A relatively early reference to a contemporaneous medical work occurs in 1586, following the appearance of Bostocke's *Difference* in the previous year. The author, who is identified only as I.W., springs to Bostocke's defence under the guise of a letter to a friend: 'it seemeth that you neuer read many of *Paracelsus* his workes, nor yet that booke lately set forth by master B. in our mother tongue.' This pamphlet may have been written in the first place as a reply to attacks on Bostocke, but it is essentially a defence of Paracelsus, and includes a brief and already familiar argument in favour of the use of the vernacular. The author is contemptuous of 'you great clarkes with al your learning' and of the 'foggie mists and bogges of Aristotle and

Galen'. It apparently took the influence of Paracelsus to rattle the complacent dignity of non-productive members of the medical establishment, and to oblige them to notice current issues in their discipline. This was a fitful beginning, but the existence of these books may indicate a lively professional discussion, at least in some quarters, as well as a realization that the printing press might be used in the service of theoretical progress, in addition to popularization. In this England was a long way behind the rest of Europe. Such works, alongside the practical sense of Clowes and presumably some of his fellow surgeons, are the first real indications that open discussion of medical developments is taking place.

The list of contemporaries generously cited by William Clowes in 1585 is, like Bullein's, a list of both physicians and surgeons, authors and non-authors, some of whom were already familiar from earlier sources, but not surprisingly a large percentage of them are surgeons. His references to certain surgical colleagues, probably ones with whom he regularly consulted, notably Baker and Banister, appear frequently. Later still in the century, citations appear less frequently in the medical literature, but John Gerarde mentions Turner, Baker, Lyte, and Priest; Peter Lowe acknowledges Gerarde. A.M., the translator of Gabelkhover and Guillemeau, is conspicuous for mentioning no Englishman in spite of having lived in England, only alluding to his master, Baumann of Dort. Nevertheless, by the latter years of the sixteenth century it is clear that credit is accorded to Englishmen for writing in English far more extensively than for writing in Latin.

It does not seem to be those prominent in the Royal College of Physicians who are generally published in English. On the other hand, the more prominent surgeons did publish, so much so that they seem quite self-supporting and even self-congratulatory in these efforts, and were only too willing to make cross-references to each other and to write laudatory epistles and verses for each others' volumes. Vicary and later Gale and Baker were masters of the Company, and Clowes and Banister were among its more prominent members.

If the number of references to an author can be taken as a rough guide to the extent to which he was read, then clearly Turner was the most widely read English writer in the medical field. Perhaps given that herbals were of prime importance to medical practice, and that his held the field for nearly half a century, this is not so surprising;

what may actually be more so is that his contemporaries clearly recognized his importance. It is of course possible that personal acquaintance and known repute account for some citations of him, but references do persist until the end of the century. Most citations fall in the period 1560–85, and it is also noteworthy that both physicians and surgeons make use of him.[40] He is cited by five different authors, Bullein, Llwyd, Jones, Gerarde, and Clowes, sometimes frequently, Llwyd, among the physicians, specifically mentioning his contribution to nomenclature. A number, though not all of these citations are laudatory, suggesting that he was widely regarded as indispensable, and probably original. His personal reputation was considerable in spite of his having produced only two works in Latin, and those by no means major ones—the modest herbal of 1538 and his work on birds of 1544—but it is not as a physician that he was primarily recognized. Neither did he produce an out-and-out medical book, the bulk of his work being encyclopaedic natural history in English. His repute in this area is shown by the fact that he is mentioned approvingly by Gesner more than once. The man whose particular achievement it was to regularize, modernize, and to supply his discipline with a working nomenclature in English was quickly lauded for his achievement, and this fact emphasizes the seminal role of herbals and of botany in the mid-sixteenth century, not just in medicine, but in taxonomy generally.

On the whole translators are not especially noticed, but the author they translate may be very frequently cited, cases in point being Lanfranc and Vigo, who are copiously quoted especially by surgeons, while their vernacular translators, Vicary and Traheron, are infrequently mentioned. Vicary is noticed only by Bullein, and Traheron by Clowes. It is also apparent that Englishmen writing in Latin are cited quite infrequently. Linacre, Caius, and Wootton, whom one might have expected to be widely used, are referred to only by four authors between them. Only Caius is cited by two, Bullein and Jones. It is difficult to know whether this represents a preference for vernacular works or a lack of repute in their own country. Neither should it be forgotten that this study entirely ignores the continuing availability and circulation of medical manuscripts throughout the sixteenth century. Thus a conspicuous absentee by contrast with Vigo and Lanfranc from those English authorities cited in printed works surveyed here is John of Arderne, who was frequently cited in fifteenth-century manuscript surgery books and collections of remedies (Jones 1989). The first printed edition of any of his works dates from 1588, and is merely an addition to John Read's translation of Franciscus Arceus.

The widespread citation of Continental sources manifests a clear preference among vernacular English writers, which prevails throughout the century, and is interrupted principally by the large-scale citations of Bullein, Jones and Clowes. Perhaps Latin texts by Englishmen were rather lost in the ruck of European publication. The fact that they also tended to publish in Europe was probably not a factor, however, since Continental publications were often cheaper than English ones, a fact which induced governments to attempt now and then to curb the trade in books from Europe.

What is slowly but inexorably emerging from all of this evolutionary linguistic process, however, is a settled and stable medical lexicon which incorporates neologisms on the one hand, where new concepts arise and older errors are expunged, and preserves neoclassicisms on the other, carefully preserving where possible their original form and pristine signification, and setting such terminology aside from the potential degradation into hopeless polysemy which widespread vernacular use would imply. It is very apparent that from about 1560 there is a spectacular increase in the scope and sophistication of vernacular medical texts, and therefore in the amount of terminology put into use, a fact which in itself must have had a standardizing influence, as the competing terminologies were sifted for their relevance and adaptability.

Notes

1. A statistically complete survey of this material would be of great value in illuminating an important and under-researched semantic domain in early modern English.
2. This argument was a standard one which goes back at least to Sylvius. See Saunders and O'Malley (1950: 13).
3. The process may be discovered in other areas with a specialist vocabulary; there is much research still to be done.
4. I will use the term 'classical' to apply simply to 'the source languages Greek, Latin, and less often Arabic'. Terms thus borrowed I have usually called 'neoclassical'.
5. Sager et al. (1980: 285) make exactly the same point about law: 'The retention of these phrases has little apparent justification; *de jure* and *de facto* are no more fixed or less ambiguous than *in law* and *in fact*.'
6. Practices like this make it impossible to assume that if a text declares a term to be Latin, the English term must therefore be something else.

For this reason, words contextually declared to be Greek or Latin are often incorporated in this study as unrecorded or as antedatings to *OED*; see Chapter 5.

7. See *OED* for the variants.
8. But there are inconsistencies here, too; he heads a chapter 'Of the inflammation of the tonsilles' (but then continues in the running text 'Tonsillae be inflammationes of those things which lye between the mouth and the throte' (Barrough 1583: 59).
9. The devices of pairing and of literal translation may look like the familiar appositive coupling which pervaded much prose writing, but is probably not intended as a flower of rhetoric, since glossing a difficult term seems to be its primary function; e.g. in the injunction to 'vse oyle solutiue and loosing' (75), or in describing that which provokes a cough in 'the instruments of respiration and breathing' (63). Similarly 'an instinction or tickling to lecherie' (158); but these are surely glosses rather than glozes.
10. See *MED*, **antrax**.
11. But note that the *OED*'s citations are no earlier than the seventeenth century.
12. It is explained by Jones 1566, Iiii$^{r–v}$.
13. *OED*, 2, (fig.) = **declination,** 5.
14. This partially explains the eminence of Turner, who had established himself as an authority not so much on medicine itself as on botanical nomenclature, in which area the classical models based on Dioscorides were already patently inadequate.
15. Banister or his printer has used the following plates from Vesalius: 1. On Biiii^{v}, *De humani corporis fabrica*, bk. 1, plate 21, the background altered from a barren landscape to a plant on the right and a barren tree on the left. 2. On Nii^{r}, *De humani corporis fabrica*, bk. 1, plate 23, again with the background altered. 3. On Niii^{v}, *De humani corporis fabrica*, bk. 2, plate 24, with a rural scene in the background changed to a tree trunk and a bush. The detail of the legs is poor. 4. On Siii^{r}, *De humani corporis fabrica*, bk. 2, plate 32, with an alteration similar to 3. 5. On Hhiiii^{v}, *De humani corporis fabrica*, bk. 1, plate 42.7, an assortment of surgical instruments on a table. See Saunders and O'Malley 1950.
16. An intriguing side issue is the question of why Banister and his publisher chose not to use more of the illustrations of Vesalius. They had already been extensively employed, by Udall in his translation of Geminius of 1553, and had been very well reproduced in that work. Perhaps they did not possess the technological means to do them justice.
17. There is also a citation for *appendancy* from Helkiah Crooke; again a medical sense (Crooke 1615). I can find no reference to **appendance** in Norri 1992.

18. See **appendo**, Lewis and Short (1969); Du Cange (1937); Anon. (1990). **Appendance** itself appears to be a French borrowing with no direct antecedent in Latin, but it is listed with the potentially medical sense 'appendage' and dated *c.*1115 in Latham (1965).
19. *OED*, 12, 'a projection from the main body of something, esp. a natural appendage, extension, or outgrowth ... *Anat.* ... of a bone.'
20. Lewis and Short (1969: III, transf, A).
21. Although it is outside the immediate scope of this work, there is an example of the reverse process in the anatomical lecture notes by William Harvey. In the sections on muscles especially, he frequently inserts the English term after the Latin, even giving alternatives in some cases; e.g. 'Carpi flectentium inferior, the nether wrest-bender, the pillow muscle, scribentes innitinur' (Harvey 1964: 406). These lectures may be presumed to have been delivered, as commentary on actual dissections (Harvey 1964: p. xxv), as part of his duties as the Lumleian lecturer in surgery, which commenced in 1615.
22. It is usual in other prose texts as well, and has a long history in English prose. The motivation for appositive coupling and its interpretation has been surveyed at some length (Mueller 1984: 147–51). Mueller uses the term 'doubling,' but since they are sometimes triple or even quadruple, and not always intended as synonyms, 'coupling' or simply 'apposition' is preferred here.
23. Pahta and Nevanlinna (forthcoming) survey the occurrence of such appositions in some medical texts in the Helsinki corpus, including Clowes's 1602 text *Treatise for the artificiall cure of struma*, showing that this technique spills over into purely native, rhetorical appositions as well.
24. Note the reverse process in a fifteenth–century manuscript; that is, Arderne's glosses in English or Anglo-Norman for many of the terms in his Latin text (Jones 1989: 69–70).
25. See Koskenniemi (1968: 75–112) for an extended discussion.
26. 'Mentula, varia nomina, penis a pendendo, virga; viginti greca nomina sexdecim latina apud Laurentium. Signum foecunditatis gignendum sibi tot nomina' (Harvey 1964: 208).
27. Other explanations suggest themselves—humbler ingredients given exotic names, recipes used as guides to confection rather than as strict rules (the tendency to multiply ingredients rather than isolate active principles would certainly lead to this), and we may simply know insufficient about the extent of trade in simples at the time.
28. See e.g. Sir Hugh Plat's compilation, mentioned in Chapter 5. A similar collection is to be found in Ffecknam (1990).
29. The will, proved on 15 July 1568, states 'to Peter Turner my sonne all my writen bookes and yf he be a preacher all my divinitie bookes yf he practise Phisicke all my physicke bookes' (Britten et al. 1965: 24–5).

30. For some insight into the position in the mid-century as reflected in the contents of the libraries of John Caius, Thomas Lorkin, and Roger Gifford, see Nutton (1979: 380).
31. 'I must confess that his doctrine hath a more pregnant sence, then my wit or reach is able to construe ... I have practised certaine of his inventions Chirurgicall, the which I haue found to be singular good' (Clowes 1602: preface).
32. Falconer is mentioned again in the *Herbal* under **Glaux** ('sea tryfoly' Bv^{v}), and Gesner in his book on fishes mentions Falconer's assistance (Hodgson 1831: 82).
33. *STC* 13175.13c; this edition, n.d.
34. Thomas Moffett published works in Latin, beginning with *Nosomantica hippocratea* (Frankfurt, 1588), as well as two later works, but he is not noticed by contemporaries writing in English.
35. Wotton (1552).
36. It is tantalisingly referred to as 'a litle boke of mine, printed about a dose[n] yeres past, which is intituled: A gret Galley lately com into England out of *Terra noua*, laden with phisitions, poticaries, & surgio[n]s, .&c. made in form of a dialoge'. *STC* has no record of this work.
37. Clowes (1596: 48, 73, 75, 111, 113). Foster, a London practitioner, seems also to have variously spelt his name as Forster or Forrestier.
38. There is no evidence of this work in *STC*.
39. Compare with Banister's views discussed earlier.
40. I have not recorded the actual number of references to him in each individual work, but in some they are frequent.

4

The Early Lexicographers: Elyot to Bullokar

Thus far we have examined the users of this terminology and some of their actual practices. Although this study concentrates on the actual contextual use of the medical lexis, our understanding of where medical terminology fitted into the language of the sixteenth century may be furthered by looking at the dictionaries of the period, since it is the lexicographers who are the first-level codifiers and interpreters of the contemporary lexicon. Their prescriptive judgements and editorial decisions have affected what was recorded in their works and exactly how it was registered. It is not to be presumed that they were on the whole comprehensively descriptive, but, since medical terminology incorporates a significant peripheral element of the English lexicon, it makes an interesting test case for the practices of these lexicographers. It is frequently the case that we must learn from their omissions rather than from their inclusions.

Although the interrelationships between dictionaries of the sixteenth and early seventeenth centuries are complex, they may for convenience's sake be grouped into bilingual; that is, usually Latin–English, and multilingual dictionaries, or monolingual; that is, English–English dictionaries. This seemingly neat arrangement is, however, cut across by the fact that the newer monolingual dictionaries derive from the well-established bilingual tradition, and were compiled from them.[1]

It is also complicated somewhat by the existence of other kinds of dictionary, including the 'double dictionary' of Latin–English, English–Latin, but particularly the English–vernacular dictionaries such as the English–French works of Hollyband and Cotgrave, Thomas's and Florio's Italian–English dictionary (O'Connor 1990), Wyllyam Salesbury's Welsh–English, and Minsheu's English–Spanish, Spanish/English (Stein 1985; 1986: 219–27). There was also Ridley's unpublished English–Russian dictionary (Stone 1987). Another type is represented imperfectly but uniquely by the so-called Rawlinson lexicographer, who attempted, apparently unsuccessfully, to compile a comprehensive monolingual English dictionary in the late sixteenth century.[2] It was not until the early years of the seventeenth century that the first monolingual dictionaries in English appeared in print. Lexicography in the sixteenth century, except for the Rawlinson lexicographer, was bilingual or multilingual in England, the majority being Latin–English. The earliest English–Latin was that of Huolet (1552), who alphabetized the English entries of an earlier Latin–English work (Osselton 1983: 15). His work was succeeded by those of Peter Levins in 1570 and John Rider in 1589. Finally there are the many other lexionaries[3] of the period, large and small, which contributed in some way to the ever-developing production of dictionaries of all kinds.[4]

In attempting to assess the treatment of English medical terminology, it is necessary to make some analysis of the contemporary dictionaries, leaving aside for the moment the glossaries in medical works themselves provided by Llwyd and others, which are specialist productions taking for granted the value and immediate contextual necessity of a compendium of such terms. The recognition of a body of medical terminology is better assessed by reference to the more general dictionaries, and the bilinguals at least attempt a reasonably comprehensive coverage of the lexicon, unlike the early monolinguals, which seem to have appeared in response to different needs, as will appear later in this chapter.

1. BILINGUAL AND MULTILINGUAL DICTIONARIES

It has been assumed here that Latin–English dictionaries were primarily intended for students and scholars of Latin, and that Latin will have been of primary importance in their compilation. There was presumably an attempt to find native English words for Latin medical terms where they occurred, but there must also have been some neologizing; that is, anglicizing Latin terms to fill lacunae in the English lexicon, even though such words may have had no actual contemporary use in English, the Latin terms being preferred in the English textbooks. It was unfortunately beyond the scope of the present research to investigate this interesting problem in sixteenth-century lexicography in depth. The assumption about what was acceptably English in an English context would be too obviously distorted in such works, and the textbooks themselves will yield a more accurate picture of usage.

The precedent for including medical terms in a dictionary was established early. Thomas Elyot, in the preface to the 1538 edition of his Latin–English lexicon, specifically mentions that he includes 'proper termes belonging to ... physicke' as well as 'the names of diuers herbes knowen among vs', and in the 1542 proem, this principle is expanded and refined a little further to include 'the proper termes belonginge to physicke and surgery' in what may be the recognition of surgery as a separate and worthy craft. A further distinction in the selection of terms is incorporated in the title-page of the 1552 edition of the *Bibliotheca Eliotae*. According to Thomas Cooper, the reviser, the list will now include 'the proper names of most herbes that be agreed of among Phisicions', suggesting a more discriminating selection of terms. Starnes draws attention to the fact that Elyot had studied medicine, even though he had not taken a degree in it, and remarks:

> Names and descriptions of diseases occupy a relatively large place in the Elyot–Cooper dictionaries. Having compiled the *Castel of Helth* Elyot early became familiar with many medical writers and books, including Galen, Aëtius, Aegineta, Trallianus, Mesue, and Celsus, to mention a few. The *De medicina* of Celsus, Elyot knew well. Phrases from this book abound in Stephanus. (Starnes 1954: 99)

Not only had Elyot a working familiarity with the terminology of the subject, but his reviser, Thomas Cooper (1517(?)–1594), apart from a distinguished career as a divine, was trained in medicine, having been admitted Bachelor of Physic at Oxford in 1556. He petitioned the university that he had 'studied Philosophy 12 years and Physick 5', and seems to have practised in Oxford during the reign of Queen Mary (*Ath. Ox.* i: 713). His interest in lexicography began with his revision of Elyot's dictionary published in 1548, but his most important work was the compilation of a major Latin–English dictionary which was an immediate success, and was revised three times before the end of the century.[5] The Coopers report that 'It was much esteemed by queen Elizabeth, and led to the author's promotion in the church.'[6] Cooper's medical sources include both Elyot himself and, indirectly, Celsus.[7]

Cooper was a serious lexicographer, and his treatment of medical terms shows his care. He frequently gives both medical and non-medical senses of words, recognizing their polysemy. Herbal entries are usually informative; for example, **dictamus** is defined as 'An hearbe hauing leaues like penie royall, but greater and somewhat hoare. It biteth the tongue like ginger, and draweth out any thing fastened in the bodie.' **Betonica**, in an entry reminiscent of herbals, is described as 'Betaine: of this name is an other kinde called *Tunica*, whereof there be two sortes one *sylvestris*, an other called *Betonica altilis, vel Coronaria*, and is our cloue giloflower.' He helpfully recognizes looser and less specialist uses of words; e.g. **præcordia** is 'the fleshie skinne called the midriffe, that separateth the heart and lungs from the stomacke: the liuer, and other bowels' as well as 'Sometimes all the numbles, as the hart, lungs, the splene, &c.' His explanation of **cholera** shows a similar sophistication: 'The humour called choler. Also a sicknesse of the stomacke, with a troublous flixe and vomite ioyned with great daunger: the choleric passion.' Many obscure terms occur, such as **chœnicon** 'An instrument of surgerie, called also *Modiolus*, wherewith they cut out little bones', and this surgical sense of **modiolus** is duly noted under that lemma.

The practices of the herbalists is of some importance to the development of medical lexicography. The most significant figure of this era was William Turner, whose herbal, the first part of which appeared in 1551, was crucial to the development of scientific botany in England. He had previously published a little work in 1548 called *The names of herbes in Greke, Latin, Englishe Duche & Frenche* (*STC* 24359) which, as the title suggests, is a quadrilingual herbal showing as much interest in the lexicon of the subject as in the herbs and their medical qualities. Alternative names in English are often given, corrections to commonly accepted usages offered as well as to the usages of other compilers of herbals, attention is drawn to the 'barbarous' professional usages of apothecaries and to the differing uses of these practitioners in different countries, and he suggests names in English for plants for which he knows none.[8] He also records plants not found in the works of the ancients. He has been claimed as a significant neologizer, but his everyday professional work on sorting out the proper names for herbs was more influential. His major work is built on this lexical interest, though it does not materially advance it. This concern also appears in his *A new boke of the natures and properties of all wines that are commonly vsed here in England* 1568 (*STC* 24360). There is an extended discussion of the terms to be used in classifying wines by taste (Diii^{r}–Div^{v}), as well as some adverse criticism of Cooper's *Thesaurus*. He even suggests the setting up of a committee to initiate the compilation of a revision of Cooper's dictionary.[9] Turner was, if the references to him and his work are any guide, the most influential botanist and physician of his time in England, and he maintained lively communication with scholars on the Continent such as Cardan.[10]

John Baret, the compiler of another dictionary entitled *An Alvearie* 1573 (*STC* 1410), received his M.D. from Peterhouse, Cambridge, in 1577, and although there seems to be no evidence that he actually practised medicine, he obviously petitioned on the basis of long study, perhaps, as in many other cases, in order to legitimize an existing practice. The dictionary is an English–Latin–French one, with some Greek as well.

Thomas Thomas (1553–88) was printer to the University of Cambridge from 1582, and compiled a Latin dictionary, the *Dictionarium linguae latinae et anglicanae* of 1587, which was frequently reprinted, the fourteenth edition appearing in 1644. His work became a source for Cawdrey and others. Many terms from Thomas were anglicized and incorporated into the early monolinguals, sometimes irrespective of whether contemporary vernacular usage justified the inclusion, in order to make lists larger and more impressive in a period where copiousness was admired. His two main sources were Cooper's *Thesaurus* and a dictionary by Morelius, the *Verborum latinorum cum graecis anglicisque coniunctorum* (*STC* 18101), which was itself a derivative of Cooper, published originally in Paris, and later in an English version of 1583. The 1616 edition of the Thomasius includes a substantial supplement by the translator and physician Philemon Holland. Francis Holyoke, who both edited Rider and compiled his own dictionary, wrote in 1633:

> Thomas first compiled his dictionary from Calepine and Cooper, traces of whom are still discernible in the Thomasius. Afterward, he augmented his dictionary with matter from the *Nomenclator* of Junius and from certain glossaries and herbals. Finally, the reverend Philemon Holland, the learned physician and philologist, so wonderfully enriched the Thomasius from the works of reputable authors that no dictionary in that kind yet exists which, in the number of terms defined and in the illustration of meaning by selected phrases, is equal in merit to the Thomasius.[11]

What is especially interesting is the alleged contribution of medical science to the work, through both the additions of Holland and the claim that herbals and a scientific compilation like Junius' nomenclator had provided some of the original materials.

John Rider (1562–1632), realizing the need for both decoding and encoding in lexicography, compiled a popular dictionary in both Latin–English and English–Latin format. He claimed to have included four thousand more words than any other dictionary, but his claim to have published the first English–Latin dictionary was unjustified. Rider's dictionary was used as a model by at least two other seventeenth-century English–vernacular lexicographers, the physician Mark Ridley and later the Irishman Ristead Pliuncéad, though the works of these men both remained unpublished. Pliuncéad also used Thomas. Rider's work plagiarized Thomas extensively, a suit for plagiarism being brought against Francis Holyoke, the reviser of Rider, by Thomas's executors as late as 1617.

Apart from the major Latin–vernacular dictionaries, nomenclators were also used as sources of information. Nomenclators were the successors of earlier glosses consisting of large lists, often of technical words classified according to different branches of knowledge. The most significant was the nomenclator of Junius (Higgins 1585), essentially a class vocabulary on the old models, which appeared in mid-century, and was extensively used by later lexicographers (Osselton 1983: 15).

A survey of the dictionaries of the sixteenth century, however extensive, would not suggest much as to the lexicographical sources of the *OED* for this period. In the results of this study reported in Table 6.1, none of the major Latin–English dictionaries is a significant source of antedatings. By far the most important is another bilingual work by John Florio published originally as a glossary in *First fruites* in 1578 (*STC* 11096), as *Second frutes* in 1591 (*STC* 11097) and subsequently revised and reissued as *Queen Anna's new world of words* in 1611 (*STC* 11099). The latter certainly constituted a major achievement in bilingual vernacular lexicography (O'Connor 1990: 22). The *OED* editors left us no assessment of their views of the relative merits of their dictionary sources, but if citation is a guide, then they regarded Florio highly. Wood also singled it out as an especially meritorious work in its scope; a dictionary which in his view 'for the variety of words, was far more copious than any in the world'.[12] Florio had certainly had comprehensiveness in mind as a goal in compiling this work, while admitting that it was ultimately unattainable:

If any man aske whether all Italian wordes be here? I answere him, it may be no: and yet I thinke heere be as many, as he is likely to finde (that askes the question) within the compasse of his reading; and yet he may haue read well too, I should thinke that very few wordes could escape those auctors I haue set downe, which I haue read of purpose to the absolute accomplishing of this worke, being the most principall, choisest, and difficult in the toong; especially writing in such varietie not onely of matters, but of dialects. (Stein 1986: 224)

This also seems to anticipate the 'hard words' principle of the monolingual lexicographers, with the exception of including the 'most principall' terms.

Thus if the lexicography of the sixteenth century was dominated by Elyot, Cooper, Thomas, and Rider, their contribution as sources of the present list of antedatings in Appendix 1 hardly corresponds with this dominance. Of the present list by far the largest number, no fewer than twenty-eight (1.09 per cent) are from Florio, indicating his importance as a source for the *OED*. Of Schäfer's 635 antedatings, twenty-two are ascribed to Florio, all of them from Nashe. Although it is not clear from Schäfer's lists how many more there are, it cannot be more than seven, so that his registered contribution is 3.46 per cent, and his potential contribution no greater than 4.56 per cent (Schäfer 1980: 83–6).[13] In any case his contribution is well in advance of any of the other lexicographers, and especially of those Latin–English dictionaries of the sixteenth century which generally were so much more sophisticated than the modest monolingual productions of the early seventeenth century; indeed Rider, Thomas, and Cooper do not appear on the list at all (see Table 6.1). Of course there was no possibility of turning up an antedating from Elyot in this study, but the monolingual dictionaries are of a later date than the present texts, with the sole exception that Cawdrey predates Cotta. Thus very few of my antedatings are from Latin–English dictionaries, in spite of the fact that Cooper, Thomas, and Rider are all listed as sources.

Another expectation is that, in a list dominated by medical terms, the work of lexicographers who either were physicians or who had studied the subject extensively might also dominate, but in spite of the professional knowledge of Elyot, Cooper, Levins, and Baret, this is certainly not the case. Medical interest in the compilation of dictionaries was continued by Philemon Holland, as we have seen, Holyoake commented on Thomas's use of herbals and of Junius, but Starnes (129) suggests that in any case his work contains few references to physicians: 'We might expect frequent citations of classical physicians. There are in this edition a few to Celsus and fewer to others.' Many of the authors cited are those he translated, as one might expect, but he translated little of medical importance, and so a paucity of medical reference would actually hardly be surprising. It is interesting that in his preface Holland refers to Thomas Linacre, among a list of lexicographers. Starnes (135) continues, however, with the claim that

> As Holland himself was a learned physician, it was but natural that he should supply medical terms from earlier writers of the same profession. Hence the increased number of references to Dioscorides, Celsus, and Paracelsus in the 1631 edition. To judge from the number of citations of Paracelsus and the numerous Latin quotations from him, one would infer that he was greatly admired by Holland.

Nineteen examples are given by Starnes; apparently there are others. Holland also used English material, including the *Catholicon Anglicum*, so that he must have had access to a manuscript of that work. The fact is, however, that although Holland is one of the authors most cited as antedated in this study, all these citations are from Holland's translations, so that his supplement to Thomas is virtually unrecognized by the *OED* as a source.

2. MONOLINGUAL DICTIONARIES

Reasonably high lexicographical standards had been set by the bilingual dictionaries of the sixteenth century. When we come to the first monolinguals however, the situation is rather different. It is apparent that the scope of these works is severely restricted, and that attention to sound lexicographical practice was wanting, so that the monolinguals were less sophisticated and orderly than their predecessors. Not that the lineal descent is very direct, Cawdrey, for example, relying not only on Thomas but also on the schoolmaster Coote, as well as other minor sources.

The monolingual lexicographers concentrated on a specific market for their books, and hence on a particular and limited field; the so-called 'hard words'. The difference between the relatively unplanned, ad hoc, non-theory-based practice of English monolingual lexicographers of this period may be contrasted with the systematic approach of their German contemporaries, Henisch and Schottelius. Henisch deliberately omitted French borrowings, preferring to treat the German rootstock exclusively. Hard words as such were therefore of no concern to him (Henisch 1616).[14] Their readership was largely unspecified, and the linking of the lexicon to grammatical theory was strongly evident in their attention to root words, to the morphological potentialities inherent in the German language, and to comparisons with Hebrew (Hüllen 1990: 189–96).[15] The German rejection of borrowings is paralleled elsewhere by the work of the Swedish lexicographer Johannis Schroderus (*c.*1608–39) in his unpublished *Dictionarium Quadriliguae*. Schroderus was interested in the Swedish lexicon, not merely its hard words (Haugen 1983: 99–105). 'Det är alltså i första rummet ett svenskt lexikon och utgör i själva verket det första avslutade ordboksarbete i Sverige, för vilket huvudinteresset har varit ett så vidt möjligt fullständigt insamlande av det i bruk varande svenska ordförrådet' (vi). (It is thus primarily a Swedish lexicon and is in fact the first finished lexicographical work in Sweden, whose main interest has been to make as complete as possible a compilation of the Swedish vocabulary currently in use.) The 'hard words' tradition seems to have been idiosyncratically English.

The attention of English monolingual lexicographers to a segment of peripheral vocabulary rather than to a core, and to a tightly specified market for this kind of dictionary, seems to suggest that they were marginal to a mainstream lexicographical tradition in spite of having used its material. That Cawdrey's introduction (and perhaps even the word-list itself) was so derivative does not point to a really serious linguistic interest, or to a pioneer in this field, except by default. It is perhaps only with the introduction of literary reference with Blount's *Glossographia* of 1656, the reintroduction of other areas of special and technical terms, and specifically the rather disorderly introduction of material from herbals in Bullokar's *Expositor* that the English monolingual dictionary takes the first steps toward the scholarly status which the Latin–English dictionaries had long since achieved. But progress was slow: by the middle of the seventeenth century, Thomas Blount undertook to record words for a rather more specific area of medical reference, terms particularly for 'the seuerall parts of mans body ... the names and qualities of at least twenty ordinary diseases ... fit for the knowledge of many, who neither profess in the study of *Physick*, *Anatomy*, nor *Chirurgery*' (Blount 1656), but it hardly seems to be a significant advance over the claims in Elyot–Cooper.

It is rather surprising, then, that the early monolingual lexicographers make a relatively larger contribution to the present list of antedated *OED* authors[16] in Table 6.1 than do their bilingual betters. Blount comes first in the list of mid-century monolingual lexicographers with seventeen (0.66 per cent), but he does not belong to the early group. Cockeram is the most significant of the early monolingual lexicographers with sixteen, and Cawdrey has seven, but considering that this represents 0.63 per cent and 0.27 per cent respectively, it is hardly a major contribution.[17] The very low figure for Cawdrey might suggest that on any measure this dictionary had relatively little to offer. Being so derivative of course implies that the wordstock is easily and obviously antedatable. Bullokar appears only twice in the complete list, a negligible 0.08 per cent, so that he is quite unrepresented in Table 6.1, which is all the more surprising since he was himself a physician.[18] From the middle of the seventeenth century *Blancard's Physical Dictionary* and Blount provide thirty-eight and seventeen respectively. The 1706 edition of Phillips edited by J.K. is the most significant source of all, but there is not so much from the earlier editions. Some of their contribution is probably concealed under the rubric 'Eng dicts'. There is no problem of their missing chances to be represented, since Cotta is the only medical author in this study who postdates a lexicographer (Cawdrey). It might be suggested that these lexicographers had a relative lack of interest in the language of medicine, which, given the large number of medical texts available to the reading public from the middle of the sixteenth century on, would seem a curious omission. There may also be criteria involved in this state of affairs which have escaped our notice; for example, the criteria for the selection of 'hard words', which the lexicographers themselves did not enunciate, and which have not subsequently been ferreted out from the mass of available material. To hazard a guess, an emerging body of words of a specialist nature may have been of less inherent interest to the readership of Cawdrey or Bullokar than, say, those fashionable coinages which formed the elegant alternatives for familiar words. It is also possible that the tendency to keep medical words out of the mainstream lexicon already noted, and particularly evidenced in the re-encystation of many terms, means that lexicographers simply did not regard many of them as legitimately English.

Neither was it the practice of these early lexicographers to include other than the primary sense of their hard words for the most part.

More obscure senses were generally ignored. Many medical terms were polysemous words with a more familiar primary meaning, and their specialist senses were simply not recorded in the early monolinguals. These lexicographers may have felt that to include monosemous esoteric terms or ones with newly acquired second senses might have been taking the 'hard words' principle beyond the limits of practical application, so that words of limited specialist use may have been overlooked as being beyond the capacity or indeed the usual notice of the 'ladies, Gentlewomen, or any other vnskilfull persons' who were their intended readership (Cawdrey 1604: title-page).

It is also possible that this relative uninterest may ultimately be reflected willy-nilly in the *OED* itself, and that works like Chamber's *Cyclopedia* (1728–51) and the *New Sydenham Society Lexicon*, published in the late nineteenth century, inevitably became important supplements to a relatively meagre stock of terms. Neither has it been the practice of recent commentators to inquire into the nature of 'hard words'. Both Starnes and Noyes and Hayashi[19] have been content to accept the fact of the inclusion of hard words and the primary interest of the early lexicographers in them without asking in what, precisely, they might consist. In fact we know as much from Cawdrey and Bullokar themselves about the nature of these words as we do from the enquiries of later researchers.

It has generally been supposed that the words concerned are for the most part latinate,[20] but that was not always the case, and it cannot be supposed that such words were the only ones seen as causing problems to readers. Peter Levins's *Manipulus vocabulorum* of 1570 (*STC* 15532) refers to terms 'either barbarous, straunge, or fallen out of vse'. He appears to have been the first specifically to give a field marker to such words and notes particularly in his preface **kirk**, **murk**, and **ken**.[21] A full list of words marked by Levins as obscure may be found in Kerling (1979: 254–8). It is notable that some medical terms appear in this dictionary; e.g. **coloquintida** glossed as 'an herbe'; **fistula** and **oncome**, both glossed as 'disease'. It could not be supposed that a reader could be greatly enlightened by what are merely assignments of semantic category rather than definitions, but this was common enough at the time. Levins lists about 187 in all, not a large sample,[22] and all his medical terms are common enough in the medical literature. Stephen Batman also compiled a short list of 'hard words' which were mainly Old English in origin (McNair

1984: 317–19). Bullokar also has a fairly high percentage of words which had become obscure or archaic—marked as such in the *Expositor*—which are almost exclusively from Speght's Chaucer glossary, which provided by far the majority, and from Spenser's *Shepheardes Calendar* (Kerling 1979: 54–8). Hüllen tentatively suggests that about one-third of Bullokar's words fall into this category (Hüllen 1990: 194).

Problems are also created by the fact that lexicographers depended heavily upon each others' work, especially in the early dictionaries. Lexicographers rarely shied away from plagiarism and paraphrase, and the lineage of early dictionaries, whether monolingual, bilingual, or polylingual, shows a considerable degree of inbreeding. Not that this is necessarily a bad thing entirely; as Starnes and Noyes aptly put it, 'the best lexicographer was often the most discriminating plagiarist' (Starnes and Noyes 1991: 183). Indeed, reliance on earlier, reputable dictionaries was seen as admirable.[23] The result of this interdependence for the present study is that the ascription of a term or group of terms to a particular lexicographer may be nominal only, since they may well have been borrowed. It cannot be assumed that a lexicographer was necessarily practically acquainted with the more obscure words appearing in his pages; indeed, some may have been quite unfamiliar to him aside from his source. It is also the case that errors were both created and perpetuated by this practice and were not corrected. Blount complained bitterly about precisely this problem following the appearance of Phillips's derivative *New World of Words* in 1658, incorporating as it did many of his own errors (Blount 1673). There is no evidence to suggest that the early lexicographers used empirical methods to ascertain meanings and usage; even Blount's references to learned sources are in many cases spurious (Starnes and Noyes 1991: 43–4). The use of literary or scholarly names was designed more to convince potential purchasers of the wisdom of their investment than to ensure readers of a sound scholarly basis for the work.

Thus in considering the inclusion of medical terms it cannot be assumed that the inclusion of such a term means anything more than that it appears in the pages of a certain lexicographer—it need not be his own original inclusion. The exclusion of such terms may, as will appear, be as meaningful as their inclusion. Exceptional circumstances such as apply to Bullokar will need to be considered separately.

Robert Cawdrey's *A table alphabeticall* (1604) (*STC* 4884) is generally regarded as the first monolingual dictionary of English (see Peters 1968). In at least one respect, however, it would be dangerous to assume that the earliest such work was also the most original and the least derivative. Cawdrey in preparing his word-list drew heavily on at least two works—Edmund Coote's *The english schoole-maister* of 1596 (*STC* 5711) and Thomas Thomas's *Dictionarum linguæ Latinæ et Anglicanæ* of 1587 (*STC* 24008), and there were also others of lesser importance. His debt to these two works is very heavy.[24]

It is in practice rather difficult to sort out what Cawdrey's editorial practices might have been from the comments he has left us. There is at least one clue in his identification of his 'hard' words with 'vsuall' words, which might indicate some perception of the naturalization of earlier borrowings giving a word more right to recognition than more obvious neologisms. But it is clear enough that the values implicit in his designation of the market for the book, which were probably more important to him than lexicographical principles, belong to areas of social nuance not easily recoverable except as gross generalizations, and certainly not reducible to the systematic tagging of lexicographers.

What then does he tell us? Assuming for the moment the bona fides of Cawdrey's preface, he does at least indicate that he disapproves of 'straunge ynkhorne termes' (Cawdrey 1604, A3^{r})[25] especially in the mouths of preachers. He apparently shared with many others in this period the view that men of God had a particular influence and responsibility in matters of vernacular speech. He inveighs against the use of 'over-sea language', but is approving of 'words translated, from one signification to another (called of the Grecians *Tropes*) vsed to beautify the sentence as precious stones are set in a ring to com[m]end the gold' (Hayashi 1978: 32–47).[26] Whether this latter category encompasses the better part of his 'hard words' is unfortunately not clear. The distinction between these and inkhorn words might be muzzy indeed. It is difficult to generalize on the basis of such slight evidence, but at least it does seem fair to suggest that his intended readership had no particular use for the special terms of a craft like medicine. The situation is in fact even less clear than it seems, however, since the text in question cannot be taken at face value. Much of Cawdrey's 'To the Reader' is itself plagiarized from Thomas Wilson.[27] One may suppose that he plagiarized because, among other things, he substantially agreed with Wilson. It does, however, make it impossible to ascribe what nuances there are and their application to lexicographical principle to Cawdrey himself. The 'ring' metaphor, for instance, is Wilson's alone. One may still presume that the title-page is Cawdrey's. The reference to preachers was also his own, but phrases like 'over-sea language' and 'straunge ynkhorne termes' are Wilson's. It must also be said that such expressions, even prior to 1550, were common enough (Jones 1953: 103–14).

Some indication of Cawdrey's practice can be gained from a detailed examination of his text, though its very brevity is something of a limitation. There are some words included in it which were clearly medical in application, and rather more which may be so. Of the latter, a number can be identified in other texts of the period as having a specific medical application. Among these are **adustion**, **confection**, **debility**, **fume**, **imbecility**, **imperial**, **judicial**, **obstruction**, **ministration**, **reduce**, **resolve**, **tertian**, and **vehement**. Consideration of the definitions shows that in most cases he did not think of them in their medical senses.[28] In none of these cases does he employ a definition which clearly stipulates a medical usage, and almost all of them have other non-medical significations, the only obvious exception being **quartan**, which along with **tertian** appears to be something of an oddity in as much as any non-medical sense seems unlikely. For **tertian**, Cawdrey gives 'belonging to every third day', and the *OED* identifies this very common contemporary usage specifically with fever characterized by a paroxysm every third day. Other uses are to do with different measurements. For **quartan**, *OED* records only the medical sense (a. and sb.). Thus Cawdrey's omission of a specific reference to or a field marker for medicine in defining these terms does seem strange.

In all, terms of the latter kind amount to about 6 per cent of his total corpus. The actual number is insignificant to the extent that there would be legitimate disagreement about the inclusion or exclusion of many items on such a list—to take particular instances, **suppress**, **vicious**, **mixture**, and **humid** seem arguable, although they frequently appear in medical texts. The particular case of **suppress** is dubious because it often occurs in medical texts in special phrases concerned with the suppression of urine, or the suppression of mentruis ('woman's flowers'), but appears to have no special significance in medicine beyond such contexts and should be regarded as enactive rather than truly specialist.

Other words are given a definition which in some way suggests a medical meaning. These include **antidote**, **catarrh**, **decoction**, **gargarize**, **flux**, **instinct**, **nerve**, **putrefy**, **spleen**, **ulcerate**, and **vapour**. Such words represent about 3.4 per cent of the whole corpus. Again, there must be argument about specific cases, so the business of getting some realistic measure of the number or proportion of medical terms in Cawdrey must rely on a choice of some more limited range of words about which there is a high measure of agreement, and which will provide some firm basis for comparison. Two obvious choices seem to be the names of diseases and the names of bodily organs or constituent parts. An examination of these categories reveals a total of seven in each case. The diseases are **catarrh**, **epilepsis**, **fever**, **flux**, **frenzy**, **lethargy**, and **pest**. Two possibles, **ulcer** and **vertigiousness**, have been omitted as being, at least in sixteenth-century usage, symptoms rather than diseases, though as elsewhere there may be dispute, not so much about these two terms as about the nature of the contemporary distinction between disease and symptom. The bodily constituents listed by Cawdrey are **entrails**, **genitals**, **nerve**, **ossicle**, **sperm**, **spleen**, and **ventricle**. In neither case does the list seem very large given the possibilities for further inclusions, each representing a negligible 0.023 per cent of the total.

At the same time, it is impossible to identify an area of technical language to which Cawdrey did particularly address himself, apart from the odd term, so that medicine is in this respect no exception. His categorization of words as 'hard' and 'usuall' seems then to carry the very particular implication that specialist terms on the whole were to be excluded, especially those with no wider area of denotation. In this he differs from Bullokar (see below), who makes a statement of the principle of including technical terms.

It is possible to make some comparison with the usage of Cooper, if only to illustrate the disparity. For the term **splen**, Cooper gives two terms, 'the Spleene: the milte'; **catarrhus**, he defines as 'A rewme or stilling downe of humors from [th]e head'; and the entry for **lethargus**, while lengthy to the point of being encyclopaedic, is not untypical of his work:

> A drousie and forgetfull sickenesse rising of impostumation of colde fleugme putrified, especially in the hinder parte of the braine, whereby memorie and reason almost vtterly perisheth, and the power sensitive is greatly annoyed. In it men commonly forget their owne names, & also to shut their mouthes after they haue gaped, ne can they by any meanes be stayed from sleeping.

The difficulty here as elsewhere in this study is the lack of comparative information from which to draw conclusions. The obvious yardstick is John Bullokar (*c.*1580–*c.*1641), especially since he was himself a physician,[29] and one might expect therefore a rather more extensive coverage of the subject area.[30] Nevertheless he saw himself, like Cawdrey, addressing a limited audience with no great pretension to learning, consisting of those whose education was not learned. Unlike Cawdrey however, Bullokar also undertook to include medical terms as well as other words specific to particular fields of knowledge. He mentions 'diuers termes of art, proper to the learned in Logicke, Philosophy, Law, Physicke, Astronomie, &c, yea and Diuinitie it selfe, best knowen to the seuerall professors thereof'. He further hoped to 'open the signification of such words, to the capacitie of the ignorant' (Bullokar 1617: A3[v]). It is certainly true that law terms are an obvious feature of his lexicon, and that he takes trouble to explain them at length. The fact that hunting terminology is also extensively registered is not, however, anticipated by his preface. He also included older and obsolete terms, marking them as such, the majority being taken from Speght's Chaucer glossary (Speght 1598). The work contains approximately 4,000 entries, of which 318 (7.95 per cent) are medical in the sense that they either have a clear field marker (52), or that they are obviously medical by Bullokar's own definition.

The most immediately striking feature of his use of medical terms is that the names of herbs are well represented and copiously explained, in the tradition of the herbals rather than in the dictionary tradition, and that some account of their origins, nature, properties, and use in medicine are usually included. The same applies to other substances used in the preparation of medicines, e.g. **oringes** or **copall**.

A closer look at the terms registered reveals little or no systematization, although it does seem that certain editorial decisions have been taken. One is to exclude names of surgical instruments. Only one, **trepaniron**, appears, and it is difficult to see any convincing reason why this, of all terms for surgical instruments, should be the sole inclusion. There are not very many anatomical terms, and what there are form a curious mixture. Twenty-three are included: **arterie**, **cullion**, **filme**, **membrane**, **meninges**, **matrixe**, **midriffe**, **muscle**, **nerue**, **palate**, **pia mater**, **pores**, **prepuce**, **pulse**, **scalpe**, **secundine**, **sperme**, **splene**, **umbilike**, **ventricle**,

vreters, **vuula**, and **whirlebone**, many of which have lengthy encyclopaedic entries. But there is no field marker for anatomy at all. Some are non-classical, and the emphasis in this list is by no means on specialist terms, some of which might well have been registered instead; e.g. **œsophagus** or **testes**. Some of these terms are obvious (**muscle**, **nerve**), and others less so (**meninges**, **secundine**). There is a mixture of both generic (**artery**, **ventricle**) and specific (**prepuce**, **uvula**) terms. There are manifest omissions—for instance none of the major bones of the body is listed—as well as inconsistencies; **pia mater** is listed while **dura mater** is not. Even more quirkily, the latter does appear in the text, but not as a main entry. He has not had before him in the preparation of this element of the dictionary even so much as an anatomical fugitive sheet, let alone a medical textbook.

Thus the list is quite haphazard; clearly it was not Bullokar's intention to incorporate into his expositor a list of the more basic anatomical terms, such as might be extracted from fugitive sheets or a household medical textbook. Bullokar's list is not therefore a useful guide to the reading of a medical textbook; rather, its anatomical terms are a collection of lexical curiosities. Neither does usage suggest itself as a criterion for his selections.[31]

Those words which describe the *realia* of the subject are the most apparent in the *Expositor*. The most frequent class of words is those for herbs and simples, the largest subgroup of these by far being the words beginning with **dia-**, from **diacatholicon** to **diaturbith**, sixteen in all. The entries for these terms are usually like those of a herbal, giving the plant source, the degree of the herb's quality, and its medicinal use. The names of diseases are as follows: **apoplexie**, **canker**, **carbuncle**, **cataract**, **catarrhe**, **consumption**, **fluxe**, **gangrene**, **hemorrhodes**, **lethargie**, **lunacy**, **migraine**, **mother**, **noli me tangere**, **ophthalmie**, **pleurisie**, **pose**, **saint Antonies fire**, **sciatica**, **shingles**, **squincy**, **strangurion**, and **tympanie**. The majority of these terms are familiar and anglicized in form but, as with the list of anatomical terms, he did not apply a consistent rule as to form. It is odd that a physician should have used the form **strangurion**, which *OED* suggests is a confusion of **strangury** and **strangullion** (a disease of horses). But he is in good company, Turner having made the same error in his herbal.

There is another numerous class of words which appears in the *Expositor* describing the processes of medical phenomena and the results of those processes (e.g. **putrefy**, **putrefaction**, **mollify**, **mollifaction**) as well as generic concepts such as **superfluity**, **confection**, and **vehemency**. This class also includes those words used for states or conditions such as **stupefaction**, that is, the enactive terms of the lexicon of the discipline. The great majority of them are not identified as medical at all. Bullokar only gives them field markers very infrequently, and in many instances, the single-term definition offered gives no indication whatever of medical use. Examples are **adust**, **eiection**, **euacuation**, **ingredience**, **putrifaction**, **rupture**, **tertian**, and **ventositie**. There are also some which are marked as medical, e.g. **collyry**, **conuulsion**, **criticall**, and **purgatiue**, but they form only about one-eighth of the identified medical terms, and are heavily outnumbered by the words for the *realia*. In some instances of the unmarked words scanty definition probably produces this odd state of affairs; e.g. 'swelling' for tumour might be understood to describe a bodily symptom, but it is by no means clear. Along with the hunting and legal terms which figure so largely in the *Expositor*, such terms give the whole an encyclopaedic rather than strictly lexicographical appearance.

Scientifically accurate nomenclature ultimately necessitates an exact and practical record in the lexicography, and herbals from Turner's on maintained a glossarial function. The gulf between these and dictionaries, on the other hand, remained very apparent in the way in which Bullokar clumsily inserted his herbal items without regard to an overall pattern of entry structure.

There was no lack of precedent for the inclusion of the names of herbs. Elyot had incorporated them, and the interest in such compilations had received a great boost from the influential work of William Turner. The compilers of dictionaries of 'hard words' seem, however, to have had a different readership in mind. Cawdrey's 'hard words' on the whole exclude the terms special to medical practice, and probably those of other areas of specialism, presumably with a shrewd eye to the market for his book.

Thus there is a sense in which the early monolingual tradition represents a step backwards both for natural philosophy and for lexicography in England. At precisely the time when the awareness of the Latin language as facilitating scientific taxonomy and having the potential to provide what the vernaculars could not was emerging—an unambiguous description of natural phenomena—the lexicographers of English were abandoning this function.

Convincing reasons other than neglect to explain the relative lack of attention to the medical lexicon by sixteenth- and early seventeenth-century lexicographers are not easy to find, but perhaps the sense that its words were not proper to the English lexicon was the most likely. This might be a result of the process of encystation inasmuch as such terms are usually in the context of teaching in Latin and Greek, and are strictly non-anglicized in form, even in the few works in the vernacular on the subject. Stein points out, while offering no hard evidence for, the relative absence of terms of rhetoric in English–vernacular dictionaries. Similar considerations may explain the relative lack of medical terms (Schäfer 1980*b*: 7–17; Stein 1986: 225).

The early monolingual dictionaries therefore offer little insight into the resources of contemporary medical terminology, having tended either to avoid it or to deal with it unsystematically, both tendencies being sufficiently clear in spite of the small scope of the works involved. The bilingual ones have more, being in any case more substantial, but they seem not to have been used extensively by the *OED* as sources, and may not have reflected contemporary English usage accurately. The *OED*'s practice has related inversely to the lexicographical weight and seriousness of these dictionaries, and it is clear that the bulk of the data for sixteenth-century medical terminology came from other prose sources rather than from dictionaries of the period. For a more detailed and comprehensive view of medical terminology we must look at the English textbooks and handbooks themselves, the yardstick for this aspect of the study being the *OED* itself. It is essential to understand how well or ill the *OED* covered the lexical material available in the medical works of the period, especially since it made use of those dictionaries less able to provide data, while scanting those with more potential.

Notes

1. The best coverage of these interrelationships is still to be found in Starnes (1954).
2. Osselton (1986: 175–84) suggests a late sixteenth-century date for this compilation, leaving the reader with a choice between the last quarter of the century, *c.*1570 (the Bodleian's date for the MS), and post Rider (i.e. 1589), if this is indeed the major source of his compilation as is claimed. In any case, it almost certainly precedes Cawdrey, and is quite different in scope and intention, as well as being unusual in employing an English–Latin rather than a Latin–English source.

3. I have used the word 'lexionary' as a general term to cover any dictionary, glossary, or word-list, whether separate or appended to another work.
4. Schäfer (1989) contains a very full review of these glossaries in its vol. i, *A survey of monolingual printed glossaries and dictionaries*. At the same time many of these glossaries in medical works are small, Llwyd's for example containing only 46 lemmas, Recorde's 39, and Barrough's, consisting only of weights, 10. Traheron's on the other hand was far more extensive, containing 426.
5. First published 1565. His dictionary was alluded to both unkindly and inaccurately during the Marprelate controversy: 'To go forward, his Lordship of Winchester is a great Clarke, for he hath translated his Dictionarie, called Coopers Dictionarie verbatim out of Robert Stephanus his Thesaurus, and ill fauoured so they say' (Penry (or Penrey; see also Marprelate, Martin) 1588: 46).
6. (*Ath. Cant.* 1858–1913: ii. 166). Thomas Cooper was successively Bishop of Lincoln and of Winchester.
7. 'Cooper, in the *Thesaurus*, draws from both sources. Sometimes he carries over what was in the *Bibliotheca*, as under *Attalus emplastrum*, *hyposarcha*, and *psylli*; sometimes he draws from Stephanus, as under *atrophia, cancer, cardia, cardiacus, lien*, and *tabes*. In many entries, Cooper, citing Celsus, has a composite of the two sources, as under *angina*, *lethargus*, and *febris*. There is no evidence that Cooper gathered illustrations directly from the *De medicina* of Celsus' (Starnes 1954: 99).
8. He uses German words, for example, as models from which to coin new English terms; e.g. *Solidago saracenica* (229), which 'is called in duch Heidnishe wuntkraut [and] may be called in english Woundwurte', as well as *Perfoliata*, which 'the Germans call Durchwassz. It maye be called in englishe Thorowwax, because the stalk waxeth thorowe the stems' (227). There are other names which he provisionally suggests; e.g. **opulus**, for which he knows no English name but which he thinks may be called **opier** after the French word 'tyl we find a better name' (199).
9. 'Wherefore I wishe, to the ende that the booke may be in dede as it is called: that one learned phisition & philosopher like vnto *Lineker*, one gram[m]arian like vnto *Clemond*, and one perfite Englishman like vnto *Sir Thomas Moore*, had the amendment and making perfite of this booke committed vnto them.'
10. See Wheeler (1986: 291–305) for text and discussion. Gesner saw fit to publish the letter in *Historia Animalium*, 1558, lib. iii.
11. Starnes's translation, in Starnes (1954: 115).
12. *Ath. Ox.*, i. 423. Wood also points out that the collecting of material went on up to Florio's death, and was subsequently carried on by Giovanni Torriano. It finally appeared in print in 1659 as *Vocabulario*

Italiano e Inglese. Wood also notes that these additional words were those 'relating to Arts, Sciences, and Exercises'.

13. Schäfer's list stops at ten irrespective of the fact that those with the same percentage of contributions whose names are further down the alphabet do not appear. The Shakespeare list ends with Holland (two), so that Florio can have contributed no more than one antedating to this list.
14. Only A to G was ever published. Henisch, like so many of his counterparts in English lexicography, was a physician, signing himself 'B. medicinæ Doctoris' on the title-page. Adrian Junius, whose *Nomenclator* was published in English by John Higgins in 1585, was another physician.
15. See Top (1603) for somewhat similar theorizing in English.
16. 'Author' is used here to include works not ascribed to a particular author, in order to avoid confusion over the use of the term 'source' both for the sources of my new data and for the *OED* 'authors' antedated.
17. See Table 7.3 for a full list.
18. See Bullokar (1617: title-page), 'By I. B. Doctor of Physicke'.
19. Starnes and Noyes (1991: esp. 8), where the authors content themselves with 'those [words] of foreign origin which offered difficulty to the reader'; also (Hayashi 1978).
20. 'The earliest English dictionaries were modest lists of 'hard'—generally Latinate—words that posed problems to "Ladies, Gentlewomen or any other unskilfull persons" as Cawdrey's title-page shows' (Kerling 1979: 1).
21. Preface. Kerling points out that it is Levins's intention to 'warn his readers against using' these words, and also that it is 'hard to say which he would have found "barbarous", and which "straunge" or "obsolete"' (Kerling 1979: 45), but the meaning of 'barbarous' was clear enough at the time, referring to medieval rather than classical Latin usage. We are thus left with 'strange' and 'obsolete'; if he wished to reform uncultured usage, then 'obsolete' was hardly a fitting description. Could it boil down to 'unfashionable'?
22. There are words included because they are homophones or near-homophones, which he marks, but these referred to are not included for that reason.
23. Note for instance Wood's praise of Florio's continuing to collect words and phrases 'out of other Dictionarys and Italian authors'. (*Ath. Ox.*, 423).
24. Starnes and Noyes (1991: ch. 2).
25. Neither was there anything especially striking about Cawdrey's concern for the usages of preachers. Paul's Cross had already been a favourite forum for regaling the public with such sentiments, and criticism usually took the form of remonstrations against the unintelligibility of

those whose duty it was to put God's word to the people plainly.

26. Hayashi does not appear to understand what this passage means. His discussion of Cawdrey (34–5) is rather misleading, since he has assumed that inkhorn terms are borrowings, but this is incorrect since on the whole they are neologisms.
27. Wilson (1553: 86^{r}–88^{r}). The debt has already been noticed by Kerling (1979: 6), but he did not discuss the matter at any length, merely noting the fact, and describing it as 'largely an adaption'.
28. Cooper has such entries as '*adustio* . . . Burning or rosting', and '*obstrictus* . . . A straight or harde wringing.' For some words there is nothing medical, e.g. **confectio**.
29. Admitted MD, Caen, 1612.
30. *An English expositor* 1617. It is not known how far, if at all, John Bullokar depended on the efforts of his father, William, who mentions on several occasions the compilation of a dictionary which seems never to have been printed and perhaps never completed; but John makes no mention of it. It seems unlikely therefore to have been his father's, especially considering that William Bullokar would probably have produced something more sophisticated than a bare word-list, and that it would probably have been put in his own orthography. In *Book at large 1580* (Leeds 1970: 52), he claims that he will 'not only spedily imprint the Grammar, but also put my helping hand vnto a necessary Dictionary, agreeing to the same' (original spelling regularized and modernized). This was the first grammar of English, in either English or Latin, to be produced.
31. This seems to be typical of the *Expositor* as a whole. Bullokar's unmethodical approach is also commented upon by Kerling (1979: 73) with respect to his treatment of old and obsolete terms.

5
New Data for the *OED*: Methodological Problems

Having spent some time examining attitudes to the use of English in the sixteenth century and some of the ways in which the medical profession used it and the lexicographers recorded it, we now turn our attention to the works which have been the special subject of this study and to the work which best records the vocabulary of these books, the *Oxford English Dictionary* (*OED*). We have now seen that the bulk of the sixteenth-century medical terminology in its pages probably did not come from the dictionaries of the period, and it is also probable that these dictionaries did not make a serious attempt to record this terminology. It seems possible therefore that we do not now understand the emergent terminology of the profession sufficiently well. However, the primary focus of an investigation into the recording of a particular semantic domain in the sixteenth-century lexicon must inevitably be the *OED*, and only secondarily those sixteenth- and early seventeenth-century dictionaries which were the source of some of its information. If the *OED* is inaccurate or misleading, in what ways and to what extent is it so? What are its actual deficiencies? This also leads inevitably to questions about the way in which the *OED* was put together, and to the ways in which it utilized its sources.

This book had its genesis in the fact that in the course of pursuing more literary studies than these I kept coming up against the problem of words which did not appear in its pages, as well as antedatings and other corrections to its entries. With the usual perversity of research, the compilation of lists of these became the main objective. As these lists became alarmingly and publishably long, it eventually became clear that the dictionary itself should be the object of research. Time has only served to reinforce that view; indeed, it has been apparent for some time that there is a pressing need for large-scale research into the sixteenth-century lexicon as well as into the *OED*, which has for so long dominated our view of the history of the lexicon and of the language itself (Schäfer 1980: esp. chapter 5).

For more than sixty years the *OED* has been an unparalleled source of information on the lexicon of English and, apart from the efforts of a few scholars, it has been generally assumed to provide the last word on almost all such matters. It has been used uncritically, probably because the task of finding enough material to bring it into some sort of scholarly perspective and to outline its shortcomings precisely has seemed, like Murray's, nothing short of herculean. But it is possible, without reduplicating those efforts, to prise open the gates and to make a properly documented assessment of the dictionary, as the pioneering work of Jürgen Schäfer has shown, especially in the list of something over 5,000 items of new data published in recent years (SchäFer 1989).[1] The generalized results of such research are that the *OED*'s deficiencies are in the final analysis those of any dictionary and need surprise no one—it is by definition out of date, it is not comprehensive, it reflects the biases of it editors, and the details of its presentation are inconsistent. But we need to examine the results here in much more detail.

Throughout this work, the first edition of the *OED* has been used. The new edition appeared late in the course of the task of gathering data, and it has therefore not been practical to revise all the lexical material in this study. In any case nothing prior to 1800 has been altered, since the policy of the supplements had long been to add antedatings only later than 1800, so that none of the present list can have been anticipated, and the second edition only adds to the integration of the supplement material about 5,000 new words or senses 'which have gained currency' since then (Simpson and Weiner 1989: vii). It also should be clearly understood that the object of this research is the original *OED* and certain of the policies which shaped it, not the more recent supplements or the new edition, which have been created in different circumstances, and with somewhat different policies and methods. The present research was carried out manually in the first place, and subsequently completed using commercially available word-processing and spreadsheet software.[2] The appearance of the compact disc version has also been an important supplementary source of information from the *OED* which it would have been quite impossible to retrieve any other way, such as lists of citations of individual authors.

The works excerpted for this study are:[3]

1. Anon. [Plutarch], *The gouernaunce of good helth*, 1549
2. Bailey, W., *A treatise of the medicine called mithridatium*, 1585
3. Baker, G., *The composition ... of the moste excellent and prestigious oil called oleum magistrale*, 1574
4. Banister, J., *The historie of man*, 1579
5. Barrough, P., *The methode of phisicke, conteyning the cavses, signes, and cvres of the inward diseases in mans bodie from the head to the foote*, 1583
6. B[ostocke], R., *The difference betweene the auncient phisicke ... and the latter phisicke*, 1585
7. Clever, W., *The flower of physicke*, 1590
8. Cotta, J., *A short discouerie of the vnobserued dangers of seueral sorts of ignorant practisers of phisicke in England*, 1612
9. Hester, J. [Fioravanti], *A short discourse ... vppon chirurgerie*, 1580
10. Hill, T. [Fioravanti], *A ioyfull iewel. Contayning ... excellent orders, preseruatiues and precious practises for the plague*, 1579
11. Langton, C., *A uery brefe treatise, ordrely declaring the principal partes of phisick*, 1547 (cited as *VBT*)
12. ——*An introduction into physyke, with an vniuersal dyet*, *c.*1550 [cited as IP]
13. More, P., *The hope of helth*, 1564.

Some of the lexicographical material excerpted from their works has been published previously in the form of lists of new data for *OED* (McConchie 1981; 1983*a*; 1986; 1987*a*), but in that form it does not precisely correspond to what is presented here. Lists of corrections already published vary in that new data for *OED* which is already noted in the *MED* (Kurath and Kuhn 1956–)[4] and a few which have already been noted in other similar publications, primarily in *Notes and Queries*, have been excluded. These words are, however, included here, since not doing so would distort the results for the purposes of this study, which is primarily concerned with the original *OED* and its editorial practices, and not with the compilation of some newer dictionary, whether actual or proposed. The editors of *Notes and Queries* have treated such information primarily as an accumulating resource for the *OED* editorship, and have therefore been careful to exclude duplication where possible—for example, if a word or sense has been recorded by the *MED*.

It has been normal practice over the years during which collection of antedatings, new words, new senses, and other forms of data for the *OED* has been carried out to describe them either as 'corrections' or 'additions' or as both. In order to avoid the inevitable suggestion that the collection of such material and its publication means that the *OED* was 'wrong', which is an invidious view of the circumstances of its production, it seems better to adopt a somewhat more neutral terminology. Schäfer's 'innovation units', apart from being a little clumsy, hardly a happy choice for this particular study, since it is arguable whether very much of the data can be demonstrated to be in any sense innovative, although it seems more appropriate to the verbal fireworks of Shakespeare and Nashe. It is better to regard the present material simply as supplementary to that in the *OED*, without enshrining any value judgement in the terminology, and I have chosen merely to call it 'new data'.

There have been no very rigorous selection critieria applied in choosing the works for analysis. In general, the body of texts has grown in response to my slowly increasing awareness that what appeared at first to be a few chance omissions from the *OED* was actually the early evidence of a very large and unexplored body of lexical information about early modern English. Later revision of works excerpted very early has resulted in at least one case in a very substantial increase in the data. John Cotta's work originally yielded 48 antedatings, but the number is now no fewer than 238. Robert Bostocke's contribution similarly increased from 33 to 185. As this perception grew, it seemed desirable to be more systematic; for instance, to invoke chronological limits to the study, to define the kinds of work which would form a part of it, and to expand the coverage so as to present a roughly representative sample of them. This is not really as complete or methodical as might be wished at this stage, but enough has been done to indicate the potential for research and to show the nature of the lexical material and the questions which are raised by it. The kinds of criterion which have been applied to other forms of data collection and research into historical linguistics need of course to be considered.[5] It has been felt necessary only to limit texts to those whose primary subject is medicine, but not to classify further within the selected group. The choice of medicine as a discipline is convenient and interesting, but also somewhat arbitrary. To discriminate between different areas of medicine is tempting but would be rendered problematic by having to decide whether modern or contemporary distinctions should apply; e.g. should the application of external remedies to the body be regarded as strictly surgical, as in the sixteenth century? It would also compound the already inherent difficulty of extrapolating results from the works studied to the whole lexicon and to the structure of the *OED*.

Works covered range in style, scope, and subject-matter from the relatively homely ones obviously written for the layman, perhaps intended as household reference works, such as the early translation of Plutarch, to the highly technical books intended for the practising professional, like Barrough's large textbook and Banister's anatomy. The range of dates is 1547–1612, which covers at least the better part of the century, allowing for the fact that little is available before 1530, and that the most substantial works before that date are herbals, a category which I have excluded.[6]

The contemporary popularity of a text was not considered as a special criterion, except that at least some texts incorporated into the list should be ones which were reprinted and presumably widely read. However, the reasons for popularity and the actual readership are difficult to estimate. Popular books were obviously regarded as readable rather than dauntingly technical, and so might be more useful in determining what medical jargon was acceptable to the public at large. Books with a large amount of such language, which are of great interest in this study since a greater volume of data comes from them, may have had less popular appeal to sixteenth-century readers for precisely that reason. Others may have had limited appeal for other reasons, an example being Bostocke's Paracelsian treatise. On the other hand, Barrough's long and extremely technical text, which can hardly have appealed to the general reader, went through seven editions (1583, 1590, 1596, 1610, 1617, 1634, and 1639), so that the potential professional market for such books could have been quite sizeable.

Neither has one particular type of medical text been preferred to another, although there are difficulties of definition involved here. It is instructive to look at contemporaneous classification; for example, that used by Andrew Maunsell in the second part of his pioneering bibliography (Maunsell 1595). This section of the work deals with physic and surgery as well as the 'sciences mathematicall' (title-page). The work is divided into subject headings giving some indication of informed contemporary interest, though not necessarily professional interest in the area. They are: anatomy, aphorisms, baths, distillation, herbals, mithridate, oils, plague, pox, secrets, and urines. The three further categories of dreams, planets, and prognostications seem arguable, though many physicians involved themselves in astrological writing. Maunsell obviously did not intend these categories to be exhaustive, and many well-known medical works are under none of these headings. Nevertheless, he clearly saw these as being of convenience to the informed reader. The selection here has not followed the categories indicated by Maunsell, but if the research had been more narrowly concerned with the identification of contemporary medical terminology, these categories might have been of much greater weight in taking these decisions.

Contemporary issues in the classification of texts have become urgent matters with the recent development of diachronic corpora of English, in which text-typing and considerations of genre are a crucial element. The parameters being discussed and employed now cross older distinctions, primarily external literary classifications by genre and other stylistic features, so that multidimensional linguistic analyses are able to shed new light on this question. What precisely the parameters are and how they are to be interpreted are being radically re-examined. A new development of vital significance is that many previously neglected non-literary texts such as those under discussion in this study are now being treated on an equal footing with those literary texts traditionally valued.[7]

Some classes of publication have not been excerpted; for example, the multifarious and widely-read almanacs and prognostications, many of which were prepared and published by medical men; e.g. Askham, Borde, Bright, More and others.[8] Securis produced at least twelve between 1562 and 1581. These often contained sections dealing specifically with the predictions of plagues and other diseases, appropriate times for the administration of therapeutic measures, and other medical matters. Almanacs and prognostications were widely read, and must have been a useful and perhaps profitable way of employing astrological skills.

No herbal has been included, and neither has any natural history, even though the former was regarded as somewhat less peripheral to the main interest of the study in the sixteenth century than it might seem now. A herbal was then a basic medical reference work, but became increasingly botanical and taxonomic as the century went on. It seemed better, however, to concentrate on texts about which there would be no question as to their present status as medical publications, since it is in this century that botany begins to emerge as a separate science. It is now apparent that the herbal began to diverge from the medical mainstream in England with the appearance of Turner's herbal, which is also the first major English herbal in the sixteenth century. As is explained in Chapter 6, however, the authors of such works will be included as medical authors when considering the nature of the sources of first citations in the *OED*.

Other kinds of work which are excluded are the small ephemeral works which were commonly printed during this period. These included such things as the anatomical fugitive sheets, which were usually single pages depicting the male and female anatomy, often with blood-letting points indicated (*STC* 564.2–8); however, they contain little lexical information compared with other sources. Proclamations dealing with medical matters, especially instructions issued in plague years, are also excluded, being generally too short and uninformative for the immediate purpose to warrant attention.

The most basic criterion has been that a text should be primarily medical; that is, its medical or surgical content should be the rationale for its existence, and not be an incidental feature. Thus books on husbandry, which often contain remedies and instructions for their preparation, are excluded in spite of containing some interesting material.

It is also the case that works have been analysed irrespective of whether or not they have been read for the *OED* in the course of its compilation.[9] The works by Baker, Cotta, Barrough, Banister, and More, all of which have produced considerable amounts of new data, duly appear in the *OED* bibliography among 'such works as have been most commonly quoted in the Dictionary'.[10] These latter are for the moment assumed to have been read, unless some evidence to the contrary is found, as with George Baker's treatise *Oleum Magistrale*. An analysis of entries in *OED* for George Baker reveals that his *Iewell of health*, a translation of Gesner, is cited in all 139 times.[11] His rendering of *Guydos questionary* (1579) yields a further six entries, but there are absolutely none for *Oleum Magistrale*. Presumably either it is mistakenly listed in the bibliography, or the material excerpted from it was all rejected for some reason. Whether it was intended to use material from this work is obscure, but for all intents and purposes it should be regarded as a book not analysed for *OED*. Any other unlisted work is assumed not to have been read, though it is possible that one from which there is a negligible number of quotations might be unlisted in the *OED* bibliography. In the case of John Hester, a work was read for *OED* entitled *A compendium of the rationall secretes of L. Phioravante*, published in 1582, two years after the publication cited here. It was substantially a different work, but contained virtually the same text in Book iii, where the recipes in the *Short discourse* are reproduced verbatim.

Very few of the authors whose work is excerpted here are well known. Banister and Clowes have been noticed sometimes, generally by physicians and surgeons interested in the history of their profession, and what articles there are about their lives and work usually repeat the same small amount of biographical information. Some others are quite obscure, such as William Clever, John Securis (Hatchett), and Robert Bostocke. In still other cases, these authors are relatively obscure even though they may have been well known in their own time; George Baker, for example, though a leading surgeon of his time, is scanted in the official history of the College of Surgeons (Cope 1959), of which he was master. I am not in a position to know how far this merely reflects the neglect of practitioners who are not considered to have advanced medicine significantly—perhaps a concerted search of the available records would yield some more details about their lives. It is only recently that scholars have begun extensively to study the history of the day-to-day business of medical practice rather than its momentous discoveries.[12]

Certain biographical details are obviously important to the present work in that they may illuminate the texts themselves and fill out the background to this study: whether an author was a Galenist or a Paracelsian, a popularizer or a committed professional practitioner; what kind of qualifications he had, and where they were obtained; whether conservative or progressive in outlook; whether a physician, surgeon, or some other trade—apothecary, distiller, writer. His contemporary reputation might also be of interest. Thus I will attempt to summarize what little is known about these individuals and where possible to clarify some of these matters. Biographical details in what follows have in the main come from *DNB*.

Walter Bailey (1529–1592)

A physician, born at Portsham in Dorset, became a fellow of New College, Oxford, about 1550, became the Queen's Professor of Physic of the University in 1561, and physician in ordinary to Queen Elizabeth in 1581. There is some evidence that he took an interest in botany, and had botanized near Winchester.[13] He wrote works on baths, on peppers and the medicines made from them, and was the first Englishman to write a treatise on the diseases of the eyes (Bailey 1586).

George Baker (1540–1612)[14]

Baker was representative of the generation of surgeons who became increasingly articulate and used the printing press with enthusiasm in the second half of the sixteenth century, such as Thomas Gale, William Clowes, John Banister, and John Woodall. He rose ultimately to be master of the Barber-Surgeons' Company. Although he was a Galenist, he supported the use of Paracelsian chemical remedies, and had a part in advancing their use. He claimed in a preface to a reissue of Traheron's translation of Vigo in 1586 to have had an acquaintance with Paracelsus' works—'I for my part have read and vsed his medicines this xviii yeere'—although with a circumspection typical of many English practitioners of the time claims that he 'dare not avouch to vnderstand him, and much lesse put anie parte in printe of him' (Traheron 1586: ||iii^r). Baker had made some corrections to Traheron's original, though circumstances prevented him completing the task, which he handed over to Robert Norton, 'who hath shewed his skill and paines therin' (||ii^r). Baker added a preface to the text left him by Thomas Hill at the latter's death in which he advocated the use and 'vertues of medicine [made] by chimicall distillation' (*DNB*). He wrote a treatise on mercury and its medical use which appeared appended to Clowes's work on syphilis (Clowes 1579)[15] and translated Galen's epitome of book three of the *De compositione medicamentorum per genera*, which appeared in a reissue of Guy de Chauliac in 1579. He also had a hand in Hill's translation of Gesner (Hill 1576), and englished some of Ambroise Paré (Baker 1629).[16] Another translation was the treatise on oleum magistrale, originally written in Spanish (Ungerer 1986: 203–11), which has been excerpted for this study.

He appears to have collaborated with Thomas Hill, and certainly knew John Hester, whom he mentions in a list of spagyrists (Hill 1576). Baker was not only energetic in writing his own texts but also in providing prefaces and other additions to the work of colleagues. He wrote consistently in the vernacular. The *Newe iewell* also has a picture of 'Alchymia' as a frontispiece. Some collaboration between the three of them seems a possibility, especially since Baker's work shows a consistent interest in medications and their formulation. He was an ordinary surgeon to the Queen and master of the Barber-Surgeons' Company in 1597. Both he and John Banister seem to have provoked the College of Physicians into acting against them by breaking their monopoly of medical practice. The College issued a warning to the Barber-Surgeons' Company in 1595 that the offending surgeons refrain from the practice of medicine; i.e. the administration of internal medicines (Debus 1969: 65–6; Pelling and Webster 1979: 177). Baker's inclinations seem therefore to have been towards innovation and reform, in both the practice and administration of medicine, and he used the vernacular to advance this cause.

John Banister (1533–1610)

A surgeon, he was given permission from Oxford to practise physic in 1573. He worked both in Nottingham and in London, and had been to sea as a surgeon as well. A letter of Elizabeth I (Munk 1878: 104) reports that he 'hath of long time practised the art of chirurgerie, in sundry places of this our realme, & also in some service vpon the seas'. This service was apparently on Leicester's expedition to the Low Countries (*DNB*). He finally settled in London in 1585, achieving a great repute as a practitioner. He was also a long-standing friend of Clowes. Eventually he became a licentiate of the College of Physicians in 1593. Apart from his own works, he also contributed to other works through prefaces and dedicatory material.[17]

*Phillip Barrough (*fl. *1559–1583)*

Barrough, whose brother was the much-published divine Isaac Barrow, studied at Cambridge, became both a fellow and benefactor of Trinity College, was granted a licence to practise surgery in 1559, and also took a medical licence in 1572 (Pelling and Webster 1979: 177). He seems also to have become tutor to Robert Cecil (Ward 1740/1969: 158). Barrough's substantial work went through many editions, surviving well into the seventeenth century.

R.B.

An author with an obviously Paracelsian outlook was R.B., generally supposed to be Robert Bostocke. The attribution is not absolutely certain, but it does derive from Maunsell's contemporary bibliography (Maunsell 1595: 4). Bostocke seems not to have been a physician. He saw medicine as 'the searching out of the secretes of nature', and as a task to be carried out by resort to 'mathematicall and supernaturall precepts, the exercise whereof is *Mechanicall*, and to be accomplished with labor' (Bi^r). He was evidently a thoroughgoing Paracelsian and was prepared, unusually for an Englishman, to declare his support in principle. His work appears to have elicited no response from his contemporaries and no further edition of his work is recorded by *STC*. It might not have helped his cause that he signed himself only with his initials, having no established reputation upon which to claim the reader's attention.

William Clever

Little is known of William Clever, who does not appear in the records of either university, in *DNB*, or in the records of the Royal College of Physicians. If he was professionally trained it was probably on the Continent. His book seems not to have been a great success, being printed only once. There was a William Clever described as a schoolmaster who published a book in 1576, but it is not known whether this is the same person, and they are listed separately in *STC*.[18] His book, while quite lengthy for the time, does not reveal a great depth of practical medical knowledge, being rather repetitively concerned with temperament, climate, diet, and so forth. He shows some familiarity with the medical literature, and includes many allusions to Paracelsus, but the work does not contain a relatively high percentage of specialist vocabulary.

John Cotta (1575?–1650)

Cotta lived and practised in Northampton, and is better known to posterity for his book against witchcraft, but he shows himself to be a physician of some insight and sensitivity. He clearly saw that the repeated use of mercury as a remedy for syphilis was probably as bad as the disease itself in its effects.[19] Cotta was also a participant in the controversy over Francis Anthony's use of *aurum potabile* in the early years of the seventeenth century.[20]

John Hester (d. 1593)

Hester was neither a physician nor surgeon, but was a self-professed student of the secrets of nature; he became a distiller or spagyrical chemist no later than the early 1570s, and is described on the title-page of the *Short discourse* as a 'Practicioner in the arte of

Distillation'. Thomas Hill bequeathed the text of *A ioyfull iewell* (*STC* 10880) to him to put through the press, so that there must have been a relationship of trust between them. Hester claims to have a large project in hand in the introduction to the reader in his *Short discourse*: 'I meane to set out all the workes of this Authour: which are .24. bookes, comprehended in eight volumes.' The work had been begun by Hill with his *A ioyfull iewell*, which Hester mentions as having been 'sette forth already',[21] and Hester may have inherited the idea (as well as the text) from Hill in the first place. Although he did not complete his grand scheme, he himself produced an impressive series of translations of Fioravanti, Duchesne, (Quercitanus), Hermann, and pseudo-Paracelsian writings. In the address to the reader in his *Short discourse* (*STC* 10881) he advertised his wares which the purchaser 'may haue ... at Paules Wharfe, by one Iohn Hester practitioner in the Arte of distillations, at the signe of the Furnaises' (Aii^{r}).[22] Elsewhere in a broadsheet Hester offers not only his distillations but also his skills as a teacher for sale.[23] George Baker's list of spagyrists in London in the *Newe iewell* (*iii^{v}) includes a reference to Hester, whom he describes as working 'on Powles wharfe, the which is a paynefull traveyler in those matters'. His practice at this address was of long standing. He was referred to with affectionate regard (and we are provided with an *obit.*) in Gabriel Harvey's *Pierce's Supererogation*: 'Poules wharfe honour the memorye of oulde John Hester' (80), and Harvey describes him elsewhere as a 'chimist'. Harvey seems to have been on friendly terms with him, and also mentions him in the same place in a list of 'expert artisans ... howsoeuer Vnlectured in Schooles, or Vnlettered in books'[24] and recalls fondly that he would 'often tell me of *A magistral Vnguent* for all sores' (Harvey, Gabriel 1593/1884, 80). The title-page of another work, edited by James Forrester, *The pearle of practise*, 1594, acknowledges its debt to 'I. H. (a spagericke) or distiller'. His writings show that for the most part he was interested in lists of recipes rather than Paracelsian theory as such. As Harvey's *Pierce's Supererogation* is dated 27 April 1593, it seems possible that Hester was a victim of the 1592–3 plague.

Thomas Hill (1528?–1575)

An enthusiastic compiler, translator, and popularizer of works of scientific and practical interest in the period *c.*1550–75,[25] Hill appears not to have had a medical training but was by his own evidence 'rather always rudely taughte, amonge the Smythes of Vulcanus forge' (Hill, DDiii^r). Perhaps this suggests that he was trained as a smith or a metal-worker of some kind. Miller describes him as having 'posed as an expert' on various subjects (Miller 1959: 206). He did nevertheless translate works by several scientific writers, including Bartholomeus Cocles, the influential Conrad Gesner, and the Italian Paracelsian and quack Leonardo Fioravanti. There were also vendipotent works on comets, the interpretation of dreams, and gardening. He gives the appearance in the two extant lists of his published and proposed works of being able to make a modest living as a writer, and Johnson's account of his career suggests an astute business mind as well as a lively and comprehensive scientific curiosity. He appears to have collaborated with John Hester in translating the works of Fioravanti,[26] and he left a work with Hester before his death which the latter saw through the press. Hester wrote in the preface to this work that 'that towardly and learned young man Thomas Hill' had 'committed them to my hands, requesting me to set them foorth in print, which I haue polished and filed as nye as I could according to the right sence of the Author'.[27] He also left a work to George Baker.

Hester's description of Hill seems somewhat inapposite, even though Hester may have been the older man, since Hill was perhaps 48 when he died about 1575, and his publishing career had already spanned twenty years. The estimates of the date of his birth depend on the woodcut of Hill which first appears in the 1568 edition of his translation of Cocles *Physiognomie* and bears the inscription 'aetatis suae 28'. Had it been prepared for that edition,[28] then Hill would have been about 36 at his death, making Hester's dedication read more sensibly. On the other hand, he must then be supposed to have done the Cocles translation at the very towardly age of 16.

Christopher Langton (c.1521–1578)

A physician, he was incorporated MD at Cambridge in 1552, and was a fellow of the RCP between that year and 1558. He was expelled for indecent behaviour,[29] but apparently his sexual excesses continued, since in 1563 the diarist Machin noted that 'The xvj day of June dyd ryd in a care [to the] yeld-hall docthur Langton the phesyssyon in a g[own] of damaske lynyd with velvett and a cott of velvett ... and a cape of velvett, and he had pynd a bluw ho[d on] hys cape, and so came thrugh Chepe-syd on the market [day,] and so a-bowtt London, for he was taken with ij wenchys yonge at-ones' (Nichols 1848: 309). Nevertheless, his medical practice continued, attending on such people as Sir Thomas Smith and Sir Thomas Gresham, probably until his death.[30] Both his published works were youthful productions.

Phillip More (fl. *1564–1573)*

More lived in Halesworth in Suffolk and was a friend of the physician William Bullein. It is possible that he possessed no medical qualifications as such, but he 'firmly identified with the learned physician' as Margaret Pelling puts it (Pelling and Webster 1979: 230). Certainly his work shows far less professional terminology than some of his contemporaries, such as the surgeon Thomas Gale. As well as the medical work analysed here which promotes herbal remedies, he published a series of almanacs between 1567 and 1580.

Although biographical information is difficult to come by, there does seem to be a spread of views in this list of authors from the conservative to the radical and progressive among a group including several types of practitioner, as well as a variety of motives for publishing. While it is hoped that the data excerpted from their works goes a significant way to covering the medical lexicon of the period, it cannot be claimed to represent it adequately.

1. TYPES OF NEW DATA

The words recorded in this study as new data for the *OED* have been collected as a result of the selective excerption of texts. This has been done by listing all words which have seemed to be worth checking against the dictionary whether on the grounds of date, usage, sense, familiarity, or rarity. The results appear as Appendix 1. The basic principle has been that for a word to be listed as an antedating, postdating, or new sense, it must be a lemma, sub-lemma or fine-print lemma of *OED*. Neither should it simply be a definition, or part of one, or form part of an illustrative quotation. This is not so straightforward a matter as it may seem, and examples of words appearing in definitions and citations but being unrecorded themselves do occur.[31] In general, medical terms, unusual words, words used in an unfamiliar sense, and words used in a modern sense which seems to be an early instance of that sense have been preferred, being more obvious, but attention was paid to the familiar words of the language as far as circumstances permitted. Consequently there are inherent biases in the kinds of word chosen for analysis. While it would have been desirable, it has not been possible to do a full analysis; that is, an examination as in a concordance of every word in the text against the *OED*, since the resources required to carry out this time-consuming work have not been available. Such an analysis will be referred to here as a 'concordance study'. A very limited amount of such work, the results of which are discussed below, has, however, been possible and has shown the potential of such research.

In establishing what is and what is not new data for *OED*, the most basic principle has been that *OED*'s documentation has been accepted as it is, and on its own merits. No attempt has been made to editorialize or amend, since to do so would produce distortions and raise more problems than it would solve. Any textual assumptions made by the *OED* editors have therefore also been tacitly accepted here.[32] The texts excerpted have been treated similarly—only in the case of rank or obvious errors (*u* for *n*, for example) has emendation been undertaken. It seemed preferable to accept that there will be argument about some entries by those more skilled in emendation than I, rather than to obscure the original text by well-meaning but possibly wrong-headed tinkering. Words have generally been registered as they appear in the original texts in the case of unrecorded words, except that for reasons of alphabetization and sorting with the software used, initial Æ has had to be regularized to Ae, and initial V and U have been normalized. They are thus as they appear in the *OED* lemma except for Æ.

The types of new data upon which this study is based are primarily antedatings, since they are the largest and also the most amenable to interpretation. Particular attention has been paid to those antedatings which are of words with medical uses. Significant numbers of previously unrecorded words, new senses of words already recorded, a smallish number of postdatings, and minor omissions such as words with no citation or date have also been identified. Many of the other additions are also medical terms, especially among the unrecorded group. The nature of these groups and their hermeneutic usefulness is discussed below. Antedatings are also dealt with in greater detail in the next chapter.

It should be noted, however, that determining exactly what

category a word should be entered under is not as simple as it might seem, and therefore some of the decisions made here might seem rather arbitrary. The difficulties which can arise are perhaps best illustrated by an example. Phillip Barrough makes the following remark on 227: 'Whereas in very deed /S/*ανθϱαξ*/S/ among the Greekes is the very same, that *Carbo*, or *Carbunculus* is among the Latines.' **Carbon** is listed in *OED* as deriving from *carbo*, *carbonem*, but the meaning is obviously inappropriate. The lemma for **carbuncle** also gives *carbo* as its ultimate source, by way of a diminutive form. Should the recording of Barrough's form therefore follow sense and be a form of **carbuncle**, or follow etymology and be a new sense of **carbon**, or should the difficulty be more drastically solved by making it an unrecorded, which preserves the form which Barrough has used? The solution adopted here has been the latter. Note that while an unrecorded word cannot by definition also be a new sense in Appendix 1, an antedating can and a number of these double listings occur. It has sometimes been necessary to make a best guess, often as a result of the *OED*'s definition. In Clever's work, for example, **nurse**, finally settled as [5, 1736, Swift] 2 'a bodie almost deuoured ... cannot easily be ... nursed vp' might also have been listed as **nurse up**, but the senses 'to bring up' or 'rear' were neither of them absolutely right; therefore an invidious choice has necessarily been made. Similarly **pragmatical** [3, 1601, Godwin] (94) is a good example of the problems. The word clearly antedates most listed senses, yet it was virtually impossible to determine contextually which of about four was intended. In these circumstances the necessity of recording a fairly early instance prevailed over other doubts, and the first earliest was selected.

There have also been instances where the form used in the original text has been aberrant and not easily interpreted. Two instances from Barrough will serve to illustrate the point. Barrough's **twilt** (32) in 'make a twilt with .iij. sheetes of graie paper' seems likely to be the same as **quilt** and is therefore recorded as such. *OED* records **twill**, sb^2 and v^2 as variants of **quill**, sb. and v. respectively.[33] Barrough's **fellerd** in 'fellerd leaues of sage' (56) was finally identified as **fallow** 'to grow pale, to blanch', and hence omitted from the list, being last recorded in 1584. The word **fess/fest**, recorded in both forms in Hester, appears to mean 'sediment, dregs, leavings', but was registered as unrecorded since it could not be convincingly associated with the several possible forms in *OED*.[34] The case of **absterge** will also illustrate some of the difficulties. Hill's *Ioyfull iewel* has the following: 'the *Oyle of Roses* is absterge and molificatiue' (Hiii^{v}) [1646, Browne]. There are several possibilities which might explain this form. It might be a typographical error for the adjective **abstergent**, or be a previously unrecorded adjective of the same form as the verb 'to absterge', or it might be a typographical error for the adjective **absterse**. None of these solutions is entirely satisfactory, and it has been decided to list it as the latter, as it seems to involve the fewest assumptions.

Unrecorded words

The total number of unrecorded words forms quite a large percentage of the total new data (27 per cent). The appearance of these words has, of course, a primary significance in filling out the previously known and recorded sixteenth-century lexicon which hardly needs comment, but it is possible to glean further information from this resource concerning both the wordstock itself and the registration of it in the *OED*. The existence of so many unrecorded words must in itself suggest a specific deficiency.

A considerable number of these words are the names of medicines or the simples from which they were compounded, and this is not unexpected. The *OED* did not, of course, undertake to list every obscure word of this kind, but it does list some, and it is by no means clear that those unlisted are in any sense always rarer or more obscure than many which are included. None of the criteria which might have been relevant, such as the word being in neoclassical form, or not being capable of being defined within a reasonable limit of intelligibility (both at various times invoked by the *OED* editorship), seem to apply to the question of inclusion or exclusion. Thus the commonly mentioned (and presumably commonly used) **gum edera** and **muscardini** (Hill) and **sanguis draconis** (Baker) are unrecorded, while **draconis** (Hill), **scolopendra** (Hester), **terebinthine** and **chrysocolla** (Baker) duly appear and are antedatings. Further aspects of this particular problem are discussed below, especially in Chapter 6.

Unrecorded words present particular problems in that the possibility of finding what is merely a ghost-word is always present. There have been some few instances in which it was not possible to be sure that the word concerned was not a misspelling or typographical error, and these doubtful cases have been omitted. The kind of ghost or dictionary word not infrequently found in the *OED*, often marked 'in dicts.' and often originating with early monolingual lexicographers like Bullokar and Blount, is, however, not much encountered in this study. Rare or obscure words in this study have by definition been in use, however infrequently or idiosyncratically.

Problems also arise when unrecorded words are in neoclassical form. In general the *OED* is rather inconsistent as to whether the neoclassical form or the anglicized form or both should be recorded. Extensive reading of the medical literature of the time will show that many neoclassical forms omitted from the *OED* ought, on the grounds of sufficiently frequent usage, to have been included. It is difficult to achieve consistency in this matter, however. For example, a word recorded in the *OED* in anglicized form, but recorded here in its neoclassical form is, strictly speaking, unrecorded. These forms all ought to be recorded since there is always the possibility that such pairs with distinct senses had in fact developed, as has certainly happened in some instances. But is a reference to its neoclassical form in the derivation notes, or a citation containing it, sufficient to allow us to omit it? **Stomachus**, a form unrecorded separately in *OED* but typically noted in the etymology under **stomach**, is a good example. I have tried to follow these guidelines: where a word in neoclassical form is listed in the citations as a variant of the main lemma, then it not listed as unrecorded. Where an anglicized form only is given, and there is only an etymological reference to the neoclassical form, then it is regarded here as unrecorded, e.g. **betonica**. Where a word is used in neoclassical form, and a direct link with the anglicized form is not clearly made by *OED*, I have listed it as unrecorded. Conversely, where there is an English form of a Latin or Greek name which anglicizes the ending only, I have still listed the latter as an antedating (e.g. **sanguisorb/sanguisorba**, **acetose/acetosa**). While this practice will seem contrary, allowing a borrowed word to be unrecorded where a closely analogous anglicized form which predates it is in *OED*, but to be an antedating if it does not predate it, and while it will obviously maximize the list of unrecordeds and to a smaller extent antedatings, it does nevertheless follow through the logic of the *OED*, in which many of these alternate forms are listed (e.g. **raphanus**, **dracunculus**, **scolopendrium**), even for some with little record in the language, to judge by the citations given. It also allows the maximum of data to be recorded, and this class of specialist neoclassicisms (mainly botanical) will be obvious in the full list of unrecordeds.

In the same area the *OED* shows a fundamental inconsistency in that it often uses a botanical name in the definition but does not record it as a lemma in its own right. **Lovage**, for instance, is 'b. a later bookname for the British umbelliferous genus *Ligusticum*', but neither this latter term, nor its variant **levisticum** is recorded. **Apium** (**smallage**) and **olusatrum** (**alexanders** or **horse-parsley**) are two other cases in point. To have chosen to exclude this material rather than include it would have left both the data incomplete, and the reader not knowing where the exclusions were. In the case of dual (or even triple) lemmas, such as **mithridatum/mithridate/mithridatium**, all of which are separately registered in *OED*, I have had no compunction in recording either form as an antedating if warranted by the *OED*'s lemmatization. Even then, however, the means of recording derivation in *OED* may vary very widely, so that inconsistencies are inevitable. An instance of such a difficulty is **syndesmos**. The word in this form is unrecorded, but it does occur in an illustrative quotation from Dunglison under **syndesmo-**. In spite of this, the morphological dissimilarity does seem sufficiently significant to accord it separate unrecorded status. In cases of doubt I have preferred to list an unrecorded, rather than lose the data altogether. Had only the details of the main lemmas been considered and all neoclassical forms been included as unrecorded, the list would have seemed both unduly pedantic and to have unfairly slighted the other material contained in the lemma, whether etymological and derivational, explanatory preamble, or historical illustration.

A quite different problem occurs in Hester's *Short discourse*, arising from the fact that the work is a translation from Italian, and that Fioravanti was a Bolognese. Hester uses the word **riplexione**, which, since I have been unable to consult the original Italian text, looks as if it has been left untranslated. 'The first kinde of scabbe is that which is caused of *Riplexione* of the body' (Ci^{v}). Presumably Hester finds no English or Latin equivalent. On the other hand, it is not standard Italian either, and may represent Fioravanti's attempt to coin a word, or be dialectal. It has been included as an unrecorded in spite of these difficulties.[35]

Combinations are also a difficulty, particularly for the unrecorded category. Many occur in medical texts, and some are in *OED*, but not always under their own lemmas or sub-lemmas, and the methods of recording them are diverse. Many are of course listed under sub-lemmas, but frequently these lists are exemplary rather than complete, prefaced by such rubrics as 'Examples are ...', 'Such as ...', 'as ...' and so on, indicating the possibility, indeed probability, of combinations formed on the same pattern. In some cases this possibility is particularly mentioned, obvious cases being **un-**, **-wise**, **for-**, **over-**. Another method of registration was to use *sc.* (*scilicet*) as in the case of **rectum**, for which '*sc. intestinum*' is employed. At the beginning of this research it was rather ingenuously assumed that combinations in classical form could be ignored, but this has proved to be incorrect. Thus a considerable number occur, the majority of which are or would be fine-print lemmas, but *OED* practice justifies this procedure; for example, **memoria deperdita** is listed here as an unrecorded, while *OED* itself lists **memoria technica** as a lemma in its own right. Combinations and self-explaining compounds such as **septum transversum**, **mucronata cartilago**, and **leady coloured muscle** do seem to require recording where the combination specifies a single, discrete phenomenon rather than a class of such phenomena. Some are obscurely accounted for, terms for the sensory organs being a good example. The vitreous humour of the eye is under **vitreous**, where it is sense 2b.[36] However, **vocal**, while it includes **vocal chord** (6a, 'Freq. in *vocal chord*, fold, organs, track, etc.'), does not seem to subsume Banister's **vocales nerui** (Ggi^{v}), which is not only Latin but also an obsolete sense of **nerve**. **Visible sinew** is listed as unrecorded, since **visible** has no sub-lemma indicating such a combination; hardly surprisingly, since the sense of **visible** here is also a new sense, perhaps 'serving to enable or facilitate sight'. **Faculty** and **virtue** are inadequately registered in that the virtues such as **generative**, **nutritive**, **alterative**, are not listed under their attributive adjectives, except for **expulsive**, which is cross-referenced at **virtue** 11b. An exception is **concupiscable/concupiscable faculty** under **concupiscable**, 2b. A consequence of this is that the equivalence of the terms **virtue**, **faculty**, and **power** in this sense is missed in *OED*.

Unlike antedatings, I have attempted to include doubtful unrecordeds, and have left them mainly in the form in which they appear in the original text. That such unrecordeds should be included is not necessarily to be understood as implying that a dictionary like the *OED* ought to have registered them. There are also a few words which have been registered in the supplements to the *OED* but which were not in the original edition, and these have been listed as unrecorded in spite of this.

New senses

New senses are a smaller group, and can be difficult to establish, given the often insufficiently specific contexts in which they occur, but care has been taken to err on the side of conservatism and only record those about which there can be no really serious argument. Where a new sense cannot be reasonably firmly established it has not been included, and particular note has been made of new medical senses in a few cases. A text must provide a context in which a new sense seems at least reasonably likely, although in many cases absolute certainty is of course impossible. Some are grammatical variations only, e.g. a previously unrecorded substantive sense of a participle or the verbal use of a noun. Others are increases to the known polysemy of words, and some are evidence that some kind of medical field marker probably ought to have been allotted to a particular sense.

New senses also raise questions about the lemmatization of the *OED*, there being plenty of room for argument about distinctions between and overlaps of various senses under particular lemmas. Questions arise as a result of the *OED* editors' desire to define as accurately and discriminatingly as possible and to introduce as many variables as possible. Thus the manipulation of variables such as transitivity and intransitivity or instances of action and notions of action as means of structuring sub-lemmas may produce a new sense somewhat artificially. Some of the kinds of problem encountered may be illustrated by Cotta's reference to **urinary glass**—'the looking of vnborne babes in an vrinarie glasse' (106). The *OED* records four major sub-entries for the word **urinary**, only one subdivision of which, 'of or pertaining to, affecting or occurring in, the urinary system or organs' (4b), appears to cover Cotta's usage. It lists no attributive collocations, so that we cannot assign it there, except as a new sense. The first citation under 4b refers the reader to **urinal** *a*, 1b, where, while the citation reference to 'urinary diarrhœa' seems appropriate, the definition 'marked by immoderate discharge of urine' is plainly not in the present case, though it is fine in the instance cited. I have nevertheless listed **urinary** as an antedating from 1822, and **urinary glass** as unrecorded, presuming that it would normally be listed as a fine-print lemma in an attributive and combinative sub-lemma of **urinary**. Further problems such as distinguishing past participles from the various adjectival uses of them hardly need comment, and misplaced citations in *OED* are testimony to this source of ambiguity. In the end, however, these issues are perhaps of more concern to revisers of the dictionary than to the present study.

It is essential to list a new sense which antedates all citations of that word in *OED* as an antedating. If one is done but not the other on the grounds that no word should be listed twice, information is lost. On the other hand it is impossible to list a new sense as an antedating if one citation in the lemma predates it, since it cannot be ascribed to any sub-lemma. Note that where a new sense which is also an absolute first citation is listed, as in the case of **reflecting**, *ppl. a.*, that the sense under which the antedating will be listed will be the earliest, even though that does not quite accurately represent the sense in question. At the same time it is obviously necessary to list the antedating, and it seems fairest to list the earliest date in *OED*, rather than that of the 'nearest' sense of the word, assuming that it could be unambiguously determined, since in resolving other problems the conservative figure has also been preferred.

Postdatings

The latter are probably of least significance in that it is often less easy to make a meaningful estimate of the date of disappearance of a word than it is to estimate the date (using the term 'date' for the present in a loose sense) of the first appearance of a word. The distinction between, say, archaism and outright obsolescence may in any case not be a very revealing one for the lexicographer. Neither was the *OED* intended to provide accurate information of this kind. In this study only relatively early postdatings are recorded, the *terminus ad quem* varying according to the date of the work consulted, and the number is in any case rather small, probably not representing a significant number of the total data.[37] Postdatings of less than five years have generally been left out.

Fine-print lemmas

The fine-print lemmas are those not in the heavy bold-face type used for main lemmas, and almost always occur within them, though there are exceptions. They are not listed as a separate group like those above, but they are noted where they occur. They cause some difficulties, since they may be variously recorded. Those which occur under the rubric 'Hence ...' at the end of a main lemma are usually derived participles, verbal substantives, and adverbs, and are listed here under the form of the fine-print lemma itself, e.g. **medicine-monger**, **high-coloured**. This affects the interpretation of the data to some extent, since they are frequently and indeed normally absolute first citations as recorded, only one illustrative quotation usually being given, but not so frequently absolute first citations of the main lemma itself. The *OED* often gives the former main lemma status, presumably on the grounds first of semantic differentiation, for example where an adverb cannot be seen merely as the obvious morphological derivative of its main lemma, or secondly where there is sufficient usage of the form to render its inclusion under the main lemma unnecessarily clumsy and complicated. The problem is a perennial one for the lexicographer. There are many others, placed on the left margin like a main lemma, but not in full bold type, e.g. **deglution** and **coterminate**. Since the point appears to be to indicate their rarity, rather than to stress their subordinate derivation from a main lemma, these are not noted as fine-print lemmas, although that is how they are presented typographically. Thus they are effectively treated as if they were main lemmas; that is, they can be absolute first citations as well.

Antedatings

Antedatings are words for which a date earlier than the first citation of a lemma or sub-lemma in the *OED* has been discovered. There has been a succession of reports of antedatings, which are the most common additions to the dictionary, and probably the most significant for their historical import, since the publication of the *OED*.[38] They may apply both to the absolute first citation of a word, irrespective of the sub-lemma head, as well as to particular sub-lemma heads. In the first place all antedatings of sub-lemma heads have been recorded, and if these are absolute first citations in the sense that is used throughout this work of having antedated all the dates in a given lemma (not in the sense of the absolute first use of a word), then this fact is noted separately in Appendix 1.

In some few cases, the same word can be an antedating and also a new sense; these will also appear as duplications, having been recorded for statistical purposes as if they were separate words since it is essential to record both corrections; for example, **stertor** (Cotta) is listed twice for this reason. Other examples include **croton** and **denervation** (Baker) and **monarch** (Clever). There have also been many instances in which it was impossible to determine beyond reasonable doubt that the meaning listed in the *OED* was the meaning intended in the text being excerpted itself, and not some other meaning assigned to that word which would not have been an antedating. **Bole** was a case in point, and there were many others, especially where the *OED* distinguishes particular members of classes, e.g. botanical and other *taxes*, and lemmatizes them separately. When recipes for the vast range of confections, pills, boluses, decoctions, juleps, colliries, oils, essences, etc., are given in the sixteenth century, such distinctions are very rare indeed, and many words appear to have been applied indifferently to more than one member of a class. Thus **bole** might be 'The name of several kinds of fine, compact, earthy, or unctuous clay, usually of a yellow, red, or brown colour due to the presence of iron oxide', first recorded 1641, or it might be 'an astringent earth brought from Armenia, and formerly used as an antidote and styptic', first recorded *c.*1386, but it is normally impossible to tell which is meant in a given context. These cases have all been omitted as not admitting of disambiguation in the context, except of course when they are absolute first citations. There were many less specialist terms where determining the precise meaning was not contextually possible, which were therefore excluded although there was some possibility that they were antedatings. There are also some words, however, for which it would be almost impossible to construct a definition on the basis of their appearance in a given text, which only appear once or at most a few times and whose exact meaning cannot be correlated with that in the pages of the *OED*. These are included in spite of the lexicographical difficulties where they are absolute first citations, since it is not the purpose of this exercise to provide glosses or definitions, but simply to record their presence and their lexicographical status.

In instances where the *OED* has managed to cover the relevant variant form, a term will be rather listed as an antedating than as something else, for example Barrough's **embrocha** 'make an embrocha' (4) is an antedating of *OED*'s **embroch(e)**; the spelling with *-a* is listed as a further variant occurring in the sixteenth century.

2. ANALYSIS OF ANTEDATINGS

Antedatings can tell us most about editorial practices of the *OED* and about the history of the lexicon in the sixteenth century, and have therefore been given most attention in this study. Unlike postdatings, many antedatings, especially those words with a technical, special, or restricted sense, may offer some information as to the approximate date of their first appearance, and thus teach us something significant about the development of that part of the lexicon given that sufficient words are available from which to draw conclusions. Of more immediate significance is the fact that a corpus of antedatings whose lengths in years have been calculated will suggest the extent to which the *OED* may be taken as a reliable source for the state of the lexicon in the sixteenth century.

The length of antedatings may also yield other important information. Where a sufficient number can be gathered, a graph of their lengths ought to reveal a pattern which relates to the compilation of the *OED*. Theoretically, a number of antedating lengths when graphed should form an approximately exponential curve; that is, if the *OED* had enough information to be reasonably accurate about the age of words, then there is more likelihood that many more short antedatings will be found than very long ones, and that there should be a relationship between length and frequency of occurrence determined by the probability of a word being noted by the *OED*'s readers. This is always on the assumption that the number of texts read for a given period was sufficiently large to ensure a sound statistical base in the first place, and that there were no significant variations in the amount of information available from different periods; if such variations do exist, they ought to appear on the graph as deviations from the expected curve. Neither assumption is necessarily sound, and both deserve to be tested if possible. While the skill and pertinacity of *OED* readers obviously varied considerably, it is for the moment assumed that there were enough of them to iron out individual vagaries. A further variable of great significance is the frequency of occurrence, since infrequently used words may have much longer antedating lengths; however, corpus studies are probably the only way of tackling this question, and the present study was not corpus-based.

In the case of the *OED*, texts ought to have been available for excerption approximately in relation to the period of publication; that is, the earlier the period the less available material, reckoning for the moment from the incunable period, prior to which special conditions may obtain for particular periods. If the numbers of books published can be taken as a potentially reasonable record of written English, then the availability of material for lexicographers ought to be in direct relationship; thus the chances of a word being recorded should also form an exponential curve plotted against time. This would fail to apply if, for instance, it could be shown that the *OED* editors had utilized roughly the same amount of material from, say, the sixteenth century as from the nineteenth century rather than an amount in direct proportion, in which case this would not be a significant factor in the analysis of the present findings. It would also not apply if the number of words in the lexicon also increased in direct relationship to the number of printed sources available. Clearly there has been a continual, though perhaps uneven, increase in the lexicon, so that this relationship, while beyond the scope of the present study, deserves closer examination.

The works selected for this study approximate a random sample of those medical texts available from the period, but the new data for the *OED* thus identified are therefore in no sense a random sample from those possible for the dictionary as a whole, since the corpus of text is so obviously specialized. Nevertheless there has been no attempt to select only specialist terms. Any antedating noticed in the texts excerpted has been included. It would have been highly desirable to have carried out an exhaustive analysis of the texts under consideration; while unfortunately this was not a practicable procedure given the resources available, some indication of the possible results may be gauged by a small sample which was actually carried through. The research was based on pages randomly selected from several texts. Every word on each page was exhaustively compared with *OED* entries, and a small but significant number of new data were discovered.[39] The results are discussed in Chapter 6. The data discovered in this study is shown in Table 5.1. Those authors marked with an asterisk have already been read for the *OED*.

The works of Bostocke, Clever, Cotta, and Langton have been discussed in a previous article in which 373 items of new data were

Table 5.1. *Total data extracted from texts analysed*[40]

Author	Ante-dated	New sense	Unre-corded	Post-dated	Totals
Bailey	43	7	6	0	56
Baker(*)[41]	134	15	91	4	244
Banister*	687	62	208	13	970
Barrough*	586	64	429	25	1,104
Bostocke	185	18	65	6	274
Clever	382	31	99	24	536
Cotta*	238	18	44	12	312
Hester	74	8	36	4	122
Hill	27	2	23	2	54
Langton, *IP*	60	5	13	0	78
Langton, *VBT*	65	7	6	0	78
More	53	5	51	2	111
Plutarch	24	4	18	0	46
TOTALS	2,558	246	1,089	92	3,985

notified (McConchie 1983). The information from the works now added to the list significantly expands the scope of the discussion and adds considerable weight to the statistical evidence presented in that publication. There is also a significant shift in one important aspect of the evidence, the statistics for the length of antedatings.

3. METHODS OF ANALYSIS

As already suggested, antedatings will be graphed according to length and against time, given that this study has accumulated a number large enough to show any deviations from expected norms. Clearly the potential corpus of medical terms from the sixteenth century is finite in size. That being so, it ought to be the case that as the number of texts excerpted increases, the rate of duplication of terms ought to increase in approximate relation to the percentage of the corpus which is recorded. Since the methods of excerption and the principles invoked have developed over a long period of time, and since several texts have been re-examined, no attempt has been made to assess this rate.

A finding rate will be established for each of the authors excerpted here; that is, the number of words which have to be read in order to find one item of new data. This is simply the estimated number of words in a given work divided by the total new data found. This sheds some light on the problem of an author's lexical productiveness as well as the relative treatment of different areas of the lexicon by the *OED*. Some of the analysis applied to the total lists of new data are also applied to medical as against non-medical words. Such a figure is of course affected by selective excerption, but more thoroughgoing excerption would only serve to increase the weight of evidence presented here, not diminish it. It has been possible, as explained in Chapter 6, to do a limited amount of concordance analysis from some selected pages of text, and the results of that are duly examined.

Fine-print lemmas have been treated in the following way. On the principle that all new data is inherently valuable and that its acquisition could make a significant change to the *OED* treatment, it has been decided that all fine-print lemmas should be dealt with in the same way as main lemmas, and listed with them in Appendix 1. Those fine-print lemmas given lemma status in the *OED*, for example, rare and obsolete words, are treated exactly the same as other main lemmas. Those incorporated into the running text of entries, for example, participials, verbal substantives, and derivative compounds and collocations, are also recorded, but their status as fine-print lemmas is noted in Appendix 1, and they are recorded in the form in which they appear in the running text, not under the main lemma. Thus **spermatic vessel** appears here in that form, not under **spermatic**, and **judging day** does not appear as a numbered sub-lemma of **judge** or **judging**. The provision of new data to the *OED* might in some cases change the status of a fine-print lemma to that of a main lemma.

4. OTHER PROBLEMS

The total number of new data includes all those which have been found in the texts consulted whether or not they are medical terms. The problems associated with distinguishing those words with a genuinely medical application will be discussed at length later. As has already been noted, in the absence of concordances the personal deficiencies and bias of the researcher in identifying new data and the necessary incompleteness of this task is inevitable, but any additional information would probably serve to support the conclusions reached here rather than undermine them. It is also worth remarking that, apart from the reasons mentioned alone, some indication of the frequency of terms is useful.

No attempt has so far been made to reassign the dates given for works by the *OED* editors, although it is probably desirable to do so in some cases. Needless to say there will be some disagreement as to their accuracy, for example, the dates of certain of Shakespeare's plays. There will undoubtedly be instances in which the *OED* can now be shown to be incorrect by the enquiries of subsequent researchers. There are also cases in which the *OED* was wrong in the first place; for example, there was some confusion over the date of publication of the work by John Hester excerpted here. Normally the edition of 1582 is cited, but sometimes the edition of 1590. This has presumably arisen through the work being farmed out to two independent readers, but part of it, namely Book iii, is the same text. To add to the muddle, the earliest edition is in fact 1580, and this study has revealed ten antedatings of Hester from his own 1582 edition as a result of this fact. In at least one instance, **unction**, the *OED* does cite the 1580 edition in spite of it not appearing in the *OED* bibliography. These antedatings might be thought—significantly and perhaps misleadingly—to lower the average length of antedatings for Hester in the present study, since ten antedatings of only two years' length which might be thought to be unnecessary are included. There was, however, no evidence in working through this text that changes had been made to the later edition. Similar though somewhat more complex considerations apply to Phillip Barrough, for whom at least three editions are cited: 1590, 1596, 1610. It is probable that this situation arises from a combination of the employment of different readers for this work as well as editorial inconsistency, as will appear in Chapter 7. Again, two dates, 1578 and 1576, are given for Lyte's *Dodoens*. In such cases, no attempt has been made to correct the *OED* bibliography's date, and the calculations of antedating length have been made on this basis. The alternative would have been large-scale cross-checking and collation of texts. I have also used the earlier date for calculating the length of antedatings in those cases where a range of uncertain dates is given, or where the publication spanned some years, as in the case of Holinshed's *Chronicles* or *Chambers's Cyclopaedia*. On the whole this practice will lead to conservative calculations, but not so much as to distort the final results significantly.

Other minor problems appear in the *OED* concerned with dating and with the accurate identification of authors, revisions, and reprints. An instance is Thomas Johnson's translation of the works of Paré, referred to in the case of **dartos** as being in the *Chirurgerie* but in the case of **sphacelate** referred to merely as *Works*. In this instance the identity of the two is assumed. Some other minor problems also arise; for instance, **suspensory** *sb.* includes as part of the preamble a reference to Blount's *Glossographia*, 1656, but not, it seems, as an illustrative quotation. This seems quite contrary to the usual practice. There is no obvious reason why it should not be an illustrative quotation unless it suggests that the *OED* editorial policy had by this time shied away from the Bradleian habit of citing other 'dicts.' rather too frequently. In this instance it is assumed that Blount's is the first illustrative citation. In order to complete calculations, it has been necessary to assign dates in instances where the *OED* itself does not. In those cases where no more accurate source than 'C17 dicts' or some such rubric has been used, it has been assumed, in order to facilitate matters, that this represents a quotation from Edward Phillips' *New World of English Words* of 1658, and the date has been recorded accordingly. Several of these are words beginning with **dia**-, for instance, Barrough's **diacalaminthe** (138); similarly, **diacapparis**, **dialthea**, **diasatyrion**, etc.

A further preliminary consideration is that the finding of new data for the *OED* is partly a function of the way in which lemmas were structured in the dictionary (see Zgusta 1988). A different style of lemmatization, for example, could eliminate many of the antedatings and new senses recorded here. If all chronological citations came together, and not under their separate entries for any given lemma, and if entries had tended to be conflated, perhaps a significant number of antedatings would vanish. The latter practice—the conflation of entries—and the tendency to use catch-all definitions rather than the fine discriminations used in the *OED* is noticeable in the *MED*.[42] Some may wish to argue that the *OED*'s practices are in this respect rather too finicky, creating artificial sub-divisions of entries.[43] In so far as this study depends wholly upon that method for its findings, it is a biased document.

It is naturally of interest to know in individual cases how efficiently a work was read by the original informants of the *OED* and also how great a contribution a work or group of works by some particular author might make to the historical and illustrative entries, but works have been read for this study without regard to their appearance or non-appearance in the *OED*: it has not been a criterion for selection. It is probable that a much larger sample should be made available before sensible comment on this matter can be made here, but it is obvious that works already read yield plenty of material for the researcher in all cases.

Some words appearing here as antedatings may already have been antedated in the *MED* or elsewhere, but this fact is overlooked for the purposes of this study, as previously indicated, since the *OED*, not the antedatings themselves, is the object of the research. As to new senses, the *OED* and the *MED* are not strictly comparable because of their disparate styles of definition, the nature of *MED* material requiring far less exactitude and discrimination. The *MED* almost inevitably records a longer antedating or provides an instance of precisely the sense recorded here. They do, however, appear in the present study, since their presence in the *MED* does not in the least affect their interpretative value for the *OED* or for the other matters raised here.

Having now established some ground rules, and cleared away some of the mechanical problems, I will undertake in Chapter 6 a more detailed account of the meaning of the data incorporated in this study, in particular a statistical examination of the many antedatings collected to see what they will reveal both about the state of the medical lexicon in the sixteenth century and about the way in which it has been handled in the *OED*.

Notes

1. This list forms vol. ii of this publication.
2. Primarily Microsoft Word and Microsoft Excel.
3. In these citations translators are given the primary author reference, and the original authors from whose work the translations have come are made to appear in square brackets since the major interest of this study is in the English version, not the original. *STC*, however, lists works under their original authors, not the translators.
4. For the most substantial digest of other information of this kind, see Bailey (1978).
5. See e.g. Nevalainen and Raumolin-Brunberg (1989: 67–110).
6. Cotta's book (1612) was first analysed very early, in the early 1980s, before the project took its present shape, but the arbitrary fixing of a date seemed no good reason to exclude the work, since it has proved to be a most productive one.

7. For a discussion of some of the issues involved, particularly affective features, and a bibliography, see Taavitsainen (1994). See also the handbook to the Helsinki corpus for the kinds of distinctions made (Kytö 1993). They are not fine enough to be pertinent to this discussion at present, though it is inevitable that more specialist corpus-builders will want to refine them considerably.
8. Others who produced almanacs included William Cuningham (1558, 1559, and 1566; see *Ath. Cant.* iii. 1) and Robert Watson, who authored three in 1595, 1598, and 1600; see *Ath. Cant.* ii. 310. For an account of almanacs and their relationship to medical practice, see Chapman (1979: 275–300).
9. The question of how efficiently works were read is discussed in Chapter 6.
10. *OED*, introductory note to 'List of books quoted'.
11. **Comfrey** is incorrectly listed under the date 1567.
12. Scholars such as Charles Webster, Margaret Pelling, and others have been redressing the balance.
13. Gunther (1971: 235), who identifies Bailey's handwriting as that in the margins of a BM copy of Du Pinet's *Historia Plantarum*.
14. The date is provided by Durling (1967).
15. Baker's contribution, beginning on Miii^{r}, is entitled *The nature and propertie of quicksilver*.
16. *STC* notes that bk. xxix was translated by Baker.
17. See *STC* 723, 2779, 12499, 1209, and 5447.
18. *A knowledge for kings*, 1576, a translation of a work by James Glaucus.
19. 'I might giue other instance in these well knowne and vulgar remedies of the named French disease, which by a present benumming of the sense, cousining, and easing of paine, do withall, for after time, inure and leaue behinde them such a rottennes, and a weaknesse ofttimes of the bones and sinewes, as suffereth few of our Mercurials to liue, to know their age in health, especially who throughly knew the siluer-salue in their youth. Hence toward declining age (if not before) some fall into consumptions and marasmes, some lose their teeth, some haue the palate of the mouth rotted, some the very bones of their head eaten, some by conuulsions their mouthes and faces set awry. And it is ordinary with most of this sort, long before haruest to leaue no grasse grow vpon their paued tops' (1612: 6).
20. Cotta (1623). This work is claimed by *Ath. Ox.* i. 438 to have been 'fit for the Press in 1616', as is indicated on **2^{r} of the work itself. This contribution concluded a debate which had begun much earlier (at least in the press) with Matthew Gwinne's *Aurum non aurum, sive, Adversaria in assertorem chymicae, sed verae medicinae desertorium, Fra. Anthonium*, 1611. See Ward (1740/1969: 264).
21. He also completed *A compendium of the rationall secretes, of the worthy*

knight and moste excellent doctour of physicke and chirurgerie, Leonardo Fioravanti Bolognese, 1582 (*STC* 10879).

22. Closer collaboration seems possible. There are some rare words shared between Hill's *Ioyfull iewell* and Hester's *Short discourse* which are striking—**divinely** (*Short discourse* Diii[v], antedated from Hester), **aperitive** (antedated from Hester); also shared are **feses**, **subtiliat** Fii[r], **assubtilat** (?), and **restringing** (Hii[v]). There are also two advertisements for Hester at Diiii[r] and Ei[v]. It is possible that they collaborated or that Hill taught Hester, that Hill had a hand in the *Short discourse*, or perhaps that Hester altered Hill's text of the *Ioyfull iewell*. The matter needs more detailed investigation.
23. *These oiles, waters, extractions, or essences, saltes, and other compostions* 1585[?], *STC* 13254. This pamphlet was presumably in the possession of Hester's friend Gabriel Harvey, whose autograph appears at the end of this copy with the cryptic remark 'Now M. Keymis, the great Alchymi[st] of London'. Does this mean that Keymis took over Hester's practice? It is known to have passed to the possession of the physician James Forrester in about 1594, since he alludes to the fact in the preface to *The pearle of practice*: 'The greater part of them [the oils, waters, etc.]were prepared by *Iohn Hester* of Paules wharfe, now deceased, a man, that spe[n]t much, & enda[n]gered his body, about such workes, wherof many excellent men haue enjoyed the benefite. The effect of his labour, hath and doth co[m]mend him, in Engla[n]d, and other cou[n]tries, which haue these many yeares made proofe, of these his preparations. All which as not lo[n]g since I bought of the suruiuer: so am I willing at all times, to part with any of the[m], to salue the wounded, heale the diseased' (*iiii[r]). Perhaps Keymis acquired it after Forrester's period of possession—if that is the real implication of Harvey's jotting. Forrester shares with Hester an enthusiasm for Paracelsian remedies.
24. Harvey, Gabriel (1593/1884: 289). There may also be evidence that Harvey himself had received medical training. It has been claimed that I.W.'s pamphlet was addressed to him and that he may have succeeded Lancelot Browne in a medical fellowship in Cambridge. See Schrickx (1956: 99).
25. The first record of his work is an edition of his translation of Cocles' treatise on physiognomy first dated by the *BLC* *c*.1550 and now amended, but in Johnson (1944: 329–51), it is suggested that the first work is his 1556 edition, entitled *A brief and most pleasa[n]t epitomye of the whole art of Physiognomie*, listed under Cocles, not Hill, in *STC*. Hill in his own list of writings appended to *The contemplation of mankind* 1571, itself an expanded edition of the Cocles translation, does not list a 1556 edition.
26. Not all were agreed about Fioravanti's credentials and status. Francis

Herring (1604: 32–3) went as far as to call him 'Fioravantus, that notorious Empiricke and Impostour of our time, who was banished Venice'. At the same time he was recommended to Cambridge medical students as required reading by Lancelot Browne, the sometime physician to both Elizabeth and James I.

27. Hill (1576). There is some confusion over these works. *BLC* as well as others, including Jones (1953) and Kocher (1947: 455) incorrectly ascribe *The newe iewell* to George Baker, and the error is compounded by Bennett (1965: 180). It is listed in the first edition of *STC* as being by Baker, but Hill's authorship does not seem to be in doubt. There is a disclaimer in the current edition of *STC* under Gesner. The title-page plainly declares that it is 'faithfully corrected and published in Englishe, by George Baker, chirurgian', not that it was 'englished' by him, so that this work was prepared for the press by Baker and published posthumously. See Johnson (1944: 109–35). Similarly, John Hester saw Hill's *A ioyfull iewell* through the press in 1579.
28. Johnson suggests, without giving any reason, that it was intended for the 1556 edition, *A brief and most plesau[n]t epitomye of the whole art of physiognomie.*
29. *Ath. Cant.* i. 197.
30. He attended Sir Thomas Smith in 1576, and was physician to Sir Thomas Gresham (*Ath. Cant.* i. 397).
31. Professor Richard Bailey has kindly pointed out to me that **sanguis draconis**, though unrecorded, appears under **cinnabar** 4 (quotation), **dragon's blood** (quotation), **socotrine** (quotation), and **sprinkle**, v^{1}, 1a (quotation).
32. See Schäfer (1980*a*: 17–22) for a discussion of the treatment of the Shakespeare and Nashe corpora.
33. Similarly **twitch**, v^{2}/**quitch**, sb^{1}; **twitter**, sb^{2}, v^{1}/**quitter**; **twitter-bone**/**quitter-bone**.
34. Hester (1580: Mii^{v}) 'grinde them ... distill them ... and alwayes at the last giue it a stronge fire that the fesses may remaine well burnt' and Hi^{v}: 'his common drinke was wine and water boyled on the festes of the same [decoction].'
35. Lewis and Short (1969) provide the participle **replexus**; one might expect an Italian form in *-ss-* rather than *-x-*, as in **plesso**, but there is some Bolognese dialectal influence. My thanks to Dr V. Cincotta, formerly of the University of Wollongong, for his assistance with this point.
36. **Vitreum** has been listed as unrecorded, since *OED* gives a derivation from **vitreus**.
37. There are also minor corrections to the *OED* format which have no bearing on the study in hand, but which are worth notice in any list of corrections. They include one instance of no date for an entry, and five

entries with no citation, including one with no date either, recorded from Barrough (**cypress nut, diamargariton, digestive, erysipelatoid, incourage**). There is also an instance of an extension to the last recorded date from Barrough (**inflammate**). From Banister there is the no citation **prostrate**. Although there were a number of instances of new spellings noticed, these have been omitted from the present study, in spite of their obvious usefulness to any revision of the *OED*.

38. See Bailey (1978) for a consolidated listing.
39. Thanks are due to Brigitta Flick and Sally Vickers for carrying out this painstaking work.
40. The small amount of further data including no citation, no date, etc., has been recorded in Appendix 1, but has not been subjected to any analysis, and is therefore excluded from this table.
41. Listed in the bibliography, but no citations are actually found in the dictionary.
42. *MED*, '*Plan and bibliography*', 3.
43. An early set of instructions to sub-editors indicates that this was a principle of procedure in the *OED* from the first: 'Proceed to classify the slips for each word according to meanings and constructions, dividing these as minutely as you can, with the aid of existing Dictionaries, etc.' (AOED, Misc. 91/4, 6).

6
Antedatings

The hunt for antedatings to the *OED* will seem to many to be pedantry of the most futile and pointless kind; a sort of ankle-biting at worst, and a fussy cleaning up of others' crumbs at best. But the fact is that the exercise has usually been treated as an adjunct to some more important piece of work—an edition for example—during the course of which they inevitably turn up, impede progress by their irritating presence, and are filed away for later use in some learned note. Only rarely has the collection of such information become an end in itself, and been subjected to some kind of scholarly analysis. Neither has it often been realized just how much material is potentially available to the scholar.

Gathering antedatings and other data has nevertheless occupied scholars since the *OED* first appeared, and over the years some very substantial lists have been assembled. More is at stake than a little bit of scholarly housekeeping, sufficient information having already been gathered elsewhere to justify careful analysis of the lexicon registered in the work.[1] Antedatings are the most numerous and the most interesting of the possible new data for the *OED* since, where sufficient can be gathered to make meaningful analysis possible, they may shed much light on the dictionary itself. Schäfer has already pointed out the innate insecurity of the assumption that *OED* sources have been on the whole reliably and consistently examined and excerpted (1989: 35); the data compiled here further demonstrates its unreliability and at the same time shows that sources already scrutinized, and even relatively thoroughly excerpted, may nevertheless be productive of much more material. Antedatings can also suggest much about its editorial practices and the thoroughness of its informants, as well as the accuracy with which it registers the state of the lexicon in a given area or a specific period. Even though the research may be confined to a particular field or period, antedatings can also indicate how accurate the dictionary might actually be and what its limitations are, issues of crucial importance to the many scholarly users of the work.

There are several possible ways of analysing an accumulation of antedatings. These are primarily statistical, and therefore deal with overall trends, and with the larger view of the lexicon, rather than with individual words or authors, who in many cases provide insufficient material by themselves. A number of questions suggest themselves in considering the present data, which might allow us to understand the medical lexicon of this period better, and to see what lexical resources were assembled for the *OED* and how they were used.

First, there are questions about the period and the semantic domain. What was the nature of the medical lexicon in the sixteenth century? How much of it was in exclusively medical use, and how much overlapped with the general language? How much variation was there between the sources of antedatings in their use of specialist terms? Secondly, there are questions about the *OED* itself. Which authors and what works have been antedated by the present data? How was the lexicon for the dictionary compiled and what kind of information did its readers supply? How accurately and comprehensively has the *OED* covered the medical terminology of our period? Did it note medical terminology consistently? Finally there is the tantalizing question about how much more research could be done on this subject and by what means it should be carried out. It is hoped that this enquiry will provide at least some partial answers to these questions.

The questions posed imply differing means of enquiry even though there is some overlap implied. The methods employed here are broadly as follows. First, an examination of the authors and works antedated. Secondly, an analysis of the lengths of the antedatings; thirdly, an estimate of the rate at which new data has been found in these authors; and fourthly, the classification of the antedatings into medical and non-medical categories of words.

1. AUTHORS AND WORKS ANTEDATED

Antedatings may be considered by their source as recorded in *OED*; that is, by the author listed in the *OED* as providing the first known occurrence for the lemma or sub-lemma. We would expect to find that a significant proportion of these sources were works on medicine or at least works by medical authors, and that collating the numbers of antedatings attributable to a particular author or work will indicate those sources upon which the *OED* has depended for registering this corpus. It will also be possible to make some comparisons with the disposition of sources in other research data reported. Since a sizeable proportion of the antedatings consists of medical terms, it is possible to take a measure of the extent of medical reference in the corpus to hand. Such a measure cannot be mathematically accurate, since there must inevitably be some question as to whether certain words are unambiguously medical in their reference, leaving aside the core upon which there will be agreement, but a rough estimate can be made.

Thus it is of especial interest to know whether an author may be regarded as a medical writer or not, and some preliminary discussion of this question is essential before more detailed analysis can be undertaken. It is also essential to establish what is meant by a 'medical writer' and a 'medical work' in order to determine whether an author should be included among such sources of antedatings. The most obvious category is medical textbooks, compiled for an educated and possibly professional or semi-professional readership. Most books dealing with specific diseases, for example some of the many tracts on the plague or on other diseases, are clearly medical in nature, as is any work dealing with medical theory.[2] Works dealing also with specific remedies such as the treatise on oleum magistrale by George Baker and other antidotaries as well as those books which undertake to explain the principles of medicine to the wider public, will qualify as medical works. So will books on humoral theory, and anatomies. In many other cases, however, the matter is not so simple. Tracts on baths and their healing properties are by and large medical works, though in some cases they discuss the origin and nature of the waters at length. Herbals, accounts of monstrosities, unnatural births and other similarly sensational occurrences, natural histories, physiognomy, and works on alchemy may in some cases have a close relation to the theory and practice of medicine, but in some other cases may not, and there may be considerable difficulties in classifying them. It is essential to make an individual judgement rather than to attempt to construct a workable typology, given the complexities involved. Works like Bacon's *The history of man* raise this kind of problem. Lexicographers are in some respects problematical since they could perhaps be expected to be familiar with quite a lot of medical terminology, especially those such as Bullokar and Baret, both physicians themselves. The interesting question of the extent to which this is so in individual cases has been more closely examined in Chapter 4. The guidelines used here to determine which works and authors ought to be included or excluded are looser than those adopted in Chapter 5, where works which belong to subject areas with their own lexicon were to be excluded from the list of works for possible excerption on the grounds that only works dealing with medicine and its lexicon directly should be included. Here, however, works whose subjects conduce to the practice of medicine may be included, especially if it seems likely that the author was familiar with medical terminology.

In general I have adopted the policy of including herbals because of the intimate knowledge of herbal remedies required of most physicians and apothecaries, and because herbals were usually compiled with therapeutic ends in view, rather than as taxonomies only. Herbals generally contained an account of the medicinal properties and virtues of the plants described, an aspect to which Gerarde paid particular attention. Gerarde and Lyte are therefore regarded as medical writers, although there is no evidence to suggest that Lyte received a medical training (Henrey 1975: 34–5). Gerarde, on the other hand, was apprenticed to a barber-surgeon and was eventually elected master of the Company in 1607. Lyte's ultimate original, Rembert Dodoens (1517–85), was a renowned physician (Dodoens 1554).[3]

Some genres may be excluded on the grounds that they are not primarily medical, and are not intended to assist in medical practice. I have excluded natural histories, thereby omitting Bacon, and the lexicographers are also omitted. On the other hand, some authors whose work is not usually medical may be included for a particular work. An example is Thomas Timme (d. 1640), who was an enthusiastic translator and pamphleteer, writing several treatises for the good of the souls of his countrymen. But he was also the translator of Quercitanus' (Du Chesne) *The practise of chymicall and hermeticall physicke* of 1605, from which come a number of the antedatings recorded here. He appears not to have been trained as a physician, but spent his life both as an author and as the rector of Hasketon in Suffolk. His son Thomas shared his father's interest and was admitted as a Fellow of the Royal College of Physicians in 1664 (Henrey 1975: 38). It seems that the elder Thomas was at least an interested amateur. He found inspiration in the Paracelsian philosophy, perhaps through Du Chesne's writings, and saw in these principles a justification for belief in the 'Unitie of one Hupostasis Diuine' (Timme 1605: A3–4; Debus 1965: 88). An interest in medical practice would seem to have followed indirectly from the Paracelsian theory that to comprehend manifest nature is to comprehend the Good. Timme has been listed here as a medical writer, though reservations do remain. The fact of having translated a medical work does seem to be sufficient justification for inclusion by itself.

An author who figures in the list of antedatings is the ingenious and inventive Sir Hugh Plat (1552–1611?), who began an abortive literary career with some unfortunately platitudinous verses in 1572, but who later found his *métier* in agriculture, natural science, and husbandry. His most cited work here is *The iewell house of art and nature* of 1594. In 1607 we find Plat publishing a broadsheet on nutrition and medicine for seamen, and there is a series of unpublished works including a notebook lodged in the British Library which is an anecdotal and homely collection of cures (BL Add. MS M 2197), as well as alchemical material and collections of 'secrets',[4] entitled *Secrets of physick and surgery,* which might allow us to regard him as a medical writer. On the slight evidence of the latter two he will be regarded as a medical writer here, but he is a very marginal case since his knowledge seems practical and anecdotal rather than properly professional.

There are also instances where a work is by its nature marginal, but has been written by a physician or surgeon. These cases are included, since it has been assumed that what is of interest is the likelihood that an author will be thoroughly familiar with medical terminology, and have some opportunity to use it. To take a specific instance, Philemon Holland received a medical training, probably in a Continental university, but maintained only a small practice, and devoted much of his time to translation. For the most part he englished the classics—Livy, Pliny, Suetonius, Ammius Marcellinus, and others but he also published a translation of Bauderon's *Pharmacopeia* from the original French into Latin, the *Observations* of Dubois (1639), and the much translated *Regimen Sanitatis Salerni* (published posthumously, 1649). He is therefore included as a medical writer. Tobias Venner (1577–1660) was a physician who presents a rather different case, having written on rather marginal subjects, namely a book on the baths of Bath (Venner 1620), as well as a work on tobacco (Venner 1621).

Translators of other medical works were sometimes physicians by training and sometimes not. There is no hard evidence that the popularizer Thomas Hill had any formal medical qualifications, but informal training was easily accessible from the various practitioners serving the medical needs of ordinary folk. His association with Baker and Hester suggests that he may have had a professional interest of some kind in medicine. He did nevertheless translate the works of Leonardo Fioravanti, the Italian Paracelsian physician and quack, and is thus included as a medical author in this study. He also translated some of the work of the influential Conrad Gesner, who seems to have been better known in England at this time than Paracelsus himself. Gesner was widely translated, and helped to popularize Paracelsian or iatrochemical remedies, even though his own attitude to Paracelsus was sceptical. Other works by Hill included an early translation of Cocles on physiognomy (*c.*1556) and works on both the interpretation of dreams and on comets. Edmund Topsell, a considerable source for the *OED*, has been excluded from the list in spite of the fact that his *Four-footed beasts* (1607) is based on the work of Gesner, since he was primarily a divine with an interest in zoology.

A relatively obscure figure is the A.M. who was the translator of Gabelkhover and Guillemeau. There is some slight evidence as to his identity. In the introduction to his rendering of Gabelkover, he describes himself as 'a German a long time removed from England.'[5] This hardly settles the matter of his identity or nationality, but the evidence of his work does not merely suggest a competent fluency in English; he also had a sufficient mastery of the language to provide a glossary at the end of the work in which many obscure neologisms are explained. Jones notes (1953: 96 n.) that most of his obscure terms are for directions and processes. In this he differs from say, Baker, where many words are the names of remedies or their ingredients.

In Table 6.1 the whole corpus of antedatings in Appendix 1 has been sorted by the *OED* author[6] antedated in order to compare these writers with the results obtained by Schäfer for Shakespeare and Nashe. For convenience, only those *OED* authors yielding 0.20 per cent of the total of 2,558 or higher, in other words five antedatings or more, have been noted in Table 6.1, which sets out the position fully. Where necessary authors appearing in the *OED* under variants of names, such as Ralegh/Raleigh or other designations such as 'Cawdrey' and 'R.C.', 'Thomas Blount' and 'Dicts. 1656' have been silently conflated.[7]

TABLE 6.1. *Antedated OED authors*

Author	No.	%	Author	No.	%
Shakespeare	129	5.04	*Phil. Trans.*	9	0.35
Bacon, F.	81	3.17	Salmon	9	0.35
Holland	76	2.97	Sylvester	9	0.35
Crooke	64	2.50	Taylor, J.	9	0.35
A.M.	56	2.19	Cogan	8	0.31
Barrough	54	2.11	Greene	8	0.31
Browne	47	1.84	Hakluyt	8	0.31
Phillips	45	1.76	Quarles	8	0.31
Topsell	40	1.56	Ray	8	0.31
Blancard's Phys. Dict.	38	1.48	Sandys	8	0.31
Florio	28	1.09	Arbuthnot	7	0.27
Burton	27	1.06	Cawdrey, R.	7	0.27
Cotgrave	26	1.02	Chapman	7	0.27
Chamb. Cycl.	25	0.98	Clarendon	7	0.27
Spenser	25	0.98	Digby	7	0.27
Timme	25	0.98	Howell	7	0.27
Jonson	22	0.86	Jackson, T.	7	0.27
T.B.	21	0.82	Middleton	7	0.27
Milton	20	0.78	Power	7	0.27
Donne	18	0.70	Puttenham	7	0.27
Blount, T.	17	0.66	*Syd. Soc. Lex.*	7	0.27
Hart	17	0.66	Wiseman	7	0.27
Nashe	16	0.63	Banister. J.	6	0.23
Cockeram	16	0.63	Bradley, R.	6	0.23
More, H.	16	0.63	Braithwait	6	0.23
Plat	15	0.59	Lyte	6	0.23
Willis	15	0.59	Mayne	6	0.23
Hester	14	0.55	Ralegh	5	0.20
Boyle, R.	14	0.55	Smith, J.	6	0.23
Bulwer	13	0.51	Surflet	6	0.23
Venner	13	0.51	Blundevil	5	0.20
Woodall	13	0.51	Brinsley	5	0.20
Evelyn	12	0.47	Day, A.	5	0.20
French	12	0.47	Gerbier	5	0.20
Llwyd, H.	12	0.47	Golding	5	0.20
Herbert, Sir T.	11	0.43	Grimstone	5	0.20
Hooker	11	0.43	Guillim	5	0.20
Purchas	11	0.43	Hale	5	0.20
Bailey, N.	10	0.39	Healey, J.	5	0.20
Daniel, S.	10	0.39	Heylin	5	0.20

Author	No.	%	Author	No.	%
Fuller, T.	10	0.39	Holmes, T.	5	0.20
Hall, Bp.	10	0.39	Hooke	5	0.20
Hobbes	10	0.39	Junius	5	0.20
Lovell	10	0.39	Knolles	5	0.20
Biggs	9	0.35	Lithgow	5	0.20
Dryden	9	0.35	Lowe	5	0.20
Eng. dicts.	9	0.35	Marlowe	5	0.20
Gerarde	9	0.35	Moffett	5	0.20
Harvey, G.	9	0.35	Mulcaster	5	0.20
Johnson, T.	9	0.35	Pope	5	0.20
Monro	9	0.35			

What emerges from the figures in this study is that there is a relatively high number of medical writers represented among the authors who have been frequently antedated. It will at once be apparent that the spread of sources is different from Schäfer's in several important respects. In Schäfer's work Shakespeare, a non-medical writer, took first position easily. This is largely a reflection of the particular care with which his words are treated in the *OED*, rather than of his potential as a source for the *OED*. In the present study he comfortably retains that position with 129 antedatings, but his relative contribution is greatly reduced, from 19.63 per cent to a much more modest 5.04 per cent. He is now joined at the top of the list by a group including most notably the physician and translator Philemon Holland (76), the physicians Helkiah Crooke (64) and Phillip Barrough (54),[8] the medical translator A.M. (56), and Browne (47). This relative weighting of Shakespeare, who was in no sense a medical writer,[9] against other authors seems much more reasonable in this instance, though the difference between his contribution and that of the next outright literary figure, Spenser (25), is still striking. The others who now follow reasonably closely include writers who certainly had an interest in medical matters, although they may not have been formally qualified in a medical trade, such as Bacon (81) and perhaps Topsell (40). The translator of Blancard's *Physical Dictionary* of 1657 (38), Burton (27), Timme (25), and T.B. (21), the translator of la Primaudaye, are also quite well represented. Medical contributors yielding between 10 and 20 are Hester, Hart, the surgeon John Woodall, Humfrey Llwyd, Sir Hugh Plat, and Venner.

While these figures are of considerable interest, not least because some comparative material is available, it should not be thought that a relatively high number of antedatings for a given *OED* author indicates more than it really ought to. The chronological limits of the study mean that there are many authors who can only be antedated in a restricted way; for instance, Eden (1553 and 1555), Recorde (1548 and 1557), and Skene (1568) can obviously only be antedated by Langton, and [Plutarch], and so a large number of antedatings, comparable with (say) Bacon, at least some of whose works can be antedated by all of the authors in this study, can hardly be expected. Shakespeare obviously cannot be significantly antedated by Cotta. An expanded study might reveal markedly different contributions by individual authors.

Another aspect of these figures which is particularly important here is the increasing numbers of contributions from sources other than Shakespeare. It is not merely that the significant contributors are less likely to be literary figures than those in Schäfer's list, and that they are much more likely to be physicians; it is also the case that the spread of contributors is much wider and more even towards the top of the list. The relative drop in the number of antedatings from Shakespeare probably reflects the nature of the texts being studied, but it also shows his relative lack of use of the special terminology of the medical profession. It is difficult in practice to find many words in the Shakespearean corpus used in a specialist medical sense, although of course there are many which had such a sense but were used in some other way by him, or belonged to that part of the medical lexicon in more general use rather than to those terms by and large limited to the profession.

It also clearly demonstrates that there is still much to be discovered about the lexicon of this period. The fact that such a relatively minor examination of the available corpus should so markedly drop the preponderance of Shakespearean citations serves to underline the possibilities for further research.

Thus the results presented here show a particular kind of bias which operated in the selection of texts for use in the *OED*, adding somewhat to the research by Schäfer already alluded to. Although the value judgements upon which this particular emphasis are based are not far to seek, the principles which underlay this kind of bias were not always clearly enunciated by the *OED* editorship. At least it is not always essential to search for them by examining a new corpus of terms.

2. THE LENGTH OF ANTEDATINGS

Antedatings vary in their length in years, expressed as the difference between the *OED* author antedated and the new source reported here, across almost the whole possible range, from one year to well over 300. The very longest possible in this study would be a little under 400 years; in fact the longest is 331. The possible length is determined by the date of the earliest citation used by the *OED* for that word, and by the date of the text selected for analysis in which the antedating is discovered. In itself, the length of an antedating relates to the dictionary, not in any sense to the language. The length of an antedating is purely a factor of the structure of the *OED*, a measure in a way of its accuracy and comprehensiveness. A perfect historical dictionary would never be antedated, except by the discovery of previously unknown texts. The average length of the present antedatings arranged by author reveals a considerable range, from 43 to over 80 years, as well as a substantial overall average. Table 6.2 computes averages for all authors excerpted in this study.

TABLE 6.2. *Average length of antedatings*

Author	Average length
Bailey	57.19
Baker	80.51
Banister	77.54
Barrough	71.62
Bostocke	57.83
Clever	57.89
Cotta	54.18
Hester	43.32
Hill	70.15
Langton, *IP*	56.97
Langton, *VBT*	53.68
More	61.50
Plutarch	60.33
OVERALL AVERAGE	67.35

The fact that the average length of antedatings is considerably over half a century suggests that there is a substantial margin of error in the *OED*'s overall picture of the medical lexicon for the sixteenth century, and it may suggest further that research into other semantic domains could reveal similar deficiencies. There is a sufficiently substantial body of non-medical words in this collection to indicate that the conclusions drawn here apply more widely to the whole lexicon. The average length of 67 years is considerably in excess of the findings of previous research on this subject which related to literary texts (McConchie 1983*b*: 31–2). Schäfer has already shown that the coverage of individual literary sources themselves, a semantic domain in which the dictionary might be expected to have been more thorough, can be quite inadequate.

The average reader and user of the dictionary would probably concur with assessments of successive editors that the work has basically been done, and although changes and improvements are both desirable and inevitable, they would not alter the dictionary's structure drastically (Murray 1900: 49). The presumption has been that the coverage of sources has at least been adequate. It seems a reasonable theoretical assumption that, if the *OED* had indeed done a uniformly good job of identifying the words of the language and the dates of their first appearance in writing, antedatings presented in the form of a graph whose horizontal axis plots their length in years and whose vertical axis plots their numerical occurrence within a given span of years ought to form an exponential curve, with the highest numbers in the shortest spans of years and the lowest in the longest. Schäfer found that this was on the whole true for the antedatings from Nashe and Shakespeare (Schäfer 1980*a*: 46).[10] In the case of the present collection of antedatings, it is also generally the case that an exponential curve appears, but it is by no means a regular one, as appears in Appendix 2, graph 14.

One of the marked periods of deviation from the curve is in the longer time-spans, where a significant series of humps appears between about 210 and 310 years, indicating rather more antedatings of this length than might be expected. The occurrence of variations in particular time-spans may reflect the *OED* editors' use of particularly rich sources of information having a particular importance for medical terminology, such as *Chamber's Cyclopaedia* at about 160 years, and perhaps the 1706 edition of Phillips' dictionary, rather than indicating more general trends.

The most noticeable deviation occurs in the lower range, between about fifteen and fifty years. The smallest figures, which ought to be highest, clearly are not. This is less easily explained, since there appears to be no single work affecting the figures, but it is possible that the increase in the sheer number and sophistication of medical sources from about 1580 produces this result. More detailed analysis appears in graphs 1–13 for each individual author, although these are less indicative of the overall picture. Some of the features alluded to above appear in a more exaggerated form in some of these graphs. The features of the graph mentioned are most obvious in that for Banister (graph 3), in which the shortest lengths are markedly under-represented, there are two large peaks at about twenty and forty years, and another in the late seventeenth and early eighteenth century. The mid- to late nineteenth century is also over-represented. This pattern is less apparent in the graph for Barrough (graph 4). The shortest lengths are perhaps best represented in Cotta (graph 7), and to some extent in Clever (graph 6), in whose figures there is a large number of antedatings from Shakespeare.[11]

If such variations have been caused by *Chambers's Cyclopedia*, *NSSL* and perhaps by other works and authors as well, this situation ought in reality to cause some concern. It might be argued that this heavy reliance on a few sources overstrains the reliability and accuracy of these sources, leaving the dictionary over-exposed to their possible errors, as well as to inaccuracies arising from relative neglect of other sources. Given the amount of material available in the seventeenth to nineteenth centuries, it seems that much of it has been under-utilized. It ought to be the case for example, that reliance on *Chambers's Cyclopedia*, would be counterbalanced by a reliance on a number of other near-contemporary resources. This appears not to be the case, otherwise the hump would not be so obvious. To put it another way, it would be possible to assume that for well-documented periods of the language, a good historical dictionary should show itself to be statistically subject only to variations in the lexical corpus, rather than to the availability of a particular text as a source. The *OED* in certain areas and periods does seem to exhibit this text rather than corpus dependence, even in so late a period as that in which the *NSSL* was published.

3. FINDING RATES

Some indication of the potential for new lexical material of the authors examined in this study derives from estimating the finding rates for each: that is, how much new data come from what quantities of text? A raw measure of this is achieved simply by dividing the number of antedatings found in a given author by the estimated total number of words read to find them. Schäfer's research on this area has already indicated a rate of finding new data which was very high, and in the case of Nashe higher than the rate of new data for Shakespeare.[12]

The calculation of the finding rate applied to the present data produces the results set out in Table 6.3. The number of words in a text was estimated from counting on a sample of normal pages. For the sake of comparison, the figure representing the notional number of words required to be read to find a first citation for Shakespeare based on Schäfer's slightly different principles of data selection is added at the foot of the table.

TABLE 6.3. *The rate of finding corrections*

Author	Words in text	All new data	Antedatings
Bailey	13,904	248	323
Baker	16,380	67	123
Banister	199,888	206	290
Barrough	265,065	239	451
Bostocke	23,715	87	128
Clever	28,847	54	76
Cotta	34,540	110	145
Hester	37,984	311	513
Hill	34,375	636	1,273
Langton, *IP*	17,864	229	298
Langton, *VBT*	26,400	343	406
More	24,860	227	469
Plutarch	8,190	178	341
Shakespeare			422

Some of these figures, especially those for Clever, Baker, Bostocke, and Cotta, are comparatively quite remarkable. It is immediately obvious that, for antedatings, many are lower than the figure quoted for Shakespeare; Bailey, Baker, Banister, Bostocke, Clever, Cotta, both Langton texts, More, and Plutarch all returning lower figures—in Clever's case, by a factor of a little less than six. The number for all new data returned for Clever, Baker, and Bostocke indicates the great potential for lexical material of such sources. In all this it has to be remembered that Shakespeare's figure cannot be significantly lowered by further research, but those for all other authors cited here can be. The potential for doing so is discussed later in this chapter. There is certainly truth in the claim by Schäfer that the figures for Shakespeare are inflated, but at the same time it is also manifestly clear that figures for other writers have been badly underestimated.[13]

It should be noted that there would be a potential corrigibility in such figures in that if two identical corrections were discovered and the later one eliminated the figures would alter. The fact that one work might be analysed before another should also be a factor, since finding a number of corrections in one work might reduce the chance of recording them elsewhere, but I have not deliberately avoided duplications in this work and they have all been recorded, so that the excerption of one text has not affected the excerption of any subsequent text in this respect. An attempt was also made to see if arranging the works by chronological order would reveal some pattern in the figures returned, but it did not. On the other hand it would be quite arbitrary to remove a duplicate antedating simply because one text was excerpted later than another.

It was possible in Jürgen Schäfer's study to assess the reliability with which an individual author had been excerpted by the *OED*, using the measure he called the author reliability rate. Since this measure depends on the availability of concordances or exhaustive databases for the authors concerned, such figures are impossible in the present study. The further question of how many items of new data an author produces relative to others, sometimes erroneously thought of as the linguistic creativity of an author, is also intriguing, but it should be remembered that in this study the number of items is increased, perhaps somewhat artificially, by the presence of large numbers of unrecorded specialist encysts, most of which are *ipso facto* not creatively coined, and many of which are certainly capable of further antedating. The interested reader may consult Appendix 1 for other kinds of unrecorded words.

4. CLASSIFICATION OF ANTEDATINGS

This study also raises interesting questions about the kind of terminology used and the frequency of its use. First, approximately how many medical terms are there in the sixteenth-century English lexicon? Secondly, how many of the antedatings discovered in this study are actually medical terms? Appendix 3 provides a complete list of antedatings from the works studied which appear to have a medical sense, whether or not that fact is noted in *OED*. There have been considerable problems in deciding when a word had such a sense and when it did not. Medicine sometimes included other arcane disciplines such as alchemy, astrology, distillation, chiromancy, and herbalism. Only words used as medical terms in the citations from the thirteen medical sources of this study are included. There are instances in which words had a medical sense only very much later, and these are excluded where it seems highly unlikely that they would have had such a meaning in our period. Words which were probably though not demonstrably medical are, however, included, and there has been much latitude allowed; for example, in many terms, describing body parts, which, while obviously words in common or general use, appear to be used regularly in the medical literature as well in transferred senses, such as **neck** or **face**. Terms used as couplings for neoclassical terms, such as **shiplike** are included, as are many words for bodily functions not easily separable from more general senses, e.g. **motion**.

Nevertheless many problems still occur in deciding whether a particular term is used in a medical sense, as in the case of **involuntary** where the first recorded medical sense, field marked *physiol.*, is 'concerned in bodily actions or processes which are independent of the will' (1840). Has this sufficient affinity in sense with the absolute first citation of 1531 'not voluntary ... independent of volition' to make the reasonable supposition that such a medical sense might have existed in the sixteenth century? A similar case should be noted with **stertor**, where the present antedating suggests the existence of such a meaning early, as indicated, in spite of the length of the antedating (237 years): it is therefore included. In these instances, it does not seem possible to follow hard and fast rules. **Deflation**, with an antedating length of 301 years, is an example of a word whose new antedating is clearly medical, though the *OED*'s first citation is not. A further example, this time of a word with a late and unrelated medical usage, is **engraft**, where there is a sense (3b, 1717) 'to introduce small-pox virus into', which could bear no immediate relation to the use of the word in More. **Transplantation** is included, not on the basis of the meaning (4, *surg.*) 'The operation of transferring an organ or a portion of tissue from one part of the body, or from one person or animal, to another', which is given a first citation of 1813, but rather for the sense 'the pretended magical cure of disease by causing it to pass to another person, or to an animal or plant', which is first listed as occurring in 1655. Words are also included which may have only one listed medical sense among a wide area of polysemy.

Some of the words listed here are primarily alchemical terms, including **assation** and **cohobate** (Bostocke), **rectified** (Hill), **reduce**, **quenched**, and **resolute** (Baker). There are also terms which have an extranate reference to medicine, such as **medicine-monger**, but these are included in the list for the present.

There are a number of instances in which it appears that the *OED* ought to have recognized a separate medical sense for a word. Some have appeared many times in the texts consulted here with an obviously special application which has evaded the notice of the dictionary and which needs no further justification. There are several instances of a word having a medical application by virtue of belonging to a specific collocation or group of words. A collocation I take here to mean words generally used together in similar contexts. A group, on the other hand, shares a categorical likeness but not necessarily a frequently repeated context. A particular example among many which might be discussed is **revulsive** (Baker), which, though not noted in the *OED* as a medical term, should be so since it belongs to a group employed as both nouns and derived adjectives to describe the nature of certain medicines and their actions. This group includes such words as **defensative**, **mitigative**, **mollificative**, **solutive**, **preparative**, and **carnificative**. Variants include such groups as **mollicative**, **mollificative**, **remollificative**, all potentially both nouns and adjectives, as well as **mollifying** (*ppl. a.*) and **mollifier** (*sb.*).

For another reason **declination** is properly regarded as a medical word. It belongs not to a group linked by morphological likenesses but to a collocation which describes the growth and decline of a body, organism, or disease. This process is normally spoken of as the **generation**, **auction**, (or **growing** or **growth**), (**e**)**state**, and **declination** of the entity concerned, and the collocation is of frequent occurrence. Although the actual forms used vary, a typical instance is Barrough's discussion of what he defines as **oedema** which '(as other tumours also) hath four times, the beginning the augmenting, the state, and the declination of the tumour' (246).

A more difficult instance is **stove** (Hester), which only occurs once in this text, and cannot be defined with certainty. Hester reports that 'the remedies that helpe the pockes are ... *Oriola* a stoue of hearbes', from which laconic context it is all but impossible to say precisely what is meant in the absence of some corroborating definition in the *OED* or assistance from another contemporary text, which has not so far been forthcoming. Neither is it possible to be quite sure that it is not a typographical error.

The lemmatization of the dictionary itself might also cause problems. An instance of the *OED*'s being rather finicky is under **curd**, *v.* Sense 1a '*trans.* To make into curd; to coagulate, congeal' covers the idea of blood 'curding' perfectly well. The citations here include this from *Hamlet* (I, v, 69): 'It doth posset and curd, like Aygre droppings into Milke, The thin and wholesome blood', which makes it clear that both blood and milk are substances which may be curded in sense 1a. Sense 1b specifies 'To curdle (blood)', seemingly simply to accommodate Shakespeare's use of the word in *All's well that ends well:* 'Does it curd thy blood To say I am thy mother?' (I, iii, 155). Neither of these Shakespearean examples make it clear that there really is a difference between 'curding' blood and 'curdling' it (see **curdle**, v, 1). This special and over-scrupulous attention to Shakespearean usage has provided an antedating from Barrough's 'Of bloud broken out of the bladder or curded in it', which is probably unjustified, but which I include on the principle that my antedatings ought to be based on lemma divisions in preference to illustrative citations.[14] The treatment of Shakespeare and by implication other literary figures needs still more examination. In spite of these considerations, I have chosen to keep these items in the list, preferring merely to point out the problem and to avoid playing the editor with pertinent sections of the *OED*, a practice which would create more difficulties than it would solve.

Words which are the names of remedies have been included in these lists, as have the names for the separate ingredients or simples. There are a number of these in the antedatings from Baker particularly, and this reflects my growing realization as the work proceeded that the *OED* is rather inconsistent in reporting such words. This area of the lexicon now looms rather large in the overall data reported here. The large number of unrecorded words from the more extensive sources contain many such terms. Similarly, there are a number of names of herbs in authors of smaller works with an interest in remedies, such as More's list, which includes **allium**, **brassica** and **nasturtium** among many other less well known terms. The *OED* will sometimes completely omit a word which occurs frequently, for instance **hebetonice** or **nitrispuma** (Baker), but others do occur, frequently cited from late sources such as the *NSSL*. Still others are recorded not only in their anglicized but also in their Latin and Greek forms. **Mithridatium** in its various forms is recorded as a main lemma no less than three times, the other two being **mithridate** and **mithridatum**. Some commonly used substances such as the large number of oils, normally referred to in the sixteenth century as **oleum** plus a specifiying term, is unrecorded in that form, which seems an unfortunate omission, and there are others, such as **nitrum** and **mulsum.**

Bostocke's list is rather problematical, including as it does a number of terms which seem to be philosophical, Paracelsian, alchemical, or philosophical, and indeed to cross some of these boundaries. This text is by no means orthodox or a straightforward medical textbook, attempting rather to justify a radical philosophical view of medicine. The difficult words incude **arcanum**, **cabbalistic**, **intelligent**, **magisterium**, and **tincture**.

The totals are shown in Table 6.4, with the percentage of medical antedatings, remembering that the apparent precision of the figures masks a number of arguable and probably invidious judgements about individual words. The percentage of medical antedatings from each author is obviously subject to wide variation, always remembering that the present sample is a very selective one. Clearly, authors may vary greatly in the extent to which they use specialist terms.

TABLE 6.4. *Percentage of total antedatings which are medical terms*

Author	Medical	Total	%
Bostocke	82	185	44.3
Baker	97	133	73.0
Banister	499	687	72.6
Barrough	507	587	86.4
Clever	164	382	42.9
Cotta	71	238	29.8
Hester	49	74	66.2
Hill	20	27	74.1
Langton, *VBT*	26	65	40.0
Langton, *IP*	30	60	50.0
Bailey	18	43	41.9
More	27	53	50.9
Plutarch	4	24	16.7
TOTALS	1,530	2,406	63.6

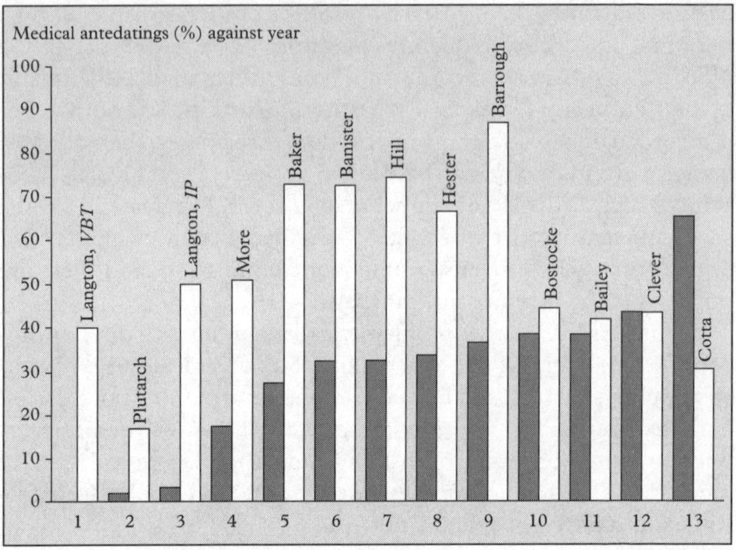

FIG. 6.1. Number of medical antedatings correlated with year of publication. Langton, *VBT* (1547) = 0.

This might vary for several possible reasons; for instance, because the author is the first to write on the subject in English, because he is addressing an unlearned audience, or because he is translating a highly technical text. Nevertheless the overall average seems amenable to interpretation and suggests a high proportion of such antedatings (63.6 per cent). At the same time, since this figure is employed without other studies of a similar kind against which comparisons might be made, it is difficult to do more than put somewhat tentative suggestions about its real significance. There is nevertheless a pattern in the percentages of medical antedatings found, charted against the years of publication, calculated here from zero for Langton *VBT* to 65 for Cotta, (see Fig. 6.1). The dotted bars are the percentages of medical antedatings, while the solid are the years from zero.

Three points emerge clearly from this chart within the limitations of the small number of texts used. The first is that the earliest of these works (Langton to More), while not yielding a large number of antedatings in absolute terms, do nevertheless have a rather high percentage of medical ones among them, suggesting either a rapid rate of introduction of terms, whether neologized, borrowed, or used formerly but now neglected, or a period of the lexicon not exhaustively treated by the *OED*. Other antedatings are in fact almost negligible. The authors of at least three of these works were physicians, again suggesting the role played by the profession in the mid-century in the growth of the medical lexicon.

Second, the most productive years, measured by the absolute percentage, are those from texts 5–9, that is Baker, Banister, Hill, Hester, and Barrough. The first four of these are not physicians, suggesting the greater interest in medical terms in English of the other medical professions, or occupations associated with it. Although this is not a significant fact in this chart by itself since it could be amended simply by adding the works of more medical practitioners from those years, it does accord with the rise in comment on the use of English which has already been noted as occurring in the 1570s and 1580s.

The third point is that between Bostocke and Cotta the columns even out and finally swap over in magnitude. From Barrough on, the percentage drops away markedly, even though at least two of the last four texts are by physicians. Again, the limited number of texts may well have produced a degree of coincidence, but the overall pattern for these four texts is markedly different from the previous two blocks, suggesting that enhancing the lexicon is of less immediate importance in itself, many terms now being firmly established. It might also mean that the most important developments in the lexicon are now taking place among surgeons and others, rather than physicians themselves, whose writings are becoming increasingly conservative. These texts correspond quite neatly with the period in which the loudest complaints about the inadequacy of the medical lexicon are heard, lending weight to the suggestion that these occur after the event, and do not necessarily accurately reflect the current state of the lexicon.

5. CONCORDANCE METHOD

The results of the concordance study mentioned in Chapter 2 are of great interest. The pages analysed were Barrough 2, Hester title-page to sig. Aiiii^{r} and 45^{r} and 24^{r}, Langton, *IP* Gii^{r} and Diiii^{v}, and Bailey Bv^{v} and Cvi^{v}, all of which had, of course, already been subjected to examination in this study. Any additions which had already been discovered were omitted from this list if they were earlier than these, so that all the words below are in addition to what had previously been found. Twenty-five items of new data, consisting of twenty-one antedatings, one postdating, and two unrecordeds were discovered from these six pages of text.[15]

Antedatings

1. **beating** [*vbl sb*, 5, 1601, Shakespeare] Barrough, 2. with the heauiness or stretching of the heade ther be beating, and as it were a pulse
2. **cinnabar** [1, 1599, Hakluyt] Hester, fo. 24. then perfumed him with ... *Scinbaber*
3. **compound** [*sb*^{1}, 2, a 1611] Bailey, B5^{v}. when the compound is fully rype, no one simple doth worke in it according to his owne nature, but by the reactions one common nature doth result
4. **crud** [*a.* 2; possibly crude *adj*, 1811] Hester, fo. 24. [th]e oyle being crud putrifieth
5. **external** [A, *a*, 4, 1651, Hobbes] Barrough, 2. headach comming of an externall cause
6. **handmaid** [*sb* 1b, 1592, Davies] Langton, Gii^{r}. generation hath thea[n] [th]e chefe rule and dominion, & the other be as handmaydes vnto it
7. **mal** [1745, Pococke] Hester, Aiiii^{r}. To helpe Mal di formica.
8. **meat pipe** [6, 1633, Fletcher] Langton, Div^{v}. the wesaunt or meate pype
9. **owe** [4a, 1591, Sylvester] Hester, Aii^{v}. The moste affectioned of all those, which owe your L. dutifull service, John Hester.
10. **perfect** [*a*, 5d, 1590, Shakespeare] Bailey, C6^{v}. the perfect kindes of Cinnamum
11. **power** [*sb*^{1}, B, 3, 1592, Shakespeare] Langton, Gii^{r}. alteration & nutrition, be but inferioure powers.
12. **public** [5d, 1641, Bp. Monagu] Hester, Aii^{v}. yet are there such ... will bear me a priuate grudge for this publique commodity
13. **quantity** [I, 1c, 1610, Jonson] Bailey, C6^{v}. in lacke of Cinnamum did sometimes substitute double qua[n]titie of Casia.
14. **reaction** [2b, 1836, Gully] Bailey, B5^{v}. See **compound**, anted.
15. **remain** [*v*, 5c, 1839, Ure] Hester, fo. 24. he was holpe of [th]e infirmitie, but the bone remained bare
16. **science** [4a, 1725, Watts] Hester, Aii^{v}. that noble and profounde Science

17. separate [*v*, II, 9a, 1638, Sir T. Herbert] Hester, fo. 24. the bone did seperate of his owne accord
18. service [9a, 1601, Shakespeare] Hester, Aii[v]. See **owe**, anted.
19. sophisticate [*v*, 4, 1598, Sylvester] Bailey, C6[v]. things were sophisticated by the monume[n]ts of old writers
20. substitute [*v*, 2b, 1620, Granger] Bailey, C6[v]. in lacke of Cinnamum did sometimes substitute double qua[n]titie of Casia.
21. tumour [3b, 1804, Abernethy] Hester, fo. 24. a certeine tumour the which had perished a great part of the skull

Unrecorded

1. cina cf. **senna**; Hester, fo. 24. I ... gaue him ... the rootes of *Cina* in decoction
2. formicola Hester, Aiiii[r]. Of formicola and his effects.

Postdatings

1. cerote [1562, Turner, *Herbal*] Hester, fo. 24. I layde ther-on our *Cerote magistrale*

What is of particular significance is that a number of the words in the list are in common use, **external**, **perfect**, **remained**, **separate**, **power**, **compound**, **reaction**, and some, such as **owe**, are among the most basic word of the language. These are not necessarily the kinds of words which a less formal and exhaustive search is likely to uncover. More detailed analysis shows the potentially remarkable nature of these findings. The number of words discovered by this method as against the number of words read for each author is shown in Table 6.5. For the sake of comparison, the finding rate reported for all new data in Table 6.4 is included in brackets in the last column.

TABLE 6.5. *Finding rates for the concordance method*

Author	Words	No. of new data	Finding rate (previous)
Bailey	446	5	89 (248)
Barrough	788	2	394 (239)
Hester	1,807	15	120 (314)
Langton	299	4	75 (298)

Although the sample is very small, there is clearly reason to infer that the possible new data found by this method might be considerable. The finding rates, except for Barrough, are very high, the highest elsewhere in this study being 52 for Clever. Thus Langton *IP*'s 17,846 words yielded 60 antedatings by the original method of this study, but a further four have been added by the re-examination of 299 words. The potential application of the concordance method to that text, found by dividing the finding rate for the concordance study into the total words for the work, suggests that, were the finding rate established here to be continued, the work would yield a further 239 potential antedatings (60 previously identified), a result which at least suggests that it is worth investigating. The last column has had the figure from the 'No. of corrections' column subtracted from it. Calculations for all four authors give the results shown in Table 6.6.

TABLE 6.6. *Estimate of new data discoverable by the concordance method*

Author	New data	Potential new data
Bailey 446	5	156
Barrough 788	2	673
Hester 1807	15	317
Langton 299	5	298
TOTAL	31	1,523

Thus it is at least possible that the numbers of antedatings cited in this study might be considerably increased, and that much more new data for the *OED*'s account of more common and less specialist words in the language of this period might be found. It is clear that the increase in data might at least for some authors be four- or five-fold. This is of course a crude calculation, which does not take account of other factors such as the relative limitations of a particular author's vocabulary or the extent to which his work may be repetitious. Obviously a work containing many recipes, to take an instance, will repeat a great deal. Nevertheless, there are enormous possibilities for further and more detailed lexicographical research into this period than have been undertaken up to now.

The relation between the finding rates and whether a work had been previously read for the *OED* provides food for thought. It might also be expected, assuming that the *OED* readers were efficient on the whole, that works previously read would generally yield significantly less material in this study; but analysis shows the results set out in Table 6.7, the asterisk indicating those works previously read for the *OED*. Baker has been left in since he is listed in the *OED* bibliography, but since there are no actual citations of this work, it should be noted that the average, excluding Baker, would be 335.

TABLE 6.7. *Finding rates for works read for OED as against not read*

Author	No. of antedatings	Total words	Finding rate
*Baker	133	16,380	123
*Banister	687	199,888	290
*Barrough	587	265,035	451
*Cotta	238	34,540	145
*More	53	24,860	469
AVERAGE			318
Bailey	43	13,904	323
Bostocke	185	23,715	128
Clever	382	28,847	76
Hester	74	37,984	513
Hill	27	34,375	1,237
Langton, *IP*	60	17,864	298
Langton, *VBT*	65	26,400	406
Plutarch	24	8,190	341
AVERAGE			213

There is some difference, with or without Baker, between the averaged finding rates for the works covered between those previously read for the *OED* and those unread, amounting to about a third. This suggests that excerpting a particular book for the *OED* editors was, in statistical terms, not likely to mean that an exhaustive study of the work was carried out. If it was supposed that the better part of the usable material from a given work or set of works was provided by the readers, then the exercise has not been all that useful, given that works already read have been on the whole not very significantly less productive than those unread. In fact, those already excerpted have still been on average more productive than Shakespeare. Those reading the works clearly extracted relatively little from them, leaving the majority of the resource untouched in many cases. The fact of a book's having already been read is simply no guide to what useful lexical data might still be found in it, unless it can be shown to have been exhaustively excerpted as in the case of Shakespeare. Taken with the results of the concordance study, these figures point to a large unused corpus of material which the *OED* editors would have found useful. Had textual resources been better employed, especially the apparently minor, insignificant, non-literary ones, the overall text dependence of the *OED* could have been considerably reduced. Scanting such resources has clearly exacerbated the situation.

The extent of this problem, and the extent to which it conceals an inherent bias, can be clearly seen if we consider the numbers of entries in the *OED* for those authors researched here as against those for Shakespeare, who is known to have been covered very thoroughly (Table 6.8). Thus, for example, the number of entries for Barrough represents only 0.62 per cent of those for Shakespeare—a negligible proportion in relation to the lexical potential of Barrough's work. It should be remembered that any antedating or other item of new data noted here would ideally be included in a thorough revision of the *OED* on the grounds of date if nothing else, so that Barrough's 204 citations would rise to 1,311, or 3.99 per cent. Many of Shakespeare's citations are of course purely illustrative rather than being first citations of senses or absolute first citations.[16]

TABLE 6.8. *Number of citations in* OED

Author	No. of citations
Baker	145
Banister	537
Barrough	204
Cotta	13
Hester[17]	90
More	12
Shakespeare	32,857

Absolute first citations, that is, the earliest citation in any given main lemma, are of value in themselves, being new data for the *OED* irrespective of sense about which there can be no argument. There is little or no guidance as to what might constitute a normal rate of finding such citations. The range discovered in this study, as set out in Table 6.9, is from 26.8 per cent (Cotta) to 64.7 per cent (Baker), a variation which, while wide, appears to show no discernible pattern, except perhaps for a tendency to rise with a later date of publication. Cotta is a notable exception to this, which may be simply explained by the fact that his text is less technical in its vocabulary than many, containing relatively little by way of pathology, anatomy, recipes, and other specialist matter, since he did not require such things in his text except incidentally and anecdotally.

TABLE 6.9. *Percentage of absolute first citations among antedatings*

Author	a 1 cit.	Total	%
Bailey	15	43	34.9
Baker	86	133	64.7
Banister	334	687	48.6
Barrough	349	587	59.5
Bostocke	117	185	63.2
Clever	168	382	44.0
Cotta	64	239	26.8
Hester	44	74	59.5
Hill	13	27	48.1
Langton, *IP*	34	60	56.7
Langton, *VBT*	29	65	44.6
More	22	53	41.5
Plutarch	9	24	37.5
TOTALS	1,284	2,559	50.2

The potential of new data to reveal something of the work to be done on the *OED* is therefore great, especially in the case of antedatings. The problem is to amass sufficient numbers to be of real use, and to find ways of interpreting the data to best advantage. The new data considered here has revealed at least some of the possibilities. To reach a better understanding of these phenomena, however, it is necessary to consider the history of the *OED* project, some policies and attitudes as they affected the work, and the practices of those volunteers assisting the work.

Notes

1. Collected from *Notes and Queries* and other sources in Bailey (1978), in which about 4,400 items were collected from publications since the first appearance of the *OED*. Schäfer (1989) has since published a further 5,000 plus, and other scholars continue to notify new data from time to time.

2. Some of the plague tracts are, however, religious in nature, being exhortations to England to repent of those sins for which the plague has been visited upon the country. Even primarily medical works containing preventative advice, remedies, and accounts of the nature of the disease are still likely to contain such an exhortation somewhere.
3. Henry Lyte translated a French version, *L'Ecluse*, 1557.
4. See *Ath. Cant.* ii, 437.
5. Cited from Jones (1953: 96n.). The *DNB* makes the suggestion that Anthony Munday—sometime stationer's apprentice, vagrant, actor, pamphleteer, and translator—was responsible for the translation of Gabelkhover, but neither the *BLC* nor the *STC* ascribe these works to Munday. He was well known for his translations of French romances for popular consumption, and the rendering of a medical text would seem to be a departure from his usual area of interest. Not that it is impossible; he may well have done it in order to claim his share of a thriving market for such texts. But I know of no evidence that he had a medical training, or any medical interests. In spite of the *DNB* attribution, Turner (1928–9: 197) has shown that it is most improbable that he was the translator either of Gabelkhover or of Guillemeau. Subsequent work n Munday has failed to reveal any evidence to change that view. The translator of Gabelkhover, according to Turner, was a pupil of 'Maximilan Boumann, an English surgeon of Dort'. It seems far more likely that the translator of Guillemeau was this same A.M.
6. Note that in order to avoid confusion over the use of the word source, 'author' here includes any work used by the *OED* whose author is not identifiable.
7. Note that the second of joint authors has not been recorded; I think the only writer to whom this does some injustice is Gervase Markham, who has four entries in his own right and a further four with Richard Surflet.
8. See Chapter 7. The great majority (48) of Barrough's antedatings are, however, references to his own works in later editions, so that he is a kind of ghost as far as this list is concerned.
9. There has been a long tradition of bardolators who would have disagreed, but his plays show nothing beyond the kind of intelligent interest in medical matters which might be expected of the educated middle-class Elizabethan. One must search for evidence of the use of arrowly specialized medical terminology, which is far more apparent in the works of Ben Jonson.
10. Note, however, the disparities which are apparent in the antedatings from Malory and Nashe on (Schäfer 1980*a*: 49).
11. A number of attempts were made to produce a graph which would show a difference between this total antedatings graph, and a plot of it without the Shakespearean antedatings. However, their total is too small to be significant overall in this form; although some formats

showed some visible difference, it was slight enough not to seem worth reproducing.

12. Schäfer (1980: ch. 4). I am using the term 'new data' to emphasize that he data Schäfer referred to as 'authorial innovation rate' is a different measure to that used here, his measure being the total of *OED* first citations, other antedatings, and parallel citations, multiplied by 1,000 and then divided by the number of words per corpus. I do not include parallel citations in any of my figures, and indeed did not register them at all.
13. Work on Shakespeare's language still presumes the historical accuracy and reliability of the *OED* for this period. See e.g. Garner (1982: 149–70) in which arguments are put about the state of the language based indirectly on the *OED*.
14. An editor might therefore remove sense 1b, probably omit the quote from *All's well* altogether, and perhaps include the Barrough citation under 1a, where it sensibly belongs. An alternative would be to create sense 1b (fig) or (trans), illustrated possibly by the Wyclif citation and one or both of the Shakespearean ones, much as was done under **curdle** (q.v.).
15. These have not been incorporated into the list in Appendix 1, so as not to alter the relative finding rates between the two sets of data.
16. Nevertheless, Shakespeare's first citations total 1,983. My thanks to Professor F. Tompa for supplying this information, as well as a list.
17. A different work to that excerpted here.

7
The Medical Lexicon and the *OED*

Much attention has been paid so far to examining what it is that a corpus of corrections to the *OED* incorporating many sixteenth-century medical terms might reveal about the dictionary and the way in which it has been compiled. The emphasis has been on what the *OED* might have incorporated had it wished, or would have incorporated had it access to the source of the data, and something has already been shown of how well the *OED* registered, or failed to register, this particular corpus. It ought to be possible to learn something from the dictionary's history as well, even though it is only partly recorded. The practices of other workers—readers, sub-editors, and other helpers—should also be considered where the evidence is available. However, a record of editorial decisions by its editors and other workers unfortunately does not exist, and in any case, even if such decisions had been minuted, it does not follow that they would have been scrupulously adhered to in the Scriptorium, let alone outside it. This chapter therefore considers the editorial practices which bore directly upon the collection of medical terms, their acceptance or rejection, their field marking, and changes to these policies which occurred during the history of the *OED*. It also considers the actual practices of the *OED* workers, from editors to readers, and the relative weightings given to various sources of lexical data as far as the present evidence will allow.

In this chapter I want also to press the point that further substantial research needs to be done, not only in the collection of data but also in other areas of the *OED*'s editorial policy not touched upon here, and to indicate what directions such research might take. The greater part of the present study has been within the terms set by the dictionary itself; in the first place, because the wealth of material was so great as to be difficult to examine on a broad enough scale and in sufficient detail to be meaningful. More recently, however, the opportunity has arisen for research based in modern technology which will be capable of extending the practical and theoretical parameters very much further. The appearance of the *OED-CD* has been of great assistance in this, opening the way for the large-scale manipulation of data. It is now possible to see clearly many of the larger patterns without relying on untestable impressions and intuitions concerning many of the details, for example, about the structure of entries, the use of sources, and so on. The position now, therefore, is one of development and change in the processes of research. With the appearance of the *OED*'s second edition scholars may now examine the first edition far more critically. We can now add to Jürgen Schäfer's remark that the '*OED*'s documentation, the richest presently available, is inadequate in the light of modern scholarship' the further observation that the light of modern scholarship has never before had the potential for a so sharp a focus (Schäfer 1987: 67).

In assessing the *OED* two important facts must be considered. The first of these, which has to do with the dictionary itself, is that it claimed a large degree of comprehensiveness for itself. In the words of its introduction:

> it is the aim of the Dictionary to deal with all the common words of speech and literature, and with all words which approach these in character; the limits being extended farther in the domain of science and philosophy, which naturally passes into that of literature, than in that of slang or cant, which touches the colloquial. In scientific and technical terminology, the aim has been to include *all words English in form*, except those of which an explanation would be unintelligible to any but the specialist; and such words, not English in form, as either are in general use, like *Hippopotamus, Geranium, Aluminium, Focus, Stratum, Bronchitis*, or belong to the more familiar language of science, as *Mammalia, Lepidoptera, Invertebrata*. (*OED*, xxviii)

We will see that the criteria here which apply to science are perhaps the hardest to comply with among the options available, since they require decisions not only as to what is 'English form' (a reasonably easy one!) but also as to what would be generally intelligible or unintelligible, what 'general use' is, and what words are scientific but 'familiar'. A litany of invidious decisions indeed, when one considers the criteria which might have been applied. Nevertheless, Murray claimed in the Romanes Lecture of 1900 that not only did the *OED* compare favourably with any other great dictionary of its time, a justifiable assertion, but also that:

> the work thus done is done once for all; the structure now reared will have

to be added to, continued, and extended with time, but it will remain, it is believed, the great body of fact on which all future work will be built ... In the Oxford Dictionary, permeated as it is through and through with the scientific method of the century, Lexicography has for the present reached its supreme development. (Murray 1900: 49)

The second, which has to do with its readers, is that since its publication most of its users have accorded it not only with the comprehensiveness which it actually claimed but with some which it did not; further, they have as a consequence accorded it an unprecedented authority as a record of the language,[1] and have generally thought it to be an unimpeachable model of objective description. A recent example occurs in a paper concerned with scientific words in the seventeenth century and the writings of Joseph Glanvill (Di Martino 1993).[2] Not only is the lexical information, apart from that gleaned directly from the works of Glanvill and a few others, derived directly or indirectly from the *OED*, but the unspoken presumption throughout is that the *OED* is right and entirely trustworthy. As is so often the case elsewhere, the author cites the *OED* by stating that such-and-such a word first occurs at such-and-such a date, not by stating that the *OED* pronounces this to be so, which is, after all, the only claim a scholar using the dictionary is entitled to make. The appearance of a first date and a citation in the *OED* is not and was never meant to be a statement of irrevocable fact about the word's use. It is a declaration of the best knowledge of the editors at the time of compilation.

The reception of the *OED* over the years has, however, reflected its comprehensiveness and scholarship—so much so that the editors of the second edition can now claim, perhaps with a touch of complacency, but certainly with the justification of history:

There is no aspect of English linguistic history that the Dictionary has not illuminated; its findings have called for the revision of many philological statements and reconsideration of many judgements on textual matters. So wide is its scope and so intensive its treatment that it ... has provided a ready quarry of material for many authors of treatises and dissertations. (Simpson and Weiner 1989: p. vii)

This reputation and authority has also passed to the smaller dictionaries derived from the *OED*. Both of these factors have tended to give the *OED* a kind of de facto immunity from rigorous analysis.

The editorial strictures which the *OED* had set out for it were not wholly adhered to; for example, it might reasonably be argued that it contains more rare and obscure words than the comments quoted above indicate, and also that it treats words not English in form with much inconsistency. It must also be said, however, in all fairness to the *OED*, that its reputation does largely reflect the magnitude of its achievement, and that if it has been accorded excessive respect, then that is a function of the relative lack of serious scholarly research on the dictionary itself. The lexicography itself has of course continued with the compilation of the various period and dialect dictionaries, many of which are now complete. It is also important to note that the analytic research needed is only partially accomplished by the continuation of the *OED* project itself, which has resulted in the publication of *OED* 2. The collection of material has of course continued on an impressive scale, and dictionaries have been improved and enlarged, but the paramount importance to scholarship of the *OED* itself demands that research be carried out independent of the strictures of publishing and of the traditions of the dictionary itself.

The instructions issued for the guidance of readers, those who supplied the raw material from which the dictionary would ultimately be compiled, are also of paramount importance in understanding the dictionary's structure. Not only is it essential to look at what the *OED* editors required of their readers, it is also important where possible to examine what the readers actually did do. This is often difficult to reconstruct; indeed, it is frequently impossible.[3] Little evidence remains, especially from the early years of the dictionary, but some of the problems presented by the management of readers by the editors have already been alluded to by Elisabeth Murray (1977: 168–9). The *OED*'s directions to its readers were brief. In the form issued in 1879 they were *inter alia* to 'Make a quotation for *every* word that strikes you as rare, obsolete, old-fashioned, new, peculiar, or used in a peculiar way ... Make as *many* quotations *as you can* for ordinary words, especially when they are used significantly, and tend by the context to explain or suggest their own meaning.' (Murray 1970: p. xv)

Jürgen Schäfer has already pointed out as a consequence of his own invaluable research that certain deficiencies do exist in the coverage of the lexicon of early modern English, and suggested that others can be assumed to exist (Schäfer 1987: 66–74). He has also suggested ways in which the *OED* can be seen as concealing rather than revealing areas of the lexicon, only the most obvious of which for the present research is the large-scale omission or, rather, the failure to identify many specialist medical terms. This seems to have happened mainly at the collection stage rather than at the later editorial stages. The concentration in this book on the medical literature of the period has several advantages. In the first place a detailed factual analysis is provided rather than a broadly impressionistic approach; next, it emphasizes for the first time a non-literary rather than a literary lexical domain, thus removing attention from those authors who had been particularly well-covered, or who have had a special claim to attention.

A problem with the present approach is that any attempts to generalize to the wider lexicon on the basis of the evidence presented here will be difficult, given the particularly full technical language used in medicine, and its especial reliance on Greek and Latin. It has been partly to offset this bias that words other than medical ones have been kept in the statistics. It will not be possible to assert with any certainty that the findings here would equate with those in some other area of technical specialism, though it is very tempting to do so.

The present bias does nevertheless at least serve to undermine the rather antiquated notion of the privileged status of the *OED* source, with its inherent value judgement, which used to dominate the *OED* editorship in the early period. Among the instructions of the Philological Society's proposal is the provision that 'when once an author, or any work of an author, shall be admitted to the rank of a Dictionary authority, all unregistered words . . . ought to be registered' (AOED Misc. 213/3, Aug. 1857, 2). The same document requests material from 'the chief classics of the present century, such as Wordsworth, Coleridge, Shelley, Byron, Walter Scott, Southey, and the leading writers of the Victorian era' (ibid.) but specifically excluded Sir Archibald Alison from this august list. He was presumably popular for his history of Europe, but not sufficiently 'leading'. The criteria for admission to this 'rank' are not explained, but are clearly concerned with literary merit, and involve a prescriptivism which is at odds with the now generally accepted norms for major dictionaries, and certainly with the *OED* itself in its finally published form. It is also at variance with the assumptions of its users. Although by the time the dictionary had been completed this notion had broken down to a considerable degree, its influence is still apparent in the final product. Murray was aware of the limitations and, in his appeal to readers in 1879, made it clear: 'We admit as authorities all English books, except such as are devoted to purely scientific subjects' (Murray: 1879: 25)[4] but as late as 1883 was under pressure from Jowett to adhere to the original policy.[5]

It will be useful now to put these considerations into an historical context. The *OED*'s policy did not remain the same throughout its long history, and neither did its practice. The way in which the project was conceived and developed, of course, had its effect on the practices of its workers at every level.

1. THE HISTORICAL CONTEXT OF THE *OED*

The *OED* began originally as a revision. The intention of the Philological Society had been at the outset in 1858 to supplement the dictionaries of Johnson and Richardson in the light of the remarks of Dean Trench about their value and completeness.[6] Neither work, the Society rumbled, should be regarded as a 'Lexicon totius Anglicitatis' (Philological Society Paper, AOED Misc. 213/3, Aug. 1857, 1). It was accordingly resolved that a search be begun for previously unrecorded words and idioms, with particular attention to the 'less-read authors of the 16th and 17th centuries' (Philological Society Paper, AOED Misc. 213/3, Aug. 1857, 2). Words should be sought which were not in Johnson or Richardson or were there but without any cited authority, antedatings of material in these two dictionaries, new senses of words already recorded, obsolete words of later date than either Johnson or Richardson, words in non-naturalized form, idiomatic and proverbial expressions missing from Johnson and Richardson, and quotations especially illustrative of meaning or etymology. Certain authors, including Philemon Holland, were singled out for attention. All that was required was 'a little care and patience' (Philological Society Paper, A*OED* Misc. 213/3, Aug. 1857, 1), and the new editor, Herbert Coleridge, confidently expected that the whole would be completed in two years (Sutcliffe 1978: 53). It is now a matter of record that it was not, the last fascicle appearing in 1928. By then the concept of the dictionary had been radically altered. The work continues still.

In the same document, however, the Society more grandly proposed that the early literature of English as a whole should be looked at, and that what was required in the end was 'a complete historical map of our language' (Philological Society Paper, A*OED* Misc.

213/3, Aug. 1857, 2). Whilst wishing to direct particular attention to the earlier periods, they would be glad to accept any information on other periods as well. The die was cast. In the end the completed map was a triumph of scholarship and had come to incorporate words from every field of knowledge, but it was literature which was the basis in the first place rather than other staple forms of writing or scientific writing.

There are unfortunately no records which tell us on what grounds books were selected for excerption, except the early requirement that they be less well-known texts of the sixteenth and seventeenth centuries. It must be presumed that the magnitude of the task was only dimly appreciated at the outset, and that the guidelines as to what should be read must have grown with experience of the project, rather than have been clearly and unequivocally conceived by the proposers. The notion of a 'dictionary authority' seems at odds with the aim of covering relatively obscure writers, but the inherent inconsistency of this would be at least partly resolved with the effluxion of time. All that we have left to inform us about these decisions is some record of what was at hand to read, and by whom it was read.

There must have been considerable problems of access to medical texts from our period, especially considering the inaccessibility of rare texts and the relative lack of bibliographical information, but the lists of books and readers prepared during Coleridge's editorship indicate that medical books were being read at a lively rate, even in the earliest period of the dictionary. Holland's *Pliny* and Burton's *Anatomy* are the first medical books 'undertaken' (AOED 213/3, 6), listed as read as early as 1857, before the project became official. It was probably the fame of Holland and Burton as a translator and a seminal prose writer respectively at the beginning of the seventeenth century which assured their place in the dictionary, rather than the fact that they wrote or translated medical treatises.[7]

Reading for the Philological Society's project was apparently well under way before the Society had resolved that a new dictionary should be compiled. By 1859 Professor George P. Marsh, the co-ordinator of the American end of the project, noted that Browne's *Works*, Burton's *Anatomy*, Gerarde's *Herbal*, and Timme's translation of Quercitanus had all been read, and that a reader was required for Norton's *Ordinal of Alchemy* (AOED Misc. 93/18/i, 8. Aug. 1859). The latter three are presumably early instances of works read primarily because they are medical or scientific texts. A notebook apparently compiled before Coleridge's death mentions that a reader is also required for Ripley's *Compound of alchemy*, and that Bacon's *Natural History* had been read (AOED Misc. 213/9). It also lists Elyot's *Castle of Health* as unread and probably therefore predates Coleridge's death in its earliest entries (Misc. 93/18/i, issued August 8th, 1859).

Coleridge died of consumption early and was succeeded by the medievalist Frederick Furnivall. By 1861 Cogan's *Haven of Health*, Lyte's *Dodoens*, Elyot's *Castle of Health*, A.M.'s translation of Gabelkhover, and Traheron's *Vigo* as well as some medical manuscripts had been added to the list.[8] Several works previously mentioned also appear on this list. The impetus may in the first place have come from Herbert Coleridge, but an early list from Furnivall's editorship shows not merely that a number of such texts were in hand or already read but also some sense that the area might require the services of a specialist. This notebook lists the following works approximately from the period of this study (with their readers) as being read or in hand (AOED Misc/182):

Book	*Reader*
A.M.'s Gabelhouer	H. H. Gibbs
Andrewe *Vertuose Boke*	W. C. Paine
Baker *Guydo's Questionarie*	W. Woodham Webb
Baker *Newe Jewel*	W. Woodham Webb
Banester *Chirurgerie*	W. Woodham Webb
Barrough *The Methode of Physicke*	W. Woodham Webb
Boke of the Quintessence	?
Bullein, W. *The Government of Health*	R. Morris
Cogan's *Haven of Health*	Fitz-Hall[9]
Copland's *Guydo's Questionary*	Furnivall, Brock
Dodoens *History of Plants by Lyte*	J. M. Cowper
Elyot *Castell of Helthe*	W. Paine
Gerarde's *Herbal*	W. C. Bromehead
Holland's Pliny	Sheppard
Hollybush *Homish Apothecarye*	W. Thompson
Hobbes's *Cornelius Philander his Chirugerie*	W. Woodham Webb
Langham *The Garden of Health*	Furnivall
Newton's Lemnius, *Touchstone of Complexions*	Furnivall

Phayer, T. *Treatise of the Pestilence* and	W. Woodham Webb
Boke of children	W. Woodham Webb
Pocton[*sic*[10]], T. *The Chirurgians Closet*	W. Woodham Webb
Optic Glass of Humours	C. M. Ingleby
Phayer's *Regiment of Life*	W. Woodham Webb
Quercitanus tr. Timme	W. M. Rossetti
Recorde *Judicial of Urines*	W. C. Paine
Turner *Herbal* and *Of Bathes*	W. Thompson
Vigo's *Chirurgery*	W. Woodham Webb
Vigo *Chirurgery* trans. Traheron	?
Vicary, T. *The Englishman's Treasure*	W. Woodham Webb

This notebook appears to be in Furnivall's hand, and was probably begun shortly after Coleridge's death. It is supplementary to and interleaved with a printed list which records his death and refers the contributors to Furnivall as the new editor. It also notes that 1,149 books had been read and that 360 were then in hand; i.e. nearly 2 per cent of all books read or being read were sixteenth-century (or nearly so) medical works. Furnivall and Coleridge had made an enthusiastic start in that area. Although some readers had one or more medical works to read among their others, including Furnivall himself and Walter Thompson, one reader in this list stands out for particular notice. Dr W. Woodham Webb, of Kirkley, near Lowestoft, in having no fewer than eleven of these works to read, seems to have been regarded as the expert on such texts.[11] Furnivall unfortunately seems to have left no records of the number of slips returned by particular readers,[12] as Murray did later, since it would be interesting to know how many Webb returned for these works. Elsewhere he is recorded as having done other medical works—Macallo's *Canons of Physick* and Harvey's *Anatomical Exercises*—as well as those already noted. He is also recorded as a sub-editor for the letter D (AOED 57/1, 1858)[13] and for I and J.[14]

The criteria applied to the selection of medical texts seem to have been in at least some cases that the writer concerned should have some claims as a literary author or be a substantial translator, e.g. Elyot, Holland, Burton, and perhaps Timme, or that the work concerned should have some special significance in the development of the sciences, e.g. Lyte's Dodoens, Gerarde, or Traheron. Merely to be a medical writer does seem, however, to have been sufficient justification for the inclusion of some of the texts included in the foregoing list.

On his appointment as editor in 1879, Murray found the state of the dictionary far from satisfactory. He promptly issued a series of lists of desiderata, and with these the concern for science was revived to some extent. One undated list (AOED Misc. 90/9, 8) emphasizes that offers to read any other 'book not yet read will be welcome, especially early treatises on any of the sciences', and a list dated April 1885 offers the revealing remark that 'earlier instances may also be found of many of the 16–17th century words from Latin, of which the exact date of introduction is very uncertain' (AOED Misc 92/17). Many of the unrecorded words listed in the present study would have been pertinent. Murray was clearly acutely aware of the problems presented by such words, and it seems reasonable to suppose that he expected slips with words still in their Latin garb to be forwarded for consideration. But it is an especially telling reflection that the same list had more confidently claimed that 'the later sixteenth-century literature is very fairly done', give or take a few outstanding texts, and had included no sixteenth-century medical works as desiderata. The texts which he had in mind to be read may have been the cluster of medical treatises of the late fourteenth and early fifteenth centuries.[15] A later list extends the appeal on science in this version to include contemporary works (Misc/90/10/1, 8).

All of this contrasts with attitudes which previously prevailed, and had in practice determined the focus of much of the labour. It was clearly understood, at least by the educated public, that the task was to unearth rare and obscure terms. Coleridge had published a work which he proposed as a methodological guide for the dictionary, by which, as *The Athenæum* reported '"each may ascertain what he is to extract, and what to reject from the author or work," in which he is seeking for examples of obsolete words.'[16] The same journal, responding to information issued by the Society, pointed out that 'great masses of English literature remain unread for the purposes of this new dictionary' and asked, 'Who will help with the work? Any lady or gentleman with a little leisure time may assist by undertaking to read with care the book of a favourite author' (No. 1933, 12 Nov. 1864, 638). The assumption was that such work could, like embroidery or sketching, fill up a few idle hours for those who could afford the pastime. It should also be noted that the lists of works read or in hand issued by the society do not read like a compilation of 'favourite authors'. Nor does Furnivall's explanatory note three weeks later on what was required suggest leisured amusement.

'Quotations are wanted from any book not solely technical for each of the three periods of English ... The last use of every obsolete word and meaning of a word is wanted, and the first use of every word and meaning introduced after 1250 AD, including therefore nearly every derivative from the classical and modern languages' (No. 1936, 3 Dec. 749). Many who worked for the dictionary obviously did so with highly professional skill and dedication, but others did not, and the languishing of the work during the latter part of Furnivall's stewardship must have arisen partly from this attitude. It must also have been the case that many medical works were to be regarded as 'solely technical'.

An appeal was issued under Dr Furnivall's editorship in 1875, which is couched in a tone which with hindsight seems almost irresponsibly insouciant. Contributors, it claims, are required

> but to scan their books carefully and pick out the plums, the scarce words and phrases ... whereas the earliest readers had a far more laborious and comprehensive task before them, inasmuch as their extracts supplied the bases of comparison ... What may be called the common words of the language ... have ... been well illustrated by extracts ... and it now remains to gather in the more out-of-the-way terms, words and phrases. (AOED Misc. 93/17/ii, Mar. 1875)

Work, obviously, for the enthusiastic dilettante. Murray was to discover not only that Furnivall's confidence was unjustified, but that the work had not been done as well as had been thought.[17] In any case, it had become clear by this time that the original desiderata for the dictionary had become outdated and superseded by a clearer vision of what the nature of the final product should be. Discussions in the Philological Society had resulted in the understanding that Murray should have a free hand as editor, and not be limited to the *Canones lexicographici* issued by the originators of the project (Murray 1977: 147).

It does seem that Murray was dissatisfied with some of the work done before his incumbency. He had the following medical or quasi-medical works reread early in the term of his editorship: the *Book of the Quintessence*, for which he had two readers; Burton's *Anatomy*; Elyot's *Castell of Helthe*; Turner's *Herbal* and *Of Bathes*; Hollybush's *Homishe Apothecary*; Lyte's Dodoens; Gerarde's *Herbal*; and Cogan's *Haven of Health*. The reasons for this rereading are unclear; it is impossible now to know whether knowledge of earlier unsatisfactory procedures, missing or defaced slips, poor quotations, or some other factor influenced his decision to have these works re-examined. One which Murray alludes to is that of reading a text only for certain letters, a practice which he found abhorrent, but which was difficult to recognize (Murray 1977: 168–9). He refers in a letter dated 10 February 1898 to a problem with Myles Davies's *Athenae Britannicæ*:

> It was one of those declared to me as read for the Philol. Soc. under Dr. Furnivall, and I, of course, did not try to get it read again. I now suspect that it was read only for one or two letters, according to the silly practice by which sub-editors were then urged to get their friends to read books for their own letter only—so as to provoke a rivalry of good works between them, the fatal result being that I never know whether a book reported as read was read as a whole or not, until some accident reveals the fact that of late we have not seen any quotes from the book in question. (AOED Misc/13/23)

It is likely that Murray only discovered some of these irregularities, and that others remain still to be found and investigated.

Problems of this kind are apparent in the case of Foxe's *Actes and Monuments* (1563–87), a crucial work of this period which is the subject of an article by Elizabeth Knowles. There is some suggestion that it was read in the first instance only to the end of the letter O, citations for later letters showing some inconsistency.[18] It may be that the citations for letters after O were the result of casual notice of the work by readers engaged on other tasks, or that some attempt was made to remedy an apparent deficiency. As Knowles demonstrates, there remains much work to be done on these aspects of the *OED*'s work practices.

Similar problems have been encountered with the citations in this study from Phillip Barrough's *The methode of physicke*, though in the case of this text, there are further complications with multiple editions. The 1583 edition, not used by the *OED*, has yielded forty-seven antedatings sourced to subsequent reprintings of the same work. The *OED* bibliography lists editions published in 1590, 1596, 1610, 1617, 1634, and 1639 respectively, and there were at least two others, in 1624 and 1583, the present antedatings coming from the 1583 edition. Listing them alphabetically, it is immediately obvious that the words A–M are mostly from 1610, while I–Z are largely from 1590. The overlapping section I–M is a mixture of both, and there is a sprinkling of antedatings with the other dates cited in the *OED*. Table 7.1 gives both the primary citation (pr. cit.), and the secondary citation (sec. cit.), which is frequently added in parenthesis and represents the edition actually available to the *OED* reader. In one case it is to another author altogether, Nares.

TABLE 7.1 *Barrough's self-referring antedatings*

Antedating	Pr. cit.	Sec. cit.	Antedating	Pr. cit.	Sec. cit.
abscession	1610	Nares	mollifying	1590	1639
asthmatic	1610	1639	moulting	1610	1639
chive[2]	1610	1639	nefresie	1590	
cholerous	1610	1639	obturation	1610	1639
commixing	1610		orthopnic	1610	1639[19]
conflate *v.*[1]	1610	1639	pretergress	1596	
deligature	1610	1639	priapism	1590	
effectrix	1610	1639	refrication	1590	1639
embrocation	1610	1639	remollition	1590	1639
evaporate	1610	1639	salvatrice	1590	1596
exquisite	1610	1639	scope	1590	1596
extenuative	1610	1639	skink *sb*[1]	1590	
exustion	1610	1634	somnoriferous	1590	1639
ilium	1590		soporiferous	1590	1639
imminution	1590	1639	strike *v*, 42	1590	1639
impertinent	1590	1639	strumous, 1	1590	1634
indicatory	1590	1639	strumous, 2	1590	1634
infrigidation	1590	1639	symptomate	1590	1639
lapidous	1610	1639	twitch	1596	
lymphate	1610	1639	ungle	1590	1596
manchet	1590	1617	unpure	1590	
mattered	1590		unulcerate	1590	1596
melancholious-ness	1610		vacuation	1590	
			yellowish	1590	1639

Since where there is an earlier edition the *OED*'s usual practice is to cite the edition actually used in brackets, it can be reasonably safely assumed that the secondary citations represent the editions actually cited, and that probably the primary citation represents the best state of knowledge at the time about the earliest edition. The most frequently cited edition of Barrough is that of 1639.

It is at once apparent that the primary list divides into two overlapping sections, one from A–O containing words mostly from 1610, and the other from I–Z containing words mainly from 1590. The middle section contains both dates. The references to 1639 occur throughout the secondary citations, though with some inconsistency. The sequence of these references down to **salvatrice** is only broken twice.

The pattern, if based on editors rather than dates, is a little different. Viewed thus, Craigie consistently cites 1590, even as early as 1903 when he was working on R–Re. Onions is also consistent in referring only to 1590. Bradley cites both dates, his earliest reference to 1590 being in S–Sh (1908–) and his latest for 1610 being in L (1901–3). Murray seems least consistent, citing both dates in M (1904–8), 1590 and 1596 in P (1904–9), and 1596 in T (1909–15). The only really discernible change in secondary citations is that 1596 is used from S on, though not exclusively.

Dr W. Woodham Webb, the early sub-editor of D, I, and J, undertook to read the work in or about 1865 (AOED 149/1, Apr. 1865), but he had the 1634 edition, to which there are only three secondary references. Little if any of Webb's material can have been used and, as this is about the time when he appears to have ceased work as a sub-editor, it may be that he produced little. The 1634 references which remain, however, are from pages 33, 250, and 258 of the work respectively, so that if these are Webb's extracts, then they may represent what was left after Murray had culled them. It seems unlikely that they represent Webb's first and incomplete attempt to excerpt the book.

The disposition of the secondary references on the whole confirms the primary reference pattern. It is set out in Table 7.2. The date 1610 does not appear in the secondary references at all. The stated practice of the editors is: 'wherever practicable, a work is dated and quoted from its first edition: if the reference is to a later edition (as has often been unavoidable), the date of this is added (within parentheses) to the reference' (*OED*, p. xxxii) The total number of primary entries in *OED* for Barrough breaks down

TABLE 7.2. *Primary and secondary references among Barrough's self-referring antedatings*

Reference	A–E	P–Z	I–O (overlap)
1639	11	7	10
1634	1	2	0
1617	0	0	1
Nares	1	0	0
1596	0	4	0
nil ref.	1	7	4

this way, again on alphabetical lines, and rather erratically overlapping each other: 1590: 89 (**fitch–writhed**); 1596: 19 (**imbecility–unsweet**); and 1610: 92 (**abscession–temperament**), suggesting that there were in all three readers or three distinct attempts to excerpt the work.

The whole matter of editions is, of course, not a difficulty in the case of Banister, the other major text in this study; nevertheless there are some strange features in his treatment, and similar considerations apply to John Cotta and William Clever. In all there are 537 citations for Banister in *OED*,[20] 481 from *The historie of man*. Thus the work is quite extensively cited but its lexical potential is very much greater, as the addition of a further 970 items demonstrates.

One of the odd features of the Banister citations is that there appear to be not very many citations apart from first citations for any sub-lemma, including absolute first citations, the proportion being about one in five. It is noticeable on the other hand that in the case of Shakespeare a great many more of the citations are other than first citations, in fact about 94 per cent in all. It may reflect on the nature of the words found in Banister, but there is no obvious reason why some of the large gaps in citations for some words could not have been filled by a quote from this extensive source. The most obvious conclusion, though there may be other reasons, is that an author such as Banister was regarded as valuable if he provided a first citation, but more generally his material could be regarded as of no special consequence. Two other ways of explaining this phenomenon suggest themselves. One is the practical reason that the editors were dependent on the productions of the readers, and assessed works as *OED* sources, particularly the lesser-known works, in that light, and generally did not return to texts themselves to check their real potential, which would of course have been time-consuming and frustrating. If a work was felt to be unsatisfactorily excerpted, it was presumably farmed out to a better reader. The other reason is that whoever read Banister was only concerned to find rare and obsolete words, thus greatly increasing the chance that such excerptions would be first citations. These two possibilities are obviously not mutually exclusive.

It is thus far from clear that the readers were always scrupulous in following the instructions issued to them, particularly the one requiring as many quotes as possible for ordinary words. In the texts examined here many words of perfectly familiar modern meaning were antedated, and many unrecorded words were found. It is apparent that the original instructions to readers proved inadequate in the light of subsequent practical experience. The principle which seemed to apply early in the compilation of the *OED* was that great literature should be exhaustively treated, but that technical lexicons like that of medicine should be treated compendiously. An imbalance was bound to be the result. Professor Max Müller, a delegate to the Clarendon Press at the time of the early negotiations with the Philological Society, had already sensed that there might be such an imbalance between rare or curious words and common words, the latter being relatively overlooked, and it is easy to see why readers might not have been enthusiastic about the recording of everyday words, which many must have thought already well-documented (Murray 1977: 151). It is apparent, however, that much work still remains to be done even in this area. To take some examples of what has turned up in this study, some antedatings from Banister of this kind include **admit**, **ample**, **basis**, **cave**, **connect**, **construction**, **contraction**, **dental**, **difficult**, **dissect**, **double**, **fibre**, **fracture**, **immediate**, **insert**, **limit**, **membrane**, **refer**, **resistant**, **scope**, **solid**, **structure**, **tooth**, **track**, and **unite**, which are used in these instances in fairly familiar modern senses. Some other examples are from Hester, **contract**, **obstruct**, **relaxation**, and **glut**; from Cotta, **course**, **fix**, **incur**, **individual**, and **tax**; **apply** from Bailey; **action**, **centre**, **loose**, **mind**, **order**, and **rise** from Bostocke; and from Clever, **active**, **black**, **stable**, **under**, and **world**. **Equal** has been recorded from several sources.

Obviously some texts were far more efficiently read than others. Further work is required, but it would be interesting to know if those texts already read for the *OED* yield a significantly different proportion of rare as against familiar words in the lists of antedatings when compared to those not previously read. It is already clear that in a general way there are many new antedatings to be found in the works already read (Cotta, Baker, More, Barrough, Banister). In the case of Baker's *Oleum Magistrale*, the current research yielded not one first citation for it among the approximately 800 words examined for this study as possible corrections, and a computer check reveals that not a single citation from this work was used in spite of its appearance in the Bibliography. It may be that whoever was deputed to examine this text originally did so extremely perfunctorily or not at all; on the other hand, it is possible that the slips returned were for some reason unusable or perhaps were lost. Firm conclusions as to whether there is a consistent disparity between the two groups in this respect will have to await a larger sample. Criteria for rarity might, however, be rather slippery, and to follow exactly the *OED*'s field markers for rarity would not be entirely satisfactory, given its inconsistencies.

The differential treatment of authors was further complicated by the relatively uncontrolled activities of readers, whose contributions could only be partly subjected to editorial management. Furnivall was obviously less punctilious than Murray in this matter, but he had the additional problems of defining the task itself and the methodology to be adopted. Close checking of readers' contributions was in any case impossible throughout the history of the dictionary, and would in itself have been self-defeating. Differences in the way authors were dealt with did not, however, stem simply from the individual characteristics of readers such as their assiduity, biases, or carelessness. It also resulted from deliberate policy on the part of the editorship.

The most obvious instance of differential treatment in the dictionary is that of Shakespeare, though undoubtedly there are many others to be found. The way in which Shakespeare has been dealt with in the *OED* has already been handled intensively by Jürgen Schäfer, but more remains to be said about this subject. In the first place the *OED* contains 32,857 citations from Shakespeare's works. By comparison there are only 537 from Banister, and a mere 204 from Barrough. Banister's therefore represent only 1.63 per cent of Shakespeare's and Barrough's 0.62 per cent. If the present findings from these two were added to the *OED*, the percentages would rise to about 5 per cent and 3.56 per cent respectively, allowing always for the fact that such additions are first citations only, and that the addition of other illustrative citations would be justified as well. Full concordance analyses of these two authors would certainly raise the figures higher again.

Let us assume for the moment that all other considerations are equal; that is, Shakespeare and the texts in this study are of equal linguistic value from a lexicographic point of view, and that a similar relationship between the number of rare words and common words obtains in all these texts. Since Shakespeare's corpus yields 1,983 absolute first citations, representing 6.04 per cent of his total of 32,857, then Banister, who yields 334 or 16.8 per cent of Shakespeare's, ought to be represented in the *OED* by 5,519 citations. Similarly Barrough, who yields 349 (see Table 6.9), ought to be accorded 5,782 and Clever (168; not cited in the *OED*) should have 2,782 to be regarded as equally well represented.[21]

The way in which Shakespeare dominates this period of the dictionary can also be seen by looking at the structure of individual entries. **Strict**, for instance, has in all seventeen numbered lemmas, and a total of thirty, including the lettered divisions of numbered sub-lemmas. First citations for no fewer than six of these are from Shakespeare. In **distraction** there are thirteen sub-lemmas, and four of these have first citations for Shakespeare; **motion** (*sb*) has thirty-five sub-lemmas, nine of which begin with Shakespeare; under **dismiss** there are five out of sixteen, and for **amazement** three out of four. I am ignoring here for the moment the other citations, since these first citations are obviously far more influential on our understanding of both Shakespeare and the history of the lexicon. Many other entries provide instances of the differential treatment of Shakespeare, **motive** providing as an addition an instance of a possible error in the structure of an entry. Under sense 6 we find two quotes, Richard II I. i. 193, 'My teeth shall teare The slauish motiue of recanting feare', Troilus and Cressida IV. v. 57, 'Her wanton spirites looke out At euery ioynt, and motiue of her body', and it is claimed that this sense, 'a moving limb or organ', is found only in Shakespeare. Neither of these quotes, however, clearly establishes the suggested meaning. A quote from Cotta, however, shows that a previously unrecorded sense 'physical motion' is quite possible: 'her imagination still lead her hands vnto many and diuers continuall actions and motiues.' (63) **Conception** accords Shakespeare special (*fig.*) notice under sense 1a; one wonders if other poets using the same metaphor would have received the same attention. A combination occurs for example in Donne's 'First Anniversary'—'And false-conceptions fill the generall wombes'—which has not been registered and is therefore an antedating from 1662.

These details should be considered in the light of the fact that Shakespearean citations represent 1.91 per cent of the total number of citations in the dictionary. It seems clear that the *OED* would look different if such attention had been paid even to the major figures in English literature, let alone writers concerned with other areas of knowledge, and would have provided a more truly descriptive account of the lexicon.

2. THE PROBLEM OF NATURALIZATION

The approach adopted here which maximizes the amount of data, especially in unrecorded words, inevitably raises the particular problem of the naturalization of words in the English lexicon. Since a large proportion of the unrecorded words discovered are non-naturalized but well established, it seems appropriate to discuss the problem at length, since in the medical discipline especially the difficulty is more perplexing than for other specialisms. The term encyst is used here to describe words which retain their non-English form, and is preferred to such terms as 'borrowing' or 'foreign term' or 'neologism', since in many cases such words would already have had a long life in, the English language by the sixteenth century reaching back in some cases as far as Old English. Many appear to have been introduced during the course of the Middle English period, and are frequently cited in the *OED*. More fully and more recently they are recorded in the *MED*, where they are cited in considerable numbers from the works of Lanfranc, Chauliac, Arderne, and others. Words of this class in medical literature are frequently debarred by the nature of medical discourse itself from full naturalization. We have already seen that much of the medical lexicon was kept isolated from the language at large for various reasons—obviously, maintenance of epistemic purity, maintenance of meanings free of obscuring polysemy, and mere intellectual snobbery and elitism being among them.

How to deal with encysts was a thorny problem the *OED* editorship had to face. There is evidence, as we shall see, that they wanted to recognise such words, but also evidence that they preferred not to include them, at least early in the history of the dictionary, though the policy subsequently changed. The pages of the *OED* are inconsistent in recording these words, and it is difficult to see any pattern, officially sanctioned or otherwise, in the way the data was used. The editors of the *OED* were concerned to see that justice was done to scientific terms in general, many of which fall into the above category. In an appeal for assistance to the scientific community in 1880 after Murray had taken over, the editor requests that 'for the investigation of the history of scientific words (as to which Dr Johnson was avowedly incurious, but to which the new Dictionary will do full justice) special help is asked from the Fellows and Members of the various Scientific Societies'. Attention is also drawn in this advertisement to the kinds of words which are of particular interest: 'the early occurrence of any name of plant or animal which has been (in whole or in part) naturalized in English, and of early instances of every word of the special terminology of the biological sciences.' The kind of information required was quite specific, and there was an assumption, not an unreasonable one, that many such terms could be given the kind of lexical history which is usually impossible for all but the most ingenious and idiosyncratic coinages. 'We want to know when and by whom *Armadillo* and *Wombat*, *Teak* and *Tulip*, were first used in English; who invented (introduced or translated) *acinaciform*, *achene*, *marsupial*, *mesoblast*, *parthenogenesis*, *biology*, and all the other words of scientific nomenclature',[22] rhetorically underscoring the eclectic nature of the information solicited. In many instances these words had retained and still retain their classical forms in the medical lexicon, e.g. **dura mater**, **foetus**, **glaucoma**, **cornea**, **patella**, **pinguicula**, **schirrhus**, **uvula**, and **cholera**.

What is less clear to the student of the completed *OED* is that hard-and-fast rules governing the treatment of such words were ever devised or put into effect. Not that final consistency would ever have been more than a pipe dream; but the practice, as it is now enshrined in the pages of the dictionary, is a cacophony of indecision. It is certainly not that the editors were unaware of it—it simply seems to have been a problem that always evaded a final solution, and it still might have to be said in defence of Murray and his co-workers that where in practice no clearer solution was attainable, flexibility was in itself the best answer. Rules were nevertheless invoked from time to time. The Philological Society issued as part of its 'Explanations' for the Dictionary the following instructions for the material to be included in the 'treatment' of words. It requested:

> The History of how the word became English within square brackets [ ], stating concisely whether the word is an *adoption* or *adaption* of a Fr., Lat., Gr., Sp., It., or other word; an English formation from a Fr., Lat., Gr., or other word, or parts of words; a formation from English words or elements; or an analogical formation in imitation of other words ... but no equivalents from foreign languages which are merely cognate with the English word, and have in no way influenced its formation or history. (AOED Misc. 91/A, 3)

It is not at all clear from this how the proper English word ought to be identified. From the initial and deceptively simple question as to whether a word of this class should be included or not, down to the last details of a particular entry, difficulties abound. Should one, for instance, include a word for which there are a small number of quotes all contextually suggesting that it is the Greek or Latin term for the phenomenon in question? This situation arises frequently with words found in Barrough and others in whose writing it was normal to state that such-and-such is the Greek, Latin, or Arabic term and then to use it without further comment in the running text. Would the addition of a single quote using it without this proviso, but employing the Greek alphabet, or the Greek or Latin form, or italics, justify its inclusion? Italics were in any case used with ineffable inconsistency in the sixteenth century, and scholars and authors were sometimes wrong about the derivation of a term. Having decided that a word should be included, which form is appropriate where contemporary quotations disagree as to its Greek or Latin form? Medicine is an area which is especially rich in such terms, many of which were achieving currency in the sixteenth century. Both Greek and Latin endings were apparently sometimes sprayed indiscriminately about the same text. Not even the employment of the Greek alphabet in sixteenth-century texts requires the reader to regard the word in question as wholly foreign. Should a dictionary entry be reconstructed on the basis of what is known about its original form or on the basis of contemporary usage? If a word has an anglicized form, should the Greek or Latin forms be incorporated under the entry-head, or be listed separately? Is the decision to do the latter merely one based on frequency of occurrence? The difficulties bristle disconcertingly from every thicket, and the solutions which the *OED* adopted were as various as the questions themselves.

It is probable therefore that practical considerations were foremost in making these decisions, rather than principles. Some instances of the apparent inconsistencies include, apart from the case of **mithridatum/mithridatium/mithridate** already discussed, the English **marasme**, which is accorded a lemma, but only as a by-form of **marasmus**, the larger lemma. The lemma for **dittany** encompasses references to such forms as **dictamnus**, **dictamen**, and **dictamion**, some of which are very common in the medical texts, while **enula campana** is given a separate lemma, with a cross-reference to **elecampane**. Other words receive a kind of preamble to the definition, a striking example being **mesentery**. In a special sub-lemma division marked with ||b, it is noted that the word occurs 'in Latin and Greek forms **mesenterium**, **mesenterion**, (†**mesentereon**)' and examples are cited. There is also a completely separate lemma for **mesenteron**. Yet another instance is the citation set aside in square brackets under **optic nerve** of **nervi optici** cited from Vicary (1548), which is not a common practice.

The question of which words to omit during the dictionary's compilation bears upon this study, since unrecorded words in the present list represent editorial decisions in many cases, not merely a lack of information. It is, however, difficult to determine in some cases which are deliberate omissions and which were missed altogether by the readers. Our knowledge of the practices of *OED* readers is very sketchy and can only be partially reconstructed; thus an attempt was made in this study to try and gain some sense of what had been done. A selection of 168 unrecorded words from Barrough was matched against the *OED*'s original slips. Where a slip for an unrecorded word was found this was presumed to mean that there had been an editorial decision to exclude it from the *OED*. Of the list, only fifteen (8.9 per cent) were matched—**anagallis**, **apium**, **aranea**, **empirica**, **epolotica**, **hemitrice** (in which instance the old slip was a reference to Barrough), **laserpitium**, **lapis hæmititis**, **leucanthemus**, **leuce**, **morbus comitialis** (under **morbus**), **nitrum**, **nux indica**, **mulsum** (under **mulse**), and **releasing** (*ppl. a.*). There were two others possibly identifiable under other forms, **rubia** (under **rubee**) and **serica** (under **sericon**). Some of these had several slips; indeed, **nitrum** and **apium** had no fewer than ten each, which makes their non-appearance in *OED* the more difficult to explain. In the case of Barrough therefore the reason for non-registration of most of these words is simply their absence from the original slips, which is presumably attributable in the first place to the reader acting on the original instructions in the dictionary's early period. In cases such as **mulsum** and **nitrum**, there was obviously an editorial decision to place them under **mulse** and **nitre**, and not to split the forms into separate lemmas, as has been done with other words such as **balsam**, **balsamo/balsamum**, **empyema/empiem**, **mithridatum/mithridate** (also **mithridatium**), and **acetabulum/acetabule**. **Basilica/basilic** have been completely separated, some substantive forms appearing under **basilic** (marked *a*), and **basilica** appearing as a separate sub-lemma of **basilica** ('royal palace') with no cross-referencing between them. A separate lemma appears for **basilic** *sb.*, cross-referenced to **basilica**, however. The picture is complicated even further by pairs such as **sternon/ sternum**. Many words are listed in the *OED* as separate lemmas, as we have seen, but instances of a neoclassical form being concealed in the dictionary under an anglicized lemma are also available, for instance **diaphragma**, which is commonly used in the sixteenth century but which is subsumed under **diaphragm**, even though the first three citations are all in the form **diaphragma**. Another variant occurs in **medulla**, where sense 1b has 'more fully *medulla oblongata*'—a means of incorporating fuller Latin forms not often used. The *OED*'s first citation for **ancyroid** is '1706 Phillips has Ancyroides'; which form is also given in the derivation. The word is commonly used in Banister and elsewhere in sixteenth-century texts, but the Latin form is not lemmatized. Banister's use of **suspensores** also illustrates some of the problems. While Latin and Greek words are often clearly cited from classical sources, it is not always the case. The context in which Banister uses **suspensores** shows him using the Latin term in an explanatory passage rather than directly as a quote. The *OED* has not recorded the word, but it does list **suspensor** and **suspensory** separately; this kind of example, showing that the word is clearly functional in an English context, gives grounds for arguing that such examples should have been included, especially when sheer weight of citation of a foreign term by itself may be sufficient to ensure inclusion: 'The auncient writers haue called these *Muscles Cremasteras*; as it were *Suspensores* or hangers vp: made as it seemeth, that the testicles should hang by them, and not sodainly slippe downe.' (Qiiii^{v})

Words from whatever source with anglicized forms were generally included in the *OED*, e.g. **canker**, **epithem**, and **imposthume**, but there are instances such as **fistule**, which is not listed as a lemma at all, but instead as an anglicized by-form of the preferred form **fistula**, to which the reader is referred. Presumably the stated preference for anglicized forms has in this case been waived in the face of the evidence, and perhaps that policy could have been applied a little more flexibly. The existence of an anglicized form alongside the neoclassical form hardly necessitated the desuetude and loss of the other, and the word in foreign form may still have a legitimate place in the lexicon. As is often the case pairs could develop with differentiated uses, as with **cancer–canker**, and the omission of one of a pair from the *OED* helps to obscure this process. Neither was desuetude inevitably followed by loss—as new observations were made, a word might be revived or reborn to fit the new circumstances. Neither did any of these circumstances prevent a particular author from reconstituting the classical forms of known terms, as we have seen in the discussion of Phillip Barrough and John Banister's terminology in Chapter 3. These considerations greatly complicate the editorial choices involved with such terminology, and less than full attention to them masks elements of the very adaptable morphology of the language at this time.

The principle of excluding non-anglicized forms, even though it was abandoned, may also be partly responsible for the non-inclusion as lemmas of terms which do appear in definitions. Barrough provides a couple of examples; **laserpitium**, 'put into ther mouth *Castoreum*, or *laserpitium* with *oxymell*' (32), is used in the definition of **laser** but not given a lemma, even though, as we have seen, a slip for the term was to hand, and **asarum**, employed in the notes on **asarine**, is not listed itself; 'these thinges that provoke vrine, as anyse, *daucus, asarum, smirinon*' (37). A further example is **rubia**, '*rubia maior*, ana' (261). The *OED* records *rubia* in the definition of **rubiaceous**, but not as a lemma. No doubt a systematic search of the *OED-CD* would turn up other examples. On the other hand, botanical names, frequently used in definitions, are a class to which a principle of exclusion obviously applied, albeit inconsistently.

Problems frequently arise with the *OED*'s lemmatization which, in the light of what appears in the medical texts, may appear deficient or inappropriately apportioned. For example, should **natural**, as in **naturall vertues** (Banister, Uii^{v}), really be given a separate sub-lemma? It appears closely related to the senses II, 8a and b, and to the collocation 12a, but this collocation is not specifically acknowledged. Antedatings also reveal other potential problems, for instance **cuticular**, where the citation for the adjective precedes that for the noun, an inevitable difficulty in a historical dictionary. In this case, the noun was also found in Banister.

The difficulty of naturalization is acute for sixteenth-century medical language, particularly because there was a range of practices among the authors themselves. Just as some chose to write in Latin rather than the vernacular, so, presumably for similar reasons, some who chose to use the vernacular retained the original form of the technical terms, usually Greek or Latin. Still others used the anglicized forms. Jonas apologizes for leaving some Latin and Greek words untranslated in his *Birthe of mankind* of 1540. Phaer, on the other hand, argues for the use of vernacular terms instead in the introduction to his book on the diseases of children, *The boke of chyldren*. Turner adopted an innovative procedure in his influential herbal, inventing or reviving an English name where there was no equivalent in Latin or Greek. Many of these have remained standard since.

The *OED* editors tackled the problem of whether a word should be identified as fully naturalized in English or not by introducing a discussion of the difficulties involved into the introduction to the dictionary, and by employing a field marker in their text. The problem will nevertheless remain for future lexicographers since it is by nature intractable, and it is particularly awkward in the case of medicine, for whose technical purposes the *NSSL*'s solution seems more appropriate, if less obviously vernacular. The discussion of the problem in the *OED* is, however, more sophisticated than the labelling system finally adopted. The *OED* merely indicates the words considered to be non-naturalized or partially naturalized in the text with the field marker ||. Within this category three subcategories are defined in the introduction: denizens, aliens, and casuals. Denizens are those words 'fully naturalized as to use, but not as to form, inflexion, or pronunciation'; aliens are those words which are the 'names of foreign objects, titles, etc. ... for which we have no native equivalents'; and casuals are similar words not in normal use, but occurring only in special circumstances. The introduction points out succinctly, however, that it is often easier for an alien or a casual to become naturalized than for a denizen, especially where the denizen is from a learned, familiar language and therefore likely to retain its original form or pronunciation or both. Clearly it is difficult to draw a dividing-line here between naturals and denizens, and that which designates all words with non-anglicized form as non- or partially naturalized might be felt to be arbitrary. Perhaps unfortunately, the editorial practice was not to identify these three categories, but merely to lump them together under a single symbol. Neither was there any further assistance in recognizing what partial naturalization might actually mean. Did it mean that a word not fulfilling all of the requirements—naturalization as to pronunciation, spelling, and usage—was in this category? Exactly what did the 'use' criterion cover? What was to be done, to take an example, with a word with a long history in the English language like **dura mater** (first recorded Lanfranc, *c.*1400) which was not naturalized as to form, but wholly naturalized as to use? The circumstances of use in such cases implicitly require the preservation of neoclassical form. The editors raised as many questions as they answered.

In the case of the medical terms in question here, less consistency is found in the *OED* itself than the editors suggest applies. The following antedatings are marked as non- or partially naturalized: **aerugo**, **brassica**, **dartos**, **ejaculator**, **id est**, **lixivium**, **lues**, **mithridatum**, **oxoleum**, **oxybaphon**, **periosteum**, **raphanus**, **rhagades**, **sagapenum**, **sapa**, **scrotum**, **stertor**, and **tetrapharmacum**. Several of these are perfectly familiar and in general if not common use. Among those not given a field marker however and hence regarded as naturalized we find the following: **calx vise**, **dracunculus**, **epiplocele**, **fraxin**, **hemina**, **meatus**, **pandect**, **scolopendra**, etc., along with the more familiar **abdomen**, **dialect**, **epiderma**, **femur**, **hydrocele**, etc. In other words, all terms on our list given this field marker (||) are non-naturalized as to form, but not all such words are given this field marker. The further qualification given in the *OED* introduction, that the field marker be assigned to all words which 'approach or formerly approached' the status of words in these classes clarifies little and leaves the situation ambiguous in practice.

For the works cited in *OED* for Banister, Barrough, Cotta, Hester, Phaer and Securis, a search of *OED-CD* yields the following results. Of the 537 words from Banister cited in the *OED*, **bregma**, **diastole**, **gomphosis**, **humerus**, **pericardium**, **scapula**, **sphacelus**, **stretto**, **struma**, **symphysis**, **synarthrosis**, and **systole** are marked ||, but it is notable that **diarthrosis**, **glottis**, **pancreas**, **occiput**, **sinciput**, **sphincter**, and **ureter** are not. For Barrough, **effectrix**, **lupus**, and **polenta** are marked, while **nausea**, **ilium**, **saluatrix**, **savin**, **soda** (except for sense 2, the prickly saltwort), and **ptisan** are not. Hester (7), Cotta (13), and Securis (6) have too few entries to be meaningful, none being marked, and none being encysts. Phaer has 15, and none marked, but the list includes **copperas**, **diarrhoea**, **lohoch**, and **ptisan**. That there is little consistency in the treatment of such words is suggested most forcibly by the pair **synarthrosis** and **diarthrosis**. There are no marked words among Baker's 144, which, however, includes **lamin**. This would appear to suggest that Baker had a preference for avoiding encysts where possible, but the list in Appendix 1 includes many such terms.

The only criterion not given a lot of attention in the comments of the editors on these editorial problems is usage itself; but one suspects that in many cases words were included in one form rather than another on the application of just this criterion, even if the fact was not publicly admitted. This conjecture is, however, a difficult one to test. A particular problem is that insufficient work was done in the discipline of medicine for adequate decisions to be made as to usage, unless of course there was an assumption that any set of usages for a particular term in medical writers was in effect equal in lexical worth to a single usage by, say, Spenser or Shakespeare, an assumption which seems unlikely on the face of it. The early instructions to reject anything not in English form was in effect rescinded by Murray, but restitution of earlier omissions was necessarily incomplete. The result is the kind of list which Baker's *Oleum Magistrale* has produced, with a large number of unrecordeds and no || markers among the corrresponding *OED* lemmas. It is also clear that in excerpting Banister, the reader has scrupulously omitted almost all encysts, as the earliest instructions required. It is these informal policy decisions, often vital in the day-to-day preparation of the dictionary, which can be so difficult to clarify and formalize.

3. THE *OED*'S SOURCES OF MEDICAL TERMS

The *OED* had, of course, many sources for its medical terms, some of which have already been identified in the list of antedated authors (Table 6.1). The potential sources of such terms fall into two classes. The first of these consists of various kinds of word-list, including dictionaries, glossaries which are often appended to a larger work, nomenclators, and encyclopaedias. I propose for the sake of convenience to call all such works lexionaries, since there seems to be no cover-all term to hand to describe them unambiguously. The other group of works is the medical texts themselves, excluding any glossaries appended to them, which would fall into the former category. It does not follow that all lexionaries of the period will register all, or even most, of the known medical terms, even taken together. Neither is it necessarily the case that their definition of terms is either accurate or sufficiently explanatory, or that the meanings suggested correspond satisfactorily to those employed in the medical texts themselves. Some of the more important lexionaries and other sources include the *Physical Dictionary* of 1659, the Kersey edition of Phillips's *New World of Words* of 1706, and *Chambers's Cyclopedia* of

1727–51; Monro, *The Anatomy of the Human Bones*, 1726, John Ray's *A Collection of English Words not generally used*, 1674, and *A Collection of English Proverbs*, 1670, as well as other works, and R. Mayne's *A Medical Vocabulary*, London, 1862. It must be noted, however, that there are discrepancies between the relative importance of works on Table 6.1 and Table 7.3 which no doubt arise from the restricted nature of the lexical evidence assembled here.

On the present evidence it seems to be the case that the seventeenth-century lexicographers gave the sixteenth-century medical lexicon rather scant notice, so that whatever was to be gleaned by the *OED* editors from this source would not have overcome other deficiencies, being no substitute for a thoroughgoing excerption of the medical texts.

Examination of the medical and dictionary sources used by the *OED* shows that, first, all fall well short of the use of Shakespeare, who provides about ten times the number of citations of the most used dictionary, Blount's *Glossographia*. It is also clear that some were barely excerpted at all, including some of the most influential of the sixteenth-century Latin–English dictionaries such as those of Rider and Thomas, the use made of Cawdrey, Cockeram, and Bullokar all greatly exceeding these. Given the variation between Rider one the one hand and Florio on the other, however, it does seem that there must have been a policy of not using these dictionaries, perhaps on the ground that they did not on the whole supply citations which were sufficiently illustrative. Table 7.3 sets out the position. As *OED* 1 contains 1,720,691 citations in all, I have also calculated the percentage of the whole represented by the figures in column 2. The comparative figure for Shakespeare is 1.91 per cent.

Analyses of these authors by letter is also revealing, showing in some cases situations which appear to relate to that encountered in the antedatings from Barrough. The letter A is missing in one case, Cooper, and probably a second, Rider, who has only one entry for A which may be adventitious, but whether this means that the excerption was begun after the completion of A, or that excerpts for A were not made at all, is difficult to say. Cooper's entries begin at **boltel** and then run more or less uninterrupted to **zoilus**. Rider's are admittedly a much smaller sample, but begin with **aduncitify** and **cur**, run from **goldilocks** to **groundsel**, and then from **lace** to **wrinkle**. Elyot's entries are a relatively complete series, except that there are very few entries for the letters A, E, and H. In the case of

TABLE 7.3. *The occurrence of citations from other medical and dictionary sources in the OED*

Source (actual *OED-CD* call-up)	Total *OED* occurrences	% of *OED* total
Blount	3,310	0.192
Florio	3,138	0.182
NSSL	2,684	0.156
Ray	2,576	0.150
Cockeram	1,266	0.074
Cooper 1565	744	0.043
Banister	537	0.031
Elyot 1538	467	0.027
Mayne 1858	382	0.022
Bullokar	382	0.022
Cawdrey 1604	377	0.022
Barrough	204	0.012
Rider 1589	72	0.004
Allbutt	70	0.004
Monro	47	0.003
Cotgrave	12	0.001
Holyoake	10	0.001
Thomas 1588	2	0.000

Mayne, the series is truncated at both ends, though it is easier to explain the lack of the last four letters, which are unlikely to yield a great number of medical terms. The series runs from **cinnamoneous** to **vigilance**, and in any case is not extensive. It is tempting to explain these deficiencies by the practice of sub-editors only farming out reading for their own letters, referred to earlier in this chapter.

As regards the antedatings listed in this study, the dictionaries appearing most frequently in Table 6.2 are set out in Table 7.4.

Large medical dictionaries, being professional by nature, tend to preserve the traditional form of encysts, and may include vocabulary which might not find its way into *OED*, so that I have looked at some entries in the *New Sydenham Society Lexicon* (*NSSL*) by way of comparison.

This lexicon began as a revision of Mayne, appearing in print somewhat in advance of the *OED*, covering the discipline rather more fully than the *OED*. It is especially helpful in assessing the *OED*'s omissions from the potential corpus of medical terminology,

TABLE 7.4. *Number of occurrences of dictionaries listed in Table 6.1*

Dictionary	No.	%
Phillips	45	1.76
Blancard's	38	1.48
Florio	28	1.09
Cotgrave	26	1.02
Blount, T.	17	0.66
Cockeram	16	0.63
Bailey, N.	10	0.39
Eng dicts	9	0.35
NSSL	7	0.27
Cawdrey, R.	7	0.27
Mayne	6	0.23

and in the treatment of encysts since, whereas the *OED* assumed (at least at first) that they should be excluded on the whole, *NSSL* clearly assumed that they should be included, and that the neoclassical form should be the basis for citation in the lemma.

The *NSSL* is a major dictionary in its own right which has fallen into undeserved neglect presumably as a result of advances in the field of medicine with the accompanying changes and expansion in modern terminology. Though extensive, it is not an historical dictionary, having no illustrative historical quotations. Definitions are generally longer and more technical than the comparable ones in *OED*. There is a very short introduction to the work, but it gives no clues as to the methods of the editors and it is impossible, regrettably, either from the introduction or from the entries themselves, to make any guess as to what kinds of sources were used by the editors. Such information would have been invaluable for the history of lexicography in this period.[23] Had it been more informative, the *OED* might have obtained better access to medical works and terminology, but in fact there is no evidence even to suggest that the editors of each dictionary were in contact with each other.[24] Nevertheless *NSSL* was a major lexicographical resource which was frequently used by the *OED* editors.

There are three substantial differences between the two works in their approach to the medical lexicon. One is that the *NSSL* frequently lists words under their classical rather than anglicized forms. Secondly, there are many words in *NSSL* which do not appear in

OED, presumably on the grounds of obscurity or of being highly specialized. Thirdly, there are a number of medical words included in *OED* which do not appear in *NSSL*, many of which appear to be older, obsolescent terms. This can be illustrated by a selection of antedatings from this study which was checked against the *NSSL* (see Table 7.5). Where they were found to be registered, the *status* column in the following list is left blank. Words not listed are noted, and those listed under a variant lemma are also noted under *status*.

TABLE 7.5. OED *antedatings in* NSSL

	OED antedating	Status
1.	absterge	Not in *NSSL*, but cf. **abstergent**
2.	accession	
3.	accident	
4.	alteration	
5.	anethine	Not in *NSSL*, but cf. **anethene, anethol**
6.	aperitive	
7.	benjamin	
8.	boxing glass	Not in *NSSL*
9.	bronchocele	
10.	calx vive	Under **calx**
11.	canella	
12.	colliquation	
13.	confection	Under **confectio**
14.	consistence	
15.	convulsion	
16.	decline	
17.	egestion	
18.	equal	
19.	experiment	
20.	fraxin	
21.	glutination	Under **agglutination**
22.	hemina	
23.	indisposition	
24.	indurate	Not in *NSSL*, but cf. **indurated, induration**
25.	judging day	
26.	judication	Not in *NSSL*
27.	lenticular	
28.	lixivium	
29.	luted	Not in *NSSL*, but cf. **lute**
30.	magistral	
31.	meatus	
32.	mesopleuron	Under **mesopleura**

	OED antedating	Status
33.	melrose	Not in *NSSL*
34.	misy	
35.	oxoleon	Not in *NSSL*
36.	pellagra	
37.	percolation	
38.	pompholyx	
39.	refriscative	Not in *NSSL*
40.	rhagades	Under **rhagadia**
41.	saphenus	Under **saphena**
42.	scolopendra	
43.	sorbition	Under **sorbitio**

Those twenty-eight with no note appear in *NSSL* as expected. Nine, however, do not appear in *NSSL* at all, and six are under another, usually non-anglicized form, although one is simply a case of a sub-lemma (**calx**). The tendency for *NSSL* to list words under the classical form is clear, as is the tendency for *OED* to record older, naturalized forms which were probably disused, as well as words for medical phenomena and processes which were obsolete, e.g. **boxing glass**, **judication**, and **luted**. Of this list, five contain a citation of *NSSL* in the *OED* lemma—**canella**, **colliquation**, **consistence**, **decline**, and **lenticular**. Those words which appear in *OED* but not in *NSSL* include **amper**, **indurate**, and **melrose**.

There are a number of close parallels in the actual definitions; however, the actual relation between *OED*, *NSSL*, and the other major nineteenth-century medical dictionaries remains to be investigated. In some cases the *NSSL* definition and *OED*'s are the same in whole or in part as in words such as **ascites, catabatic**, **cœliac**, **cœliac plexus**, **cœliac axis**, and **encystment**. To take an instance, the *NSSL* defines **asarin** as:

A white, crystallisable, solid, volatile, aromatic, camphorlike substance, obtained from the *Asarum europæum*. It is soluble in alcohol, ether, and volatile oils; softens to a waxy consistence at 26.6C (80F), melts at 65.5C (150F). Also, by some, applied to a bitter, nauseous principle found in the same plant.

An example like this shows what seems to be the *OED*'s characteristic approach to scientific words, not using the more technical details, providing some more information of a more linguistic but less pharmaceutical nature, presumably in the interests of its more educated but not necessarily professional readership: 'A crystallizable, aromatic, camphorlike substance obtained from the root of *asarabacca*, called also *Camphor of Asarum*, and asarone.' **Asarone** is not accorded a separate lemma, but is entered in small bold type, and is given a citation under the lemma **asarin**. **Encystation** in *NSSL* reads as follows: 'The process of becoming motionless and surrounded by a dense capsule or bag, as observed in some of the Protozoa.' In *OED* it reads: 'The process (observed in some Protozoa) of becoming surrounded with a cyst, bag or capsule.'

Presumably similar considerations apply to the use of material from other medical dictionaries used by the *OED*, but to examine this in detail is beyond the scope of the present book. Many *OED* entries for medical vocabulary must bear complex relationships to such material, and the *OED* was probably able to rely upon its historical information to distinguish obsolete and anglicized forms.

4. FIELD MARKERS

It would seem an easy matter to determine which of the terms we are dealing with had medical senses in early modern English and which did not simply by reference to the *OED*'s field markers, since a number of them are employed. It is not, however, the case that the *OED* has been consistent in this matter. An examination of the field markers assigned will soon show that, where a word was primarily a medical one, a field marker was not always assigned, in spite of the fact that the *OED* uses a number of field markers appropriate for medical terms. **Pestilent**, to take an instance, does not have a field marker for any of its senses, including 2 'producing or tending to produce infectious disease; infectious as a disease or epidemic; pestilential', while **egestion** does; **inflame** senses 3 and 7 which are clearly medical do not, and neither does **inflamed** sense 3, but **inflammative** sense 3 is marked 'path', as is **inflammatory** sense 4. **Inflammable** sense 3 is marked by the phrase 'Of disease'. **Agglutinate** *v* receives the marker 'Phys.' for sense 2, and **agglutinant** receives 'med' for sense 2. **Agglutinate,** *a* receives none for sense 1, though both of its pericopes are obviously medical. In cases where a field marker was not used, a medical sense is sometimes established by some clear reference in one or more of the word's *definienda*. **Sarcocolla** has no field marker, but there is reference in the explanatory matter to its 'reputed property of agglutinating wounds'. Sub-lemmas do not appear to be treated differently either; some clearly medical senses are duly noted while others are not.

While such means of identifying a word as medical, at least for one of its possible meanings, was accepted, it seems that the presence of one or more quotations among the examples of usage in the *OED* was not accepted as sufficient, even though this may strongly suggest that it should have been so regarded. Here the ground is more slippery, and an argument for a particular word's acceptance may seem compelling. However, the immediate consideration here is not whether the word is really medical in application, but whether the *OED* recognizes that it is so. Hence **auction** is not field-marked in *OED* in spite of the pretty obvious medical uses recorded by the dictionary from Ray and Phillips. The *OED* gives the following definition: 'the action of increasing; increase, growth.' The word does, however, have a specifically medical application and is often used in reference to other physical functions like **assimilation**, **nutrition**, and so forth. For similar reasons, **neezing** is excluded, but some other marginal cases are not, e.g. **inherent** and **corrugated**.

There are a number of different types of field marker involved. There is little point in restricting the analysis to the formal markers only, which are *Med.*, *Path.*, *Phys.*, *Anat.*, etc. There are less formal ones which, to avoid hopeless distortion of the available information, must also be acknowledged. For instance, **derive** is given the less obvious label '*spec.* in *med.*' as part of the definition rather than as a formal marker for the entry. All of these should for the moment be assumed to be field markers, in order to obtain a more reliable picture of editorial practice in this area, since it seems not to realize what may have been originally proposed consistently.

5. THE 'WEDGE' HYPOTHESIS

It has been assumed that the *Supplement* to *OED* or any substantial body of new data for it would be large in A and reduce towards the end of the alphabet, since the accumulating body of research and data as the project went on would render A the least satisfactory of the letters. This assumption, however, is not entirely borne out by the facts. The results of the present study are shown in Appendix 2, graph 16. This chart is somewhat tricky to interpret, and the relativities are clearer in graph 17, which is derived from it, representing the arithmetical differences between the percentage figures in 16. The *OED* percentages as expected are lower in the early part of the alphabet, except for B, F, G, and H, as against a higher rate in the present collection. W favours the *OED* heavily, but large numbers of medical terms are unlikely to appear in this letter. There appear to be two series, not continuous, running from A to I in the first case, and from J to S in the second. Taken together they show a wedge, but with a considerable discontinuity in the middle. It is more obviously continuous if E and I are regarded as exceptionally high. This pattern is also most clearly marked in most of those letters in which medical terms might be expected, that is, A, C, D, E, I, P and S, a result which could be understood to mean either that the medical lexicon was well done on the whole—at least well enough to show the expected pattern—or that it was rather uniformly done, except for R, and perhaps F, G, and H.[25] The first conclusion seems rather at odds with the evidence of this book, and the latter therefore is perhaps the more likely. It is difficult to see the predicted steady advance in the *OED*'s share as it approaches its notional perfection as absolutely clear. What must also be taken into account is the extent to which this graph might actually be trivial, since the antedatings in this study might represent something like the disposition of Latin, a large number of terms being latinate. This is not quite a simple matter, however, since not only are some antedatings in the present list from other than Latin sources, but the English lexicon in the sixteenth century would already show a considerable bias towards the Latin disposition among the letters of the alphabet. If, however, it is trivial in this sense, the underlying assumption must be that the *OED* may not even approach the state predicted, and that there is no perceptible 'wedge' at all. In any case the sample remains a very small one and any conclusions must be conjectural.

Graphs 18 and 19 show the unrecorded words in this study arranged in the same way. The result is even harder to interpret clearly, the wedge shape being perhaps even less clear than for antedatings. There are two short and rather steep declines from A to G and then from O to S. Overall a rather tentative curved decline might be inferred, excepting the obvious exaggeration at G, and the glaring exceptions of B, O, and V.

The editors of the second edition write:

It was recognised at the outset (1983) that the bulk of the material would lie in the early section of the alphabet. The lexical changes of the period (between ten and twenty years) since this part of the Supplement was prepared were yet to be recorded; moreover, the Supplement's coverage of the vocabulary already in use at that period was limited both by the relatively modest scale on which the work was initially planned and by the extent of the collections, which were inevitably small in the early stages. In this it resembled, though for different reasons, the earlier *Supplement* of 1933, of which R. W. Chapman wrote: 'We projected accordingly ... a wedge-shaped Supplement, designed to bring the work to an even date; it is, so to speak, all ABC and no XYZ.'[26]

But this asymmetry was a condition of the material being treated; there was no constraint on the editorial operation that confined it to one part of the alphabet. On the contrary, the storage of the material on the *New OED* database meant that very recent coinages from any point of the alphabet could be included. The other, historical aspect is that an improved *OED* does not necessarily obviate the necessity for further research. Schäfer has already recognized the fact that the existence of the Supplements and of *OED* 2 increases rather than decreases the opportunities for finding new data (Schäfer 1989: 4). The *OED*'s assumption about this can be tested, at least for the discovery of older words and senses. The dictionary was not published in strict chronological and alphabetical order, which requires some adjustments; however, the wedge predicted by Chapman appears only in a rather distorted form, and not for each letter of the alphabet. The material produced by Schäfer, on the other hand, appears to be somewhat at variance with this finding; indeed he claims that it 'supports the hypothesis ... that the *OED* became more reliable in the course of publication since more sources were more carefully excerpted as the work advanced' (Schäfer 1989: 4), although he does not analyse it in detail, suggesting only that two-thirds fall in the range A–L. Graph 16, Appendix 2, shows that for the present material this claim would not hold with any great accuracy, though the percentages for A–L are roughly the same, the actual percentage for the present study being 60.14. There is clearly a point on the graph, about the letter J, where the percentages from my material cease with some exceptions on either side to be greater, and the *OED*'s predominate, but there is no very clearly wedge-shaped pattern, since considerable numbers of antedatings continue to be found late in the alphabet. The distributions in the present material seems just as likely to reflect features of the medical lexicon itself such as the expectation that A, C, D, E, I, P and S should yield substantial amounts of material, and B, F, G, H, and W relatively less, as shown in graph 15.

6. CONCLUSIONS

Obviously there are large and virtually untouched areas of research in this field. But it is painstaking work, even with computer assistance, especially since concordances are generally available only for leading literary figures. Databases are potentially very valuable, but in order to give an accurate picture of the medical lexicon they ought to be exhaustive rather than selective. Schäfer notes that 'vast and structured documentation is necessary in order to reflect the state of the English lexicon in the sixteenth century' (Schäfer 1989: 70).

Nevertheless, it can already be seen that there were inconsistencies in the *OED*, both in general and relating especially to medical terminology. It has already been shown that different authors receive differential treatment, arising from the application of the principle that the great literature ought to be exhaustively treated. Technical lexicons such as that of medicine were, on the other hand, apparently treated relatively compendiously, and ranked with the lesser forms of literature. This particularly raises the problem of the treatment of highly specialized terms.

Although this work has not set out to examine the structure of the *OED*'s entries systematically, it seems clear that the entries for some words would by implication have to be considerably altered chronologically on the basis of the present findings. An obvious example is the word-group **dissect**, **dissected**, **dissecting**, **dissection**, in which case Banister has yielded antedatings for **dissect** *v*, sense 1 and 2; **dissected** sense 1; **dissecting** *vbl. sb*; and for **dissection** senses 1 and 2. Similarly there are two senses of **disseminate** from Banister, who also antedates **descendent** *a* and *sb.*, and two senses of **consistence**. **Lateral** has three antedatings from Banister out of ten adjectival sub-lemmas, and one out of the two substantive senses. This word has four first citations from Shakespeare at present. It is also true that the present data might introduce a new weighting in entries; for example, there are two antedatings of senses of **dispensation** in this list from John Cotta, which would form quite a significant proportion of the fifteen listed. There are no fewer than four senses of **consistence** out of eleven, of **observation** three out of fifteen, and so on. The real question is how much more material would be required to render at least most polysemous entries free from the kind of weighting we have discussed above, leaving aside the obvious constraints imposed by monosemous words. It is also possible that some entries might have to be reconstructed semantically, although new senses and previously unrecognized medical senses of words are not a large proportion of the present data.

The treatment of encysts is another area of difficulty. First, it is not consistently managed, as we have seen, and this is partly due to the change in policy from the early rejection of non-English terms to the acceptance of all information on early forms without reference to their naturalization. Even allowing for this, however, there are inconsistencies of detail which persist, and are probably the result of day-to-day changes of mind, insufficient information, and so on.

The *OED*'s coverage of the available texts of the period is a problem, not so much because of the range of texts, many scientific and medical texts being assigned for excerption, but because problems arose with the readers. Many of the texts were inadequately done as we have seen, even to the point where their being excerpted has added nothing substantial to the dictionary's database, and much lexical material of value remains undiscovered in these texts to this day. It would clearly be worthwhile to revise comprehensively many of the texts on which the *OED* has been based, and also to use the computer facilities now available to identify texts only partially excerpted.

The *Supplement* to the dictionary, while exhibiting the benefits of a widened approach to the lexical material of the language, also perpetuates some of the assumptions about the *OED* which we have already noted. Thus, for example, the policy of only including information from the post-1800 period left early modern English untouched by more recent research. It remains a serious gap, after the completion of the *MED*, which needs serious attention, and a large research effort. The appearance of the second edition of the *OED* has not solved the problem, having provided further information only selectively; for example, **oleum**, an unrecorded word in *OED* 1, would now be, if antedated from Baker (1574), an antedating of *OED* 2 of 331 years.

Seen in this context, the commonly received idea of the *OED* as a monolithic scholarly edifice must be modified to some extent. It is obvious that the *OED* must also be thought of as a very large, somewhat inconsistent compilation, limited by the activities of its workers, to some extent hamstrung by its own policies, and evolving further policies as the project grew. It has inbuilt biases, errors, and omissions of various kinds. Perhaps most importantly, its work of recording the historical lexicon of the English language was left incomplete, though it is not possible following the present survey to suggest how incomplete. Notwithstanding the foregoing considerations, sixteenth-century medical terminology has to this stage never been better surveyed than in the *OED*, though it seems certain that the *NSSL* would have done this better had it been a historical dictionary.

Complete concordance studies have been shown here to have the potential to yield fruitful results, and they ought to be the basis of future lexicography as well as historical lexicography. A prerequisite for databases ought to be comprehensiveness, rather than the selection of certain word classes for special attention; only thus can good and reliable coverage and a statistically reliable representation of lemmas and sub-lemmas be achieved. Some of the *OED*'s difficulty in deciding what was a rare medical term and what was not seems to have arisen from a relative paucity of material in the first place. Lexicographers engaged on large comprehensive dictionaries need to know the lexicon as completely as possible before deciding how to treat it and what to omit.

The present study certainly indicates that we cannot be confident about the present view of the sixteenth-century lexicon if medical terminology is in any sense to be seen as representing the wider lexicon. The average margin of discrepancy for antedatings is large enough to indicate a substantial shift of half a century or so in the chronology of word acquisition in this period, and there is also a considerable body of unrecorded words.

The notion that English had available to it too many words from the three languages to which it owed the bulk of its medical terminology rather than too few also deserves notice. This is not to suggest that they were all satisfactory and appropriate, or that no new ones were produced; but the problem was not so much to find new terminology as to choose among the competing claims of old, rival terminologies, and to try to dispel obscurity where possible. Perhaps we should allow Andrew Borde to have the last word on the subject for the time being from his *The breuiary of helthe*. Instead of regarding English as a language struggling to keep up with a rapidly increasing need for new terminology, we may instead have to take seriously his suggestion that 'olde auncyent, and autentyke auctours, or doctours of Physicke in theyr bokes doth wryte many obscure terms, geuyng also to many and dyuerse infirmyties, darke and harde names, dyffycyle to vnderstande' (Av^r). Since then, the dust and darkness have been gathering.

Notes

1. An authority which has passed to the various dictionaries derived from *OED* as well.
2. Similarly La Rana (1992). Research in this area is still obliged to use a tool, the best we have, parts of which are over a century out of date.
3. Perhaps a good deal of material still lies in such personal and professional records of those involved as are still extant. Much archival work remains to be done. At least one potential source, the *OED*'s old slips, has received some attention from Dutton (1987). Knowles (1990) is also a valuable contribution to this area of research.
4. *An appeal to the English-speaking and English-reading public to read books and make extracts of The Philological Society's New English Dictionary*, April 1879, 25.
5. Murray (1977: 223), and the reference to Marghanita Laski's letter to *The Times* on the subject.
6. In his lecture 'On some deficiencies in our English dictionaries', first delivered to the Philological Society on 5 Nov. 1857.
7. Burton's *Anatomy of Melancholy* is mentioned (AOED Misc. 213/3, 5), but it is not positively stated that it had been read at that early period.
8. A reference to 'Andrewes works' probably means Bishop Lancelot Andrewes, not the translator of Hieronymus of Braunschweig. See AOED Misc. 92/8.
9. Fitzedward Hall.
10. Surely Bonham.
11. Webb was a graduate of Aberdeen, and became a member of several professional bodies; see the *London and Provincial Medical Directory*. By 1865 he is listed as not practising, and is unlisted from 1867. He also disappears as an *OED* sub-editor after the mid-1860s: AOED Misc. 93/17/ii, 3 (10 Oct. 1867; a cumulative account of progress on the dictionary) reports that 'For the dictionary, additional help is urgently wanted in sub-editing the letters I and J' and it is later noted that I and J are partly done, but that they had remained untouched for some three years. Since these were Webb's letters, he was presumably unable to continue work either as a doctor or as an *OED* sub-editor after the mid-1860s, perhaps due to illness.
12. e.g. in AOED Misc. 189, where only the names of readers and works

read by them are recorded. Furnivall did report, however, on the number of slips issued by him; see *The Athenæum*, 2049, 2 Feb. 1867: 14, which reports that 530,800 had been sent, and that an estimated 550,000 returned, some of which were of course slips made by the contributors themselves rather than those provided for them.

13. In AOED 57/1, Howell is responsible for the letter D. Skeat mentions that each sub-editor was responsible for one letter, but although this may have been intended, it was not true in the early period. See Skeat (1911: 176).
14. Unfortunately, the pages containing the letter W are missing from this notebook, so that his work can be traced no further.
15. e.g. Lanfranc, Chauliac, Arderne. There is no evidence so far from the AOED collection concerning the date at which these works were actually read.
16. No. 1653, 2 July 1859; review of Coleridge 1859.
17. In 1868 the Shakespearean critic Clement Mansfield Ingelby alluded in a letter to the misreading of books for the dictionary, and pointed out that reports on the project had not been issued for some considerable time. *The Athenæum* 2116, 16 May 1868: 698.
18. Knowles (1989: 15–23), where the treatment of Foxe is discussed at length. The search string used by Knowles showed variations, but not in date; the entries found later all differ in date from the search string, and may indicate the editors' reliance on dates supplied by various independent readers.
19. Listed in *OED* as an error for **orthopnoic**, which is itself an antedating from Holland, 1601.
20. One, **knag**, *sb.*, is under 'Bannister'.
21. This figure does not include those first citations from Banister and Barrough already in the *OED*.
22. AOED, Misc. 90/8, which is an unpaginated title-wrapper, (*Journal of the Linnean Society*, 17/104–5, 1880).
23. Only a detailed examination of the relationship between the *NSSL* and its immediate predecessor, Mayne's *Lexicon*, also used extensively by the *OED* editors, and a search for other sources will reveal something about the methods of its editors.
24. No record of communication between them has been found in AOED.
25. Why these should stand out is unclear; the concentration of particular sub-editors in the early period seems a possible explanation, but surely subsequent accretions to the data would have overcome such deficiencies, and the work of different sub-editors on the same letters might have cancelled out the effects in some cases. More research on the activities of readers and sub-editors is needed to shed light on this problem.
26. Cited in *OED* 2, p. xxi.

Bibliography

Primary sources

The place of publication is London unless otherwise stated. For convenience, *STC* numbers have been added where applicable for works up to 1612. Names in square brackets are those of authors whose work has been translated.

A.M. [Guillemeau] (1597), *The french chirurgerye* (*STC* 12489).

A.M. [Gabelkhover] (1599), *The boock of physicke* (*STC* 11513).

Andrewe, L. (1527), *The vertuous boke of distillacyon* (*STC* 13435).

Anon. (n.d.), *A discourse of the scorbie* [?] (See *STC* 12489.5).

Anon. (1490?), *Gouernayle of healthe* (*STC* 12138).

Anon. (1525), *Banckes herball* (*STC* 13175.1 (formerly 4720)).

Anon. (1526), *Grete herball* (*STC* 13176).

Anon. (1526), *The treasure of pore men* (*STC* 24199).

Anon. (1527), *The iudycyall of all vryns* (*STC* 14836).

Anon. (1535?), *The boke of knowledge whether a sicke person ... shall lyue or dye* (*STC* 3319.5).

Anon. (1535?), *A lytell boke of the xxiiii stones pryncipall, that profiteth most to a mans body.*

Anon. (1540), *Here begynneth the seynge of uryns* (*STC* 22153).

Anon. (1540), *The judgment of all vrynes* (*STC* 22153).

Anon. (1540?), *The practyse of cyrurgyons of Mountpyller* (*STC* 18052).

Anon. (1542), *Antidotarius* (*STC* 675a).

Anon. [Vigo, J. de] (1543), *The most excellent workes of chirurgerie* (*STC* 24720).

Anon. [Plutarch] (1549?), *The gouernaunce of good helth* (*STC* 20060.5).

Anon. [Vigo, J. de] (1550?), *Lytell practyse of J. de Vigo in medycyne* (*STC* 24725).

Anon. (1552), *The ordre of the hospital of s. Bartholomewes* (*STC* 21558).

Anon. (1563), *A worthy practise of the moste learned phisition L. Fuchsius.* (*STC* 11408).

Anon. (1587?), *A profitable treatise of the scorbie* (*STC* 12498.5).

Askham, A. (1550), *A lytel herball* (*STC* 13175.13).

B[ostocke], R. (1585), *The difference betweene the auncient phisicke ... and the latter phisicke* (*STC* 1064).

Bacon, R. (1530?), *The beste waters artyficialles* (*STC* 1179.5).

Bailey, W. (1585), *A discovrse of the medicine called mithridatium* (*STC* 1198; see 6909).

—— (1586), *A briefe treatise touching the preseruation of the eie sight* (*STC* 1192.5).

Baker, G. (1574), *The composition ... of the moste excellent and prestigious oil called oleum magistrale* (*STC* 1209).

—— (1629), *The workes of that famous chirurgion A. Parey* (*STC* 19189).

Banister, J. (1575), *A needefull, new, and necessarie treatise of chyrurgerie* (*STC* 1360).

—— (1578), *The historie of man* (*STC* 1359).

—— (1598), *An antidotarie chyryrgicall, containing great varietie and choice of all sortes of medicines* (*STC* 1358).

Barrough, P. (1583), *The methode of phisicke, conteyning the cavses, signes, and cvres of the inward diseases in mans bodie from the head to the foote* (*STC* 1508).

Blount, T. (1656), *Glossographia*.

—— (1673), *A World of errors discovered in the new world of words*

Borde, A. (1542), *Dyetary of helth* (*STC* 3378.5).

—— (1550?), *The boke for to lerne a man to be wyse in buyldyng of his howse for the helth of body* (*STC* 3373).

—— (1552), *The breuiary of helthe* (*STC* 3374).

—— (1555?), *The fyrst boke of the introduction to knowledge* (*STC* 3383).

Braunschweig, H. (1525), *The noble experyence of the vertuous handywarke of surgeri* (*STC* 13433).

Bright, T. (1580), *A treatise: wherein is declared the sufficiencie of English medicines* (*STC* 3750).

—— (1580), *Characterie. An arte of shorte, swifte and secrete writing by character* (*STC* 3743).

—— (1586), *A treatise of melancholie* (*STC* 3747).

Bullein, W. (1562), *Bulleins bulwarke of defe[n]ce againste all sicknes, sornes, and woundes* (*STC* 4033).

Bullokar, J. (1617), *An English expositor*.

Bullokar, W. (1970), *Book at large*, in R. C. Turner (ed.), *The works of William Bullokar*, iii, (Leeds: Leeds University Press).

Burton, R. (1621), *Anatomy of melancholy*.

Caius, J. (1552), *A boke, or counseill against the disease commonly called the SWEATE* (*STC* 4343).

Canutus (*c.*1485), *Here begynneth a litil boke the whiche traytied many gode thinges for the pestilence* (*STC* 4589).

Cary, W. (1583), *A briefe treatise called Caries farewell to physicke* (*STC* 4370).

Cawdrey, R. (1604), *A table alphabeticall* (*STC* 4884).

Chauliac, Guy de (1542), *The questyonary of cyrurgyens* (*STC* 12468).
Chrisman, Miriam Usher (1982) *Lay culture, learned culture: books and social change in Strasbourg, 1480–1599* (NewHaven: Yale University Press).
Clever, W. (1576), *A knowledge for kings* (*STC* 11920).
—— (1590), *The flower of physicke* (*STC* 5412).
Clowes, W. (1579), *A short and profitable treatise touching the cure of the disease called (morbus gallicus) by unctions* (*STC* 5447).
—— (1585), *A briefe and necessarie treatise* (*STC* 5448).
—— (1588), *A prooued practise for all young chirurgians concerning burnings with gunpowder* (*STC* 5444).
—— (1596), *A profitable and necessarie booke of observations* (*STC* 5445.5).
—— (1602), *A right frutefull treatise for the artificiall cure of struma* (*STC* 5446).
Cogan, T. (1584), *The hauen of helth* (*STC* 5478).
Cooper, T. (1565), *Thesaurus linguæ Romanæ et Britannicæ* (*STC* 6586).
Cotgrave, R. (1611), *A dictionarie of the French and English tongues* (*STC* 5830).
Cotta, J. (1612), *A short discoverie of the unobserved dangers of severall sortes of ignorant practisers of physicke* (*STC* 5833).
—— (1623), *Cotta contra Antonium: or an ant-Antony*.
Crooke, H. (1615) *Μικροκοσμογραπηια*: a description of the body of man (*STC* 6062).
Dodoens, R. (1554), *Cruÿdeboeck* (Antwerp).
Drummond, J. (?) [Arnold de Villa Nova] (1540), *Defence of age and the recovery of youth* (*STC* 777).
Edwards, D. (1532*a*), *De Indiciis et præcognitionibus* (*STC* 7483).
—— (1532*b*), *In anatomicen luculenta et brevis*.
Elyot, Sir T. (1539/1541), *The castel of helth* (*STC* 7643).
Elyot, T. (1552), *Bibliotheca Eliotae* (*STC* 7662).
—— and Cooper, T. (1548), *Bibliotheca Eliotæ. Eliotæ Eliotis librarie. This dictionarie now newly imprinted ... inriched [by] (T. Cooperus)* (*STC* 7661).
Ffecknam, Maister (1990), *This booke of sovereigne medicines ... collected by Maister Ffecknam late abbott of Westmynster*, ed. E. Rawson Macgill (Ann Arbor, Mich.: University of Michigan).
Florio, J. (1578), *Florio his first fruites* (*STC* 11096).
—— (1591), *Florios second frutes* (*STC* 11097).
—— (1596), *A worlde of wordes* (*STC* 11098).
—— (1611), *Queen Annas new world of words* (*STC* 11099).
Forrester, J. (1594), *The pearle of practice* (*STC* 13253).
Frere, J. (1567), *Hippocratis coi omnis medicinæ parentis aphorismi versibus script* (*STC* 13520).
Fuchs, L. (1563), *A worthy practise of the moste learned phisition L. Fuchsius* (*STC* 11408).

Gale, T. (1563), *Certaine workes of chirurgerie* (*STC* 11529).

—— (1586), *Certaine workes of Galens* (*STC* 11531).

Gilbert, H. (1898), *Queene Elizabeths achademy* (Lansdowne MS 98) EETS, extra series, 8 (London).

Gwinne, M. (1611), *Aurum non aurum, sive, adversaria in assertorem chymicae, sed verae medicinae desertorium, fra. Anthonium* (*STC* 12550).

Hales, J. (1543), *The preceptes of Plutarch* (*STC* 20062).

Harrison, W. (1577/1968), *Description of England* Folger documents of Tudor and Stuart civilization, G. Edelen (Ithaca: Cornell University Press).

Harvey, Gabriel (1593/1884), *Pierce's supererogation* in A. Grosart (ed.), *The works of Gabriel Harvey, D.L.C.*, ii, (London: Huth Library).

Harvey, William (1964), ed. *The anatomical lectures of William Harvey* G. Whitteridge (ed.) (Edinburgh: E. & S. Livingstone).

Henisch, G. (1616), *Teutsche Sprach und Weissheit* (Augusta Vindelicorum).

Herring, F. (1604), *A modest defence* (*STC* 13248).

Hester, J. [Fioravanti] (1580), *A short discourse ... vppon chirurgerie* (*STC* 10881).

—— (1582), *A compendium of the rationall secretes, of the worthy knight and moste excellent doctour of physicke and chirurgerie, Leonardo Fioravanti Bolognese* (*STC* 10879).

—— (1585?), *These oiles, waters, extractions, or essences, saltes, and other compositions* (*STC* 13254).

Higgins, J. [Junius, A.] (1585), *The nomenclator, or remembrancer of Adrianus Junius, physician* (*STC* 14860).

Hill, T. [Cocles] ([1566]), *A brief and most pleasant epitomye of the whole art of physiognomie* (*STC* 5468).

—— (1568), *The proffitable arte of gardening* (*STC* 13491).

—— (1571), *The contemplation of mankind* (*STC* 13482).

—— (1576), *The newe iewell of health* (*STC* 11798).

—— [Fioravanti] (1579), *A ioyfull iewel. Contayning ... excellent orders, preseruatiues and precious practises for the plague* (*STC* 10880).

Hilton, W., *Scala perfecionis*, MS. Bodl. 592.

Hippocrates (*c.*1545), *Prognostication drawen out of ... Ipocras, Auicen and other notable authours* (*STC* 13521.7).

Huolet (1552), *Abecedarium anglico-latinum* (*STC* 13940).

Hunton, A. (1587?), *A worthy treatise of the eies* (*STC* 12499).

Jonas, R. [Roesslin] (1540), *The byrth of mankynde* (*STC* 21153).

Jones, J. (1566), *A dial for all agues* (*STC* 14726).

—— (1572), *The bathes of bathes ayde* (*STC* 14724a.3).

—— (1572), *The benefit of the auncient bathes of Buckstones* (*STC* 14724a.7).

—— (1579), *The arte and science of preseruing bodie and soule in healthe, wisdome and catholique religion* (*STC* 14724).

Knutsson, B. (*c.*1485), *A litil boke ... for ... the ... pestilence.*

Langland, W., ed. G. Kane (1988), *Piers Plowman: The A version. Will's visions of Piers Plowman and do-well* (London: Athlone Press).

Langton, C. (1547), *A uery brefe treatise, ordrely declaring the principal partes of phisick* (*STC* 15205).

—— (*c*.1550?), *An introduction into phisyke, with an vniuersal dyet* (*STC* 15205).

Levins, P. (1570), *Manipulus vocabulorum* (*STC* 15532).

Llwyd, H. [Pope John XXI] (*c*.1558), *The treasuri of healthe* (*STC* 14653).

Lowe, P. (1597), *The whole course of chirurgerie*. (*STC* 16869.5).

Marprelate, M. [Penry or Penrey, N.] (1588/1970), *O read ouer D. Iohn Bridges*, repr. in *The Marprelate tracts* (Menston: Scolar Press).

Maunsell, A. (1595), *The seconde parte of the catalogue of English printed bookes* (*STC* 17669).

Mayne, R. (1862), *A medical vocabulary*.

Minsheu, J. (1611), *Glosson-etymologicon* (*STC* 17947.5).

—— (1617), *Ductor in linguas* (*STC* 17944).

Moffett, T. (1588), *Nosomantica hippocratea* (Frankfurt).

Monro, A. (1726), *The anatomy of the human bones*.

More, P. (1564), *The hope of helth* (*STC* 18059.5).

Morelius (1583), *Verborum latinorum cum graecis anglicisque coniunctorum* (*STC* 18101).

Mosan J. trans. [Wirzung, C.] (1598), *Praxis medicinae universalis or a generall practise of physicke* (*STC* 25862).

Moulton, T. (1539?), *This is the myrour or glasse of helthe* (*STC* 18214a).

Nichols, J. G. (ed.) (1848), *The Diary of Henry Machyn* (London: Camden Society).

Norton, T., ed. J. Reidy (*c*.1477/1975), *Thomas Norton's ordinall of alchemy*, EETS 272 (London: Oxford University Press).

Partridge, J. (1582), *The widowes treasure* (*STC* 19433.2).

Paynell, T. [Mediolano, J.] (1528), *Regimen sanitatis salerni* (*STC* 19496).

—— (1533), *De morbo gallico* (*STC* 14024).

—— (1534?), *A moche profitable treatise against the pestilence* (*STC* 24226).

—— (1534?), *A moche profitable treatise against the pestilence* (*STC* 24266).

Percyvall, R. (1590), *Bibliotheca hispanica* (*STC* 19619).

Phaer, T. [Goeurot] (1543?), *A new booke entyteled the regiment of lyfe* (*STC* 11966.5].

Plat, Sir H. (1594), *The iewell house of art and nature, conteining the diuers rare and profitable inuentions together with sundry new experiments in the art of husbandry, distillation, and moulding* (*STC* 19991).

—— (1607), *Certaine philosphicall preparations of foode and beuerage for seamen ... with some necessary, approued and hermeticall medicines* (*STC* 19977.3).

Plutarch (1549), *The gouernaunce of good helthe* (*STC* 20062.5).

Ray, J. (1670), *A collection of English words not generally used* (T. Burrell).

Ray, J. (1670), *A collection of english proverbs* (W. Morden).

Raynalde, T. [Roesslin] (1545), *The byrth of mankynde* (*STC* 21154).

Raynalde, T. (1551), *A compendious declaration of the excellent vertues of a certaine lateli inventid oile* (*STC* 20779).

Recorde, R. (1548), *The vrinal of physick* (*STC* 20817).

Reid, John (1588), *A most excellent and compendious method of curing woundes in the head ... by ... Franciscus Arceus ... with a treatise of the fistulae in the fundament ... translated out of Iohannes Ardern.*

Rider, J. (1589), *Bibliotheca scholastica* (*STC* 21029).

Salesbury, W. (1547), *A dictionary in Englyshe and Welshe* (*STC* 21616).

Schroderus, J. (1929). *Ericis Johannis Schroderus upsaliensis dictionarium quadrilingue suedicum germanicum latinum græcum* Vilhem Eckmans universitetsfond 36, ed. Bengt Hesselman (Uppsala: Almqvist & Wiksell).

Securis, J. (Hatchett) (1566), *A detection and querimonie of the daily enormities co[m]mitted in physick* (*STC* 22143).

Speght, T. (1598), *The workes of our antient and lerned English poet, G Chaucer* (*STC* 5077).

Surflet, R. (1599), *A discourse of the preseruation of the sight* (*STC* 7304).

Thomas T. (1587), *Dictionarium linguae latinae et anglicanae* (*STC* 24008).

Timme, T. [Du Chesne/Quercitanus] (1605), *The practise of chymicall and hermeticall physicke* (*STC* 7276).

Top, A. (1603), *The oliue leafe: or vniuersall abce* (*STC* 24121).

Torriano, G. (1659), *Vocabulario Italiano e Inglese.*

Traheron, B. [Vigo, J.] (1586), *The whole worke of that famous chirurgion Iohn Vigo: newly corrected, by men skilful in that arte* (*STC* 24723).

Turner, W. (1548), *The names of herbes in Greke, Latin, Englishe, Duche & Frenche* (*STC* 24359).

—— (1551), *A new herball* (*STC* 24366).

—— (1568), *A new boke of the natures and properties of all wines commonlye vsed in England* (*STC* 24360).

Udall, N. (1553), *Compendiosa totius anatomie delineato* (*STC* 11715.5).

Venner, T. (1621), *Briefe and accurate treatise concerning the taking of the fume of tobacco.*

—— (1620), *Via recta ad vitam longum, or a plaine philosophicall discourse of the nature, faculties, and effects ... of ... oure bathes of Bathe.*

Vicary, T. (1548), *Anatomie* (see *STC* 11715.5).

Wilson, T. (1553), *The arte of rhetorique* (*STC* 25799).

Wingfield, H. (1551?), *A compendious or short treatise ... of physicke* (*STC* 25852).

Wotton, E. (1552). *Edoardi Wottoni oxoniensis de differentiis animalium libri decem* (Paris) (see *STC* 17993).

Secondary sources

Anon. (1990), *Thesaurus linguae latinae* (Leipzig: B. G. Teubner).

Bacchiello, Rolando (ed.) (1994), *Historical English word-formation: Papers read at the sixth national conference of the history of English* (Urbino: Quattroventi).

Bailey, R. W. (ed.) (1978), *Early modern English: additions and antedatings to the record of English vocabulary, 1475–1700* (Hildesheim: Georg Olms).

—— (1987), *Dictionaries of English* (Ann Arbor: University of Michigan Press).

Barber, C. L. (1976), *Early modern English* (London: André Deutsch).

Beier, A. L., and Finlay, R. (eds.) (1986), *London 1500–1700: the making of the metropolis* (London: Longman).

Bennett, H. S. (1965), *English books and readers 1558 to 1603* (Cambridge: Cambridge University Press).

—— (1969), *English books and readers, 1475–1558* (Cambridge: Cambridge University Press).

Blake, N. F. (1989) 'Manuscript to print' in Griffiths and Pearsall, 403–32.

—— (1992), 'Translation and the history of English', in Rissanen, et al. (1992: 3–24).

Bosse, Wilhelm G. (ed.) (1992), *Anglistentag 1991 Düsseldorf* (Tübingen: Max Niemeyer).

Britten, J., Daydon Jackson, B., and Stearn, W. T. (1965), *William Turner facsimiles* (London: Ray Society).

Chapman, A. (1979), 'Astrological medicine', in Webster (1979: 275–300).

Christianson, Paul C. (1989), 'Evidence for the study of London's late medieval manuscript-book trade', in Griffiths and Pearsall (1989: 87–108).

Coleridge, H. (1859), *A glossarial index to the printed English literature of the thirteenth century* (London: Trübner).

Cook, Harald, J. (1981), review of Webster (1979) *British Journal for the History of Science*, **14**: 88–9.

Cooper, C. H., and Cooper, T. (1858–1913), *Athenae cantabrigienses* (3 vols., London: Gregg International).

Cope, Z. (1959), *The Royal College of Surgeons of England* (London: RCS).

Copeman, W. S. (1960), *Doctors and disease in Tudor times* (London: Wm. Dawson & Sons).

Corsi, Pietro, and Weindling, Paul (eds.) (1983), *Information sources in the history of science and medicine* (London: Butterworth Scientific).

Danielsson, B., and Alston R. C. (1966), *The works of William Bullokar*, i (Leeds: University of Leeds Press).

Debus, Allen G. (1965), *The English Paracelsans*, Oldbourne history of science library (London: Oldbourne Book Co.).

Di Martino, Gabriella (1994), '"New science": new words in the seventeenth century', in Bacchiello (1994: 239–50).

Dorland, W. A. (1988), *Dorland's illustrated medical dictionary*, 27th edn. (Philadelphia: W. B. Saunders).

Du Cange, D. (1937), *Glossarium mediæ et infimæ latinitatis*, editio nova a Leopold Favre (Paris: Librairie des Sciences et des Arts).

Durling, Richard J. (1967), *Catalogue of sixteenth century printed books in the national library of medicine* (Bethesda: National Library of Medicine).

Dutton, Marsha (1987), 'Lexicography and popular history: readers and their slips for the *New English Dictionary*', *Dictionaries* **9**: 196–210

Eisenstein, Elizabeth L. (1979), *The printing press as an agent of social change* (Cambridge: Cambridge University Press).

Fernandez, Francisco, Fuster, Miguel, and Calvo, Juan José (eds.) (1994), *English historical linguistics 1992* (Amsterdam: John Benjamins).

Garner, Bryan (1982), 'Shakespeare's latinate neologisms', *Shakespeare studies* **15**: 82, 149–70.

Gerr, (1942), 'Language and science', *Philosophy of science* **9**: 147–61.

Görlach, M. (1985), 'Renaissance English (1525–1640)', in Greenbaum (1985: 30–40).

—— (1992), 'English historical linguistics today', in Bosse (1992: 244–60).

Gotti, Maurizio (1992), 'The development of a scientific language in the 17th century', in Nocera Avila et al. (1992: 319–43).

Greenbaum, S. (ed.) (1985), *The English language today* (Oxford: Pergamon).

Greene, E. L., and Frank N. Egerton (1983), *Landmarks of botanical history* (Stanford: Stanford University Press).

Griffiths, Jeremy, and Pearsall, Derek (1989), *Book Production and publishing in Britain 1375–1475* (Cambridge: Cambridge University Press).

Gunther, R. T. (1922/1971), *Early British botanists and their gardens* (New York: Kraus).

Hartmann, R. R. K. (1983), *Lexicography: principles and practice* (London: Academic Press).

—— (1986), *The history of lexicography*, Amsterdam studies in the theory and history of linguistic science 3 (Amsterdam: John Benjamins).

Haugen, E. (1983), 'Learned lexicographers of the north: seventeenth century vignettes', in Hartmann (1983: 99–105).

Hayashi, T. (1978), *The theory of English lexicography 1530–1791*, Amsterdam studies in the theory and history of linguistic science 3, 18 (Amsterdam: John Benjamins).

Henrey, B. (1975), *British botanical and horticultural literature before 1800* (2 vols., London: Oxford University Press).

Hodgson, J. (1831), *Memoirs of the lives of ... William Turner, M.D.* (Newcastle).

Hüllen, W. (1990), 'Motives behind 17th century lexicography: a comparison between German and English dictionaries of that time', in T. Magay and J. Zigány (eds.), (Budapest), 189–96.

Johnson, Francis R. (1944), 'Thomas Hill: an Elizabethan Huxley', *Huntington Library Quarterly* **4**: 329–51.

Jones, Peter Murray (1989), 'Four Middle English Translations of John of Arderne', in Minnis (1989: 61–89).

Jones, R. F. (1953), *The triumph of the English language* (Stanford: Stanford University Press).

Kerling, J. (1979), *Chaucer in early English dictionaries* (The Hague: University of Leiden Press).

Knowles, Elizabeth M. (1989), 'First uses from Foxe's Actes and Monuments in the Oxford English Dictionary: an interim case study', *International Journal of Lexicography,* 2: 15–23.

—— (1990), 'Dr. Minor and the *Oxford English Dictionary*', *Dictionaries* **12**: 27–42.

Kocher, Paul (1947), 'Paracelsian medicine in England', *Journal for the History of Medicine* **2**, 451–80.

Koivisto-Alanko, Päivi (1997), 'The vocabulary of cognition in early English translations of Boethius from Chaucer to Preston', *Neuphilologische Mitteilungen* forthcoming.

Koskenniemi, I. (1968), *Repetitive word pairs in old and early middle English prose of the type 'whole and sound' and 'answered and said' and other parallel constructions,* Annales universitatis Turkuensis, ser. B, tom 107, (Turku), 75–112.

Kytö, M., Rissanen, M., and Wright, S. (eds.) (1994), *Corpora across the centuries: Proceedings of the first international symposium on English diachronic corpora, St Catherine's College, Cambridge, 25–7 March 1993* (Amsterdam: Rodopi).

La Rana, Silvana (1992), 'Aspects of lexical innovation in early modern English', in Nocera Avila et al. (1992: 347–57).

Lancashire, I. (1994*a*), 'The early modern English Renaissance dictionaries' corpus: an update', in Kytö et al. (1994: 143–49).

—— (1994*b*), 'The Toronto English Renaissance dictionaries' database', *Medieval English Studies Newsletter* **30**: 6–8.

Latham, R. E. (1965), *Revised medical Latin word-list from British and Irish sources* (Oxford: British Academy).

Lewis, Charlton T., and Short, Charles (1969), *A Latin dictionary founded on Andrew's edition of Freund's Latin dictionary* (Oxford: Clarendon Press).

Lingo, A. (1986), 'Empirics and charlatans in early modern France: the genesis of the classification of the "other" in medical practice', *Journal of Social History* **19**: 583–603.

London and provincial medical directory (1848–69) (London).

Mattei, Adriana (1994), 'Word-formation in 17th century English medical terminology', in Bacchielli (1994: 251–57).

McConchie, R. W. (1981), 'Additions to OED from John Cotta's *Ignorant practisers of physicke*, 1612', *Notes and Queries* **28**: 490–3.

—— (1983*a*), 'Additions to *OED* from William Clever's *The flower of physicke*, 1590', *Notes and Queries* **30**: 396–401.

—— (1983b), '"Wise and learned cunctation": medical terminology 1547–1612 and the *OED*', *Dictionaries* **5**: 22–35.

—— (1986), 'Further additions to *OED* from John Cotta's *Ignorant practisers of phisicke* (1612)', *Notes and Queries* **33**: 460–1.

—— (1987*a*), 'Additions to *OED* from John Hester's *A short discourse of … maister Leonardo Phioravanti uppon chirurgerie* (1580)', *Notes and Queries* **34**: 11–4.

—— (1987*b*), 'An early Elizabethan artificial language?', *Henry Sweet Society Newsletter* **8**: 7–8.

McLean, Antonia (1972), *Humanism and the rise of science in Tudor England* (London: Heinemann Educational).

McNair, John R. (1984), 'An early "hard word" list: Stephen Batman's "A note of saxon wordes"', *Neophilologus* **68**: 317–19.

Middle English Dictionary, eds. H. Kurath and Sherman M. Kuhn, (1952–) (Ann Arbor: University of Michigan Press).

Middle English Dictionary: plan and bibliography, eds. H. Kurath and Sherman M. Kuhn (1954) (Ann Arbor: University of Michigan Press).

Miller, E. H. (1959), *The professional writer in Elizabethan England* (Cambridge, Mass.: Harvard University Press).

Minnis, A. J. (ed.) (1989), *Latin and Vernacular: studies in late-medieval texts and manuscripts* (Bury St Edmunds: D. S. Brewer).

Moore, J. L. (1910), *Tudor–Stuart views on the growth status and destiny of the English language* (Halle: Max Niemeyer).

Mueller, Janel M. (1984), *The native tongue and the word: developments in English prose style 1380–1580* (Chicago: University of Chicago Press).

Munk, William (1878), *The roll of the Royal College of Physicians of London: comprising biographical sketches*, 2nd edn. (3 vols, London: RCP).

Murray, J. A. H. (1879), *An appeal to the English-speaking and English-reading public to read books and make extracts of the philological society's new English dictionary* (Philological Society pamphlet).

—— (1900), *The Romanes lecture 1900: the evolution of English lexicography* (Oxford: Clarendon Press).

—— et al. (1933/1970), *Oxford English Dictionary* (Oxford: Oxford University Press).

Murray, K. M. E. (1977), *Caught in the web of words* (New Haven: Oxford University Press).

Nevalainen, T., and Raumolin-Brunberg, H. (1989), 'A corpus of early modern standard English in a socio-historical perspective', *Neuphilologische Mitteilungen* **90**: 67–110.

Nocera Avila, C., Pantaleo, N., and Pezzini, D. (eds.) (1992), *Early modern English: trends, forms, texts*, Biblioteca della ricera, cultura straniera 49 (Schena: Schena editore).

Norri, J. (1987), 'Notes on the study of English medical vocabulary from the historical point of view', *Mémoires de la Société Neophilologique de Helsinki* (Neophilologica fennica) **45**: 335–50.

—— (1989), 'Premodification and postmodification as a means of term-formation in middle English medical prose', *Neuphilologische Mitteilungen* **90**: 147–61.

—— (1992), *Names of sicknesses in English 1400–1550: an exploration of the lexical field*, Annales academiae scientiarum Fennicae, diss. 63 (Helsinki: Suomalainen tiedeakatemia).

Nutton, V. (1979), 'John Caius and the Linacre tradition', *Medical History*, **23**: 373–91.

O'Connor, Desmond (1990), *A history of Italian and English bilingual dictionaries* (Biblioteca dell' 'archivum romanum' fondata da Giulio Bertoni, serie ii, linguistica, 46) (Florence: Leo S. Olschki).

Osselton, Noel E. (1983), 'On the history of dictionaries', in Hartmann (1983: 13–21).

—— (1986), 'The first English dictionary? A sixteenth century compiler', in Hartmann (1986: 175–84).

The Oxford Dictionary on compact disc (1987). (Oxford: Oxford University Press).

Pahta P., and Nevanlinna, S. (forthcoming), 'Nonrestrictive expository apposition with an explicit marker in late middle English and early modern English', in Rissanen et al. (1996).

Pelling, M., and Webster, C. (1979), 'Medical practitioners', in Webster (1979: 165–235).

Pelling, Margaret (1986), 'Appearance and reality: barber-surgeons, the body, and disease', in Beier and Finlay (1986: 82–112).

Peters, Robert A. (1968), 'Robert Cawdrey and the first English dictionary', *Journal of English Linguistics* **2**: 29–42.

Pollard, A. W., Redgrave, G. R., Jackson, W. A., Ferguson, F. S., and Panzer, Katherine F. (1976–91), *A short-title catalogue of works printed in England, Scotland and Ireland ... 1475–1640* (3 vols, London: Bibliographical Society).

Power, H., and Sidgwick, Leonard W. (1881–?), *New Sydenham Society lexicon of medicine and allied sciences* (London: New Sydenham Society).

Rissanen, M., Ihalainen, O., Nevalainen, T., and Taavitsainen, I. (eds.) (1992), *History of Englishes: New methods and interpretations in historical linguistics* (Proceedings of the IECHL 6th Conference, Helsinki, May 1990) (Berlin: Mouton de Gruyter).

Rissanen, M., Kytö, M., and Heikkinen, S. (forthcoming), *English in transition*, (Berlin: Mouton de Gruyter).

Rolleston, S. H. (1932), *The Cambridge medical school* (Cambridge: Cambridge University Press).

Rydén, M. (1985), 'Antedatings and additions for *OED* from *The vertuose boke of distyllacyon of the waters of all maner of herbes* (1527)', *Notes and Queries* **32**: 12–14.

Sager, Juan C., Dungworth, D., and McDonald, Peter F. (1980), *English special languages* (Wiesbaden: Brandstetter).

Salmon, V. (1979), *The study of language in 17th-century England*, Amsterdam studies in the history of the language sciences 40 (Amsterdam: John Benjamins).

Saunders, J., and O'Malley, C. (1950), *The illustrations from the works of Andreas Vesalius of Brussels* (Cleveland: World Publishing).

Schäfer, J. (1980*a*), *Documentation in the O.E.D.: Shakespeare and Nashe as test cases* (Oxford: Oxford University Press).

—— (1980*b*), 'Elizabethan rhetorical terminology and historical lexicography', *Dictionaries* **2**: 7–17.

—— (1984), 'Documentation in the OED: a plea for supplementary studies', *Dictionaries* **6**: 145–9.

—— (1987), 'Early modern English: *OED, new OED, MED*', in Bailey (1987: 66–74).

—— (1989), *Early modern English lexicography* (2 vols., Oxford: Clarendon Press).

Schrickx, W. (1956), *Shakespeare's early contemporaries* (Antwerp: Nederlandsche Boekhandel).

Schmitt, C. B. (1983), 'Recent trends in the study of medieval and Renaissance science', in Corsi and Weindling (1983: 221–40).

Simpson, J. A., and Weiner, S.C. (eds.) (1989), *Oxford English Dictionary*, 2nd edn. (Oxford: Oxford University Press).

Skeat, W. (1911), *Frederick James Furnivall: a volume of personal record* (London).

Slack, P. (1979), 'Mirrors of health and treasures of poor men: the uses of the vernacular medical literature of Tudor England', in Webster (1979: 237–73).

Slaughter, M. M. (1982), *Universal languages and scientific taxonomy in the seventeenth century* (Cambridge: Cambridge University Press).

Starnes, Dewitt T. (1954), *Renaissance dictionaries, English–Latin and Latin–English* (Austin: University of Texas Press).

—— and Noyes, G. (1991), *The English dictionary from Cawdrey to Johnson, 1604–1755*, new edn., ed. G. Stein (Amsterdam: John Benjamins).

Stein, G. (1985), *The English dictionary before Cawdrey*, Lexicographia series maior 9 (Tübingen: Niemeyer).

—— (1987), 'Sixteenth-century English/vernacular dictionaries', in Hartmann (1986: 219–27).

Stone, G. (1987), 'Mark Ridley (1560–1624): An Elizabethan slavist', *Journal of Russian Studies* **53**: 3–14.

Subbiondo, Joseph L. (1984), review of M. Slaughter, *Universal languages and scientific taxonomy in the seventeenth century*, *Journal of Linguistics* **20**: 199–204.

Sutcliffe, P. (1978), *The Oxford University Press: an informal history* (Oxford: Clarendon Press).

Taavitsainen, Irma (1994*a*), 'On the evolution of scientific writings from 1375 to 1675: repertoire of emotive features', in Fernandez (1994: 329–42).

—— (1994*b*), 'Subjectivity as a text-type marker in historical stylistics', *Language and Literature* **3**: 197–212.

Talbot, C. H., and Hammond, E. A. (1965), *The medical practitioners in medieval England: a biographical register* (London: Wellcome Historical Medical Library).

Trench, R. (1857), *On some deficiencies in our English dictionaries* (London: Philological Society)

Turner, C. (1928–9), *Anthony Munday: an Elizabethan man of letters*, University of California publications in English 3 (Berkeley: University of California Press).

Ungerer, J. (1986), 'George Baker: translator of Aparicio de Zubia's pamphlet on the "oleum magistrale"', *Medical History* **30**: 203–11.

Vickers, B. (ed.) (1984), *Occult and scientific mentalities in the Renaissance* (Cambridge: Cambridge University Press).

—— (1987), *English Science, Bacon to Newton* (Cambridge: Cambridge University Press).

Voigts, Linda Ehrsam (1981), 'A letter from a Middle English dictaminal formulary in Harvard Law Library MS 43', *Speculum* **56.3**: 575–81.

—— (1986), 'The Latin verse and Middle English prose texts on the sphere of life and death in Harley 3719', *Chaucer Review* **21.2**: 291–305.

—— (1989*a*), 'The character of the *carecter*: ambiguous sigils in scientific and medical texts' in Minnis (1989: 91–109).

—— (1989*b*), 'Scientific and medical books' in Griffiths and Pearsall (1989: 345–402).

—— (1990), 'The 'Sloane Group': related scientific and medical manuscripts from the fifteenth century in the Sloane collection', *British Library Journal* **16**: 26–37.

—— (1996), 'What's the word? Bilingualism in late-medieval England', *Speculum* **71**: 813–26.

Ward, J. (1740/1969), *The lives of the professors of Gresham College* (New York: Johnson Reprint).

Webster, C. (ed.) (1979), *Health, medicine and mortality in the sixteenth century* (Cambridge: Cambridge University Press).

Webster, C. (1983), 'The historiography of medicine', in Corsi and Weindling (1983: 29–43).

Wheeler, A. et al., (1986), 'William Turner's (*c.*1508–1568) notes on fishes in his letter to Conrad Gesner', *Archives of Natural History* **13**: 291–305.

Wood, Anthony (1691), *Athenae Oxonienses, an exact history of all the writers and bishops ... of Oxford* (London: Tho. Bennet).

Zgusta, L. (1988), 'The Oxford English Dictionary and other dictionaries (Aikakosyam)', *International Journal of Lexicography* **1**: 188–230.

APPENDIX 1

An Alphabetical List by Author of the Data Excerpted

Abbreviations:

a 1 cit	absolute first citation
anted	antedating
fpl	fine print lemma
ncit	no citation
nd	no date
ns	new sense
postd	postdating
tp	title page
unrec	unrecorded

BAILEY, WALTER, *A treatise of the medicine called mithridatium*, 1585

1. Antedatings

1. accession [III, 1655, Vaughn *Silex Scint.*] D6r to keepe one from often accessio[n]s of [th]e goute [a 1 cit]

2. acetic [1, 1808, Henry] E2r *acetum mulsum*, that is wine, hony and vinegar [a 1 cit]

3. allot [*v*, 5, 1598, Bacon *Sacred Med.*] C1r some difference is to be allotted: yet such, as a man exercised in these matters, may easely supplye

4. answerable [*a*, II, 4b, 1617, J. Taylor (Water P.)] B5r we may not loke for the vertues aunswerable to the composition, but that some one simple aboue the rest may shew his quality, that the compound medicine may do an effect aunswerable to that simple

5. antidotary [A, *adj*, 1599, A. M. *Gabelhouer, B. Phys.*] B2v in many antidotary bookes

6. apply [*v*, I, 7, 1628, Coke *On Litt.*] C1r these two medicines are confected of many simples, not greatly differring, they haue many things co[m]mon: so as [tha]t which is of [th]e one affirmed, may bee applied to the other

7. attribute [*v*, II, 7, 1599, Thyme *Animadv.*] A8r The first found without name is attributed to *Andromachus*

8. canella [1, 1693, Blount *Nat. Hist.*] C6^{v} Whosoeuer wil with diligence examine the sackes of Canella ... may easely finde the perfect kindes of Cinnamum [a 1 cit]
9. coct [*v*, I, B, 1605, Jonson *Volpone*] C1^{v} For if *Theriacle* being cocted in one yeare [a 1 cit]
10. confecting [*vbl sb*, 1626, Bacon *Sylva*] Av^{r} very expert in co[n]fecting of medicines [a 1 cit]
11. confectioner [1, 1606, Holland *Sueton.*] C2^{r} that the confectioner may in all pointes doe his duty [a 1 cit]
12. consistence [4, 1626, Bacon *Sylva*] C3^{r} First therefore in consistence of substance ... it ought to haue an equality of substance, not drie nor ouer liquide [a 1 cit]
13. constantly [*adv*, 2, 1651, Hobbes *Leviath.*] C5^{v} later writers do constantly affirme that in this our time
14. contemper [*v*, 2, 1605, Timme *Quersit.*] E2^{v} hauinge regarde that the liquore might contemper and mitigate in some part the quality of the medicine
15. conveniency [5, 1650, Greville *Sidney*] C8^{r} that our Apothecaries in *England*, may with as good conueniency procure the[m]
16. decline [*v*, 3c, 1615, G. Sandys *Trav.*] C3^{v} which ought to be a little rednes declining to yealownesse
17. display [*v*, 7, 1726–31, Tindal *Rapin's Hist.*] D2^{v} where *Galen* at large displayeth [th]e faculties & vertues of *Theriacle* in his bookes
18. divulging [*vbl sb*, 1604, *St. Trials, Hampton Crt.*] Aiii^{v} so doubtlesse more renowme is due vnto *Pompey* for diuulging of this medicine [a 1 cit] [fpl]
19. dormitory [*a*, 1631, R. H. *Arraignm*] B7^{v} that stupefying and dormitory power in *Opium* [a 1 cit]
20. durance [2, 1599, Moufet *Silkwormes*] D1^{v} *Theriacle* & *Mithridatium* haue their times of fermentation, of their duraunce, and ... after a certaine age they decline
21. east indian [B, 1831, *Asiatic Journal*] C7^{v} are procured from [th]e east and west *Indians*
22. equal [*a*, 4, 1661, Morgan *Sph. Gentry*] C3^{r} it must be in substance, coherent, equall, and smooth
23. exactly [*adv*, 3, 1646, Browne *Pseud. Ep.*] B8^{v} *Galen* in his bookes *de Theriaca* doth write exactly of the time of fermentation of *Theriacle*
24. examination [3, 1630, R. Johnson's *Kingd. & Commw.*] C3^{r} we will apply the same to [th]e examination of *Mithridatium*
25. fermentation [1a, 1601, Holland *Pliny*] B4^{v} And as compounds must haue a time of fermentation, and rypening
26. impaired [*ppl a*, 1611, Speed *Hist. Gr. Brit.*] D4^{r} that the wittes are dulled, the senses and discourse of reason either greatly impaired or cleane taken away [a 1 cit]

27. indication [2, 1668, More *Myst. Godl.*] E2[r] hee made choise of the liquores by indication taken of the countrey, of the time f the yeare, of the age and complexion of the patient, and of the nature and disposition of the disease

28. malignity [3, 1605, Timme *Quersit.*] B7[v] for the better correction of the malignity of [th]e beast [the viper] which hapely might remaine in the flesh

29. mithridatium [1693, *Blancard's Phys. Dict.*] Aii[r] A BRIEFE DISCOURSE OF THE MEDICINE called Mithridatium [a 1 cit]

30. obscure [4b, 1757, Woolsey–Foote (1757)] D3[v] And where oftentimes many fumes doe ascend, by the which the animal spirits are obscured, the vse of *Mithridatium* doth dissipate, extenuate, & consume the same

31. opisthotonos [1657, *Phys. Dict.*] D6[r] [th]e paulsye, the crampe, [th]e diseases called *Tetanos Ambrostonos*, and *Opistetanos* [a 1 cit]

32. pamphlet [2, 1592, G. Harvey *3rd Lett. in Shaks.*] B3[v] as the same is expressed in the second booke ... that such as shall thinke better to follow the same, may by this pamphlet knowe the ingredience

33. paucity [2, 1650, Bulwer *Anthropomet.*] C8[r] I see no cause why we should not best allow of it made heere: neither ought [th]e paucitie which we do lacke, to draw vs better to esteeme of a forrayne medicine

34. prepared [b, 1663, Boyle] C3[v] *Andromachus* ... did adde vitreoll prepared

35. reaction [1, 1644, Digby *Nat. Bodies*] B4[v] those reactions not being infinite, at the last one forme and quality must result in the compound [a 1 cit]

36. remit [*v*, II, 6c, 1615] B6[v] *Opium* may remitte the whot qualities

37. security [2, 1597, A. M. *Guill. Fr. Chir.*] B8[r] with lesse danger and more security

38. stupefy [*v*, 1b, 1691, Hartcliffe, *Virtues*] B7[r] and being certaine [th]e *Opium* doth stupefy [a 1 cit]

39. stupefying [*ppl a*, 1611, Cotgrave *Noix Vomique*] B7[v] See **dormitory**, anted. [a 1 cit] [fpl]

40. substitute [*sb*, II, 5, 1589, Puttenham *Engl. Poesie*] C7[r] the simples wanting, are few in number: [th]e substitutes for the same ... so aptly appointed

41. substitute [*v*, 4, 1778, W. Marshal, *Min. Agric.*] C6[v] and in lacke of Cinnamum did sometimes substitute double qua[n]titie of Casia

42. supply [9b, 1650, *Hist. Tom Thumb*] Aviii[r] and required many supplyes, for simples vnknowen

43. ungrateful [*a*, 2b, 1597, Gerarde *Herbal*] C3[r] In smell it must rese[m]ble the simples ... a common odoure ... not peculier to any one, nor vngratefull, but answerable to the ingredience

2. *New senses*

1. alteration B4[v] And albeit these [simples] being contrary, and repugnant, do make alteration the one with the other

2. belk [not as *sb.*] D5[v] cureth euill belks, & inflacion of the stomacke
3. ceruse [not as *a*] C2[r] they are often corrupted with ledde, and gather a ceruse matter
4. compiled Avi[v] And it may be obiected, that in *Theriacle* co[m]piled by *Andromachus* are many simples added
5. express [*v*] C3[r] the taste must not expresse any one simple
6. fertill D6[r] it doth remedy [th]e barrenness in women, & maketh them fertill
7. sophisticated [not as *vbl sb*] C2[v] the good from the bad, the sophisticated from [th]e true

3. Unrecorded
1. ambrosostonos D6[r] See **opisthotonos**, anted.
2. enunce D2[v] *Galen* ... doth not particulerly expresse the properties of this medicine: but generally enunceth, that it doth good
3. exsist E1[v] that the spirites comforted, might the better exsist and the sooner expell the venyme
4. faba aegyptia D7[r] Massarius ... saith that *Faba Aegyptia* importeth a *scruple* and a half
5. inuenting [*sb*] Aiv[r] commendation for the inuenting and compounding of *Mithridatium*
6. michelty D7[r] the michelty or bigness of a beane of *Ægypt*

BAKER, GEORGE, *Oleum Magistrale*, 1574

1. Antedatings
1. abdomen [2, 1615, Crooke] Iii[r] Except it be in the muscles of *Abdomen*, which the Prince *Auicenna* calleth *Mirac*
2. above-mentioned [1707, Freind] Ci[r] See **experiment**, anted. [a 1 cit] [fpl]
3. accomplishing [*sb*, 1581, Marbecke] Miv[r] for the accomplishing of the whiche, you shall applye vpon the wound [a 1 cit]
4. acopon [1661, Lovell, R.] Kiii[r] your Unguents such as the Phisitions call *Acopa*, that is to say taking away of werines or pain [a 1 cit]
5. actually [3, 1587, Golding] Hi[r] you shall note then that the medicins whiche be applyed in wounds of *Nerues* ... ought to be actually hot
6. aerugo [1753, *Chambers's Cycl. Supp.*] Iiii[r] *Chalcitis* & *Erugo* if they be burnt: they haue lesse sharpnes in the[m] [a 1 cit]
7. afflicted [*ppl a*, 2, 1680-90, Temple, St. W.] Ei[v] First the hurted and afflicted partie must vse this Regiment folowing
8. agglutinate [2, 1620, Venner] Ii[v] with good and conuenient rowling the musculous parts may wel be agglutinated [a 1 cit]
9. amphora [2, 1607, Topsell *Ff. B.*] Riii[r] *Amphora* of the Italy measure, dooth contain 72. pound of Oile

10. amply [4, 1651, Hobbes *Lev.*] Gi^{v} the nature and facultye of Simples whiche is amply shewed in many good Bookes

11. anethinum [1700, Sedley *Past. Virg.*] Ri^{r} See **carnificative**, unrec. [a 1 cit]

12. angelical [2, 1577, *Bullinger's Decades*] Aii^{v} many famouse Cities ... whose edifices for magnificence might seem Angelicall

13. answerable [3b, 1580, Lyly] Biii^{v} Which woork ... although [not] answerable to your honours oppinion and expectation of me

14. apostemation [1578, Lyte] Miv^{r} to defend the parte afflicted from fluxions and Apostumation

15. application [1, 1632, Sanderson *Serm.*] Pii^{r} The fourth error touching the applications of the Træpans Terebelles

16. artificially [1b, 1586, Rogers, T.] Cii^{v} him that cureth artificially obseruing the learned method and order

17. asarin [1834, *Penny Cycl.*] Mi^{v} you shall vse ... *Oleum radicis ... Aggrestis, Asari* [*sic*] [a 1 cit]

18. attic [1, 1599, *Broughton's Lett.*] Hiiii^{v} *Arsenicum* which is called in the Attique tung *Arenicum* [a 1 cit]

19. bitterish [1605, Timme] Lii^{r} they haue a bitterish tast [a 1 cit]

20. bronchocele [1657, *Phys. Dict.*] Mii^{v} for Tumours of the Throte called of the greeks, *Bronchocilas* [a 1 cit]

21. bruised [1b, 1579, Langham *G. Health*] Fi^{v} you may purge the wound of Contusion or brused blood

22. bubonocele [1615, Crooke] Qii^{r} These [hernias] are vij kindes, that is *Enterocele*, otherwise called *Epiplocele*, or *Hernie Zirbale*, *Bubonocele* or *Hernie Inquinale* [a 1 cit]

23. carvy [1648, Digby, *Closet*] Ri^{r} Seeds and hearbs, as *Semen, anisi, Carui, Fœniculi* [a 1 cit]

24. catagmatic [A, 1684, *Bonet's Merc. Compit.*] Mii^{r} Another catagmatique medicin composed by Moschion [a 1 cit]

25. caustic [1, 1582, Hester, *Sec Ph.*] Oiii^{v} it is the moste surest way to mundifye the said Vlcers and to open the Nodes with a cawstick [a 1 cit]

26. cedron [1859, Marcy, *Pr. Trav.*] Fiiii^{v} Oile of *Cedron* is of a greater and more excellent vertue [a 1 cit]

27. chalcitis [1626, Bacon *Sylva*] Fiiii^{r} See **asia petra**, unrec. [a 1 cit]

28. chrysocolla [1, 1600, Holland *Livy*] Fiiii^{r} And next to this are placed *Spodium, Pompholix, Psoicum* & *Chrisocolla*, medicens of suttle substance [a 1 cit]

29. cicatrizing [*vbl sb*, 1607, Topsell *Ff. B.*] Gii^{v} then he thought best to vse moderate drying things without *Cicatrising* or skinning [a 1 cit]

30. cluttered [*ppl a*, 1, 1577, Holinshed, *England*] Giiii^{r} when it doth chau[n]ce [tha]t there remaineth any cluttered or congeled blood to be taken away out of the wound [a 1 cit]

31. communication [6b, 1715, Desaguliers *Fires Impr*] Miii^{r} and ofte[n]

times death by reason of the communication and consent that they [Nerves] haue with the Brain and other noble partes [a 1 cit]

32. compressor [b, 1870, T. Holmes *Sing.*] Niii^v The hand and the fingers must be situated half bowing and you shall put within the hand some round Ball or compressor [a 1 cit]

33. consistence [5, 1626, Bacon *Sylva*] Kiii^r the Pich dooth make the consistance of the *Cerot* [a 1 cit]

34. contraction [5b, 1871, Holmes T. *Sing.*] Miiii^v If ... there be any contraction of *Nerve* : you shall apply speedily hot seething Oil [a 1 cit]

35. convulsion [2a, 1585, Lloyd *Treas. Health*] Fiii^r many patients suffered bothe ... greeuous conuolsions and painful cramps [a 1 cit]

36. cooling [a, 1588, Shakespeare *Tit. A.*] Fiii^v at all times drying & cooling things ought to be vsed [a 1 cit]

37. croton [1751, Hill, and ns] Qiv^r we wil begin with the [Hernia] *Aquose*, whiche is no other thing then a certain watrish tumour of *Croton* [a 1 cit]

38. dartos [1634, Jonson T. *Parey's Chir.*] Qiv^r it may be contained between *Dartos* and *heritroides* and between *Dartos* & the *Scrotum* [a 1 cit]

39. defensative [1576, Baker *Jewell*] Gii^v the Tendones or Cordes are couered with the said *Nerues, Membrana* as defensatives [a 1 cit]

40. defluxion [2a, 1576, Lyte *Dodoens*] Nii^r any Oilly or greasy medicine ... relaxeth the substance of the Muscles ... by the which meanes it dooth make the place more apt to receive defluxions [a 1 cit]

41. degeneration [1, 1607, Topsell *Ff. B.*] Aiiii^r those same Lacedemonians which afterwards by degeneratio[n] were brought to the like thraldome

42. denervation [1657, Tomlinson *Renou's Disp.* and ns] Miv^v The wounds of the ioynts are for the moste parte mortall by reason of their deneruations or Tendones and membranes [a 1 cit]

43. desiccate [*v*, 1, 1575, Turberville *Faulconrie*] Piii^v This Vnguent dooth heat moderatly, attract and dissicate [a 1 cit]

44. diabotanum [1655, Phillips] Li^v Of medicines called Diabotanum, that is to say, made of herbes [a 1 cit]

45. dracunculus [3, 1706, Phillips (ed. Kersey)] Mi^v you shall vse strong Oile as *Oleum radicis, Ficus, Aggrestis, Brionie, Asari, Dracunculi, Aristolochiae* and *Panacis* [a 1 cit]

46. egyptian [A, 1, 1646, Crashaw *Delights*] Rii^r The *Attique* and *Egiptienne* is .16. vnces

47. ejaculatores [1727–51, *Chambers's Cycl.*] Ri^v the[m] which bring the Sperme to the neck of the bladder which is called *Eiaculatores* [a 1 cit]

48. elevator [2, 1879, *Syd. Soc. Lex.*] Pii^r before that you apply the *Træpan* ... it is better ... to vse other instrume[n]t[es] as Eleviatories, Cisers, *Lenticulj* [a 1 cit]

49. enterocele [1879, *New Syd. Soc. Lex.*] Qii^r See **bubonocele**, anted. [a 1 cit]

50. entertain [*v*, 1579, Fenton *Quicciaid*] Bii^v the[m] which your honor hath entertai[n]ed into your seruice [a 1 cit]

51. epiplocele [1721, Bailey *Epiplocele*] Qii^{r} See **bubonocele**, anted. [a 1 cit]
52. experiment [1b, 1586, Cogan *H. H.*] Ci^{r} such learned iudgement as procedeth by discretion and certain knowledge of the iudications abooue mentioned, and afterwards maketh apt choise of experiments
53. fatherly [2a, 1577, Northbrooke *Dicing*] Biii^{v} one small work of the fatherly both Phisition and Chirurgion Galen
54. femur [1, 1799, *Med. Jnl.*] Niv^{r} If the wound be in the Hip, you shall vse such order that the *Os femar*, doo not come out of his place
55. folium [1848, Price, B.] Liv^{r} medicines whiche haue a mene astrictio[n] with resolute vertue and without biting as ... *Folium Malabathri* [a 1 cit]
56. foment [*v*, 1, 1611, Cotgrave] Fiii^{r} And if there chaunced any inflamation: then they fomented the afflicted place with hot water [a 1 cit]
57. fraxin [1864, Watts *Dict. Chem.*] Oii^{v} you shal vse of *Fraximus*, the which openeth obstructions of the Liuer [a 1 cit]
58. glutination [1, 1607, Topsell *Ff. B.*] Niii^{r} the glutination and consolidation shall the better and sooner be doon [a 1 cit]
59. glutinative [*a*, A, 1578, Lyte *Dodoens*] Nii^{r} the medicines ... must be dessicatiue and astringant as this ... which is bothe astringant, dessicatiue and glutinative [a 1 cit]
60. griper [2, 1587, Harrison *England*] Piv^{r} but like greedy gripers catch what they may
61. gurgling [*sb*, 1814, Southey] Qii^{v} and in the redusing you shall hear a gurguling or noise [a 1 cit]
62. hemina [1601, Holland *Pliny*] Riii^{v} The *Hemine* is of Wine and Vinagre 10. vnces of Oile 9. vnces, and of Hunny 1. pound [a 1 cit]
63. heroical [1b, 1599, Shakespeare *H5*] Bii^{r} one espetial signe of your honours heroicall minde
64. hot [*a*, 11e, 1618, Bolton *Florino*] Qi^{r} see how long any of these cutters doo tarry in a place, some a quarter of a yeere, some half, and none scant a yeer, for it wil bee to hot for them
65. hurted [1643, Steer *Exper. Chyrurg.*] Ei^{v} the hurted and afflicted partie [a 1 cit]
66. hydrocele [1597, A. M. *Guill.*] Qii^{r} the first is called *Hernie Aqueuse* and of [th]e Greeks *Hidrocele*, the second *hernie charneuse* or *Sarcocele*, the third: *Variquese*, the fourth *Venteuse*, which is called of the Greeks *Pneumatocele*, [th]e fifth *Humorale* [a 1 cit]
67. id est [1598, Florio] Fiiii^{r} some be very suttle as *Aphronitiu[m] id est* Nitrispuma, the frothy parte of *Nitrum* [a 1 cit]
68. intestine [1a, 1597, A. M. *Guill.*] Qii^{r} See **scrotum**, anted.
69. introduction [1, 1651, Hobbes *Lev.*] Riii^{r} Scrupple is as it were the beginning of all waights as an introduction
70. islandish [1577, Dee *Gen & rare*] Aiii^{r} in his co[n]quest of those Ilandish Cuntreyes [a 1 cit]
71. judication [1625, Hart *Anat. Ur.*] Ci^{r} method ... proceedeth a sure way taking iudications of the complexion of the body [a 1 cit]

72. lacedemonian [*sb*, B, 1870, Emerson *Soc & Solit*] Aiii^{r} those same Lacedemonians which afterwards by degeneratio[n]s were brought to the like thraldome [a 1 cit]
73. lenticular [B, 1658, J. S. tr. Le Dran's *Obs. Surg.*] Pii^{r} See **elevator,** anted. [a 1 cit]
74. licentiously [2, 1581, Savile *Tacitus Hist.*] Aiv^{v} eche ma[n] accou[n]ted that libertie to doo what liked him, to liue riotously and licentiously
75. lixivium [1612, Woodall *Surg. Mate*] Fiiii^{v} the licour or water of *lixivii* whiche the *Greeks* call *Stacta* [a 1 cit]
76. lues [1634, Herbert, Sir. T. *Trav.*] Oi^{r} the dissease called in Latin, *Lues Venerea* [a 1 cit]
77. membrane [1a, 1615, Crooke] Gii^{v} See **defensative**, anted.
78. mesopleuron [1848, Maunder, *Treas. Nat. Hist.*] Pi^{v} you shall doo it ... very gentely in cutting *Mesopleuria* or [th]e muscles between the ribs [a 1 cit]
79. methodical [*a*, 1, 1597, A. M. *Guill.*] Niii^{r} For the which cause the *Methodicall* Chirurgian, must haue a great respect to these wounds
80. misy [2, 1601, Holland *Pliny*] Fiiii^{r} See **asia petra**, unrec. [a 1 cit]
81. mithridatum [1603, Dekker *Wonderful Yeare*] Oiii^{v} ad thereto of fine Treacle or *Mithridatum* [a 1 cit]
82. mollifying [*ppl a*, 1590, Barrough *Meth. P.*] Oii^{r} you shall apply continually mollifying & drawing medicines [a 1 cit]
83. morisco [B, 1, 1629, Wadsworth *Pilgr.*] Civ^{r} In the Realme of Spain there inhabyted a people called in the Spanish tung *Moriscus*
84. mucilage [2, 1600, Surflet *Country Farm*] Nii^{v} So that the excrements whiche doo avoid is a glittig *Musceledge*, thin or watrish humor, which dooth commonly folow in these kindes of wounds
85. naked [2c, 1599, Shakespeare *H5*] Cii^{r} See **particularity,** anted.
86. noble [7c, 1632, Sherwood] Oiii^{r} the Region of the hart, and other noble partes
87. node [3a, 1610, Healey *Theophr.*] Oiii^{r} the vlcers be made clean or the Nodes taken away
88. outbreathing [*vbl sb*, 1831, Houghton, Ld. *Mem.*] Giii^{v} the colde dooth stop and hinder outbreathing of the member [a 1 cit]
89. oxoleon [1699, Evelyn *Acetaria*] Hi^{r} the Vinagre must be very sharp wherwith the *Oxelam* is made [a 1 cit]
90. oxybaphon [1850, Leitch tr. C. O. *Müller's Anc. Art.*] Riii^{v} The *Oxibaphus* is of Wine and Vinagre 18. Drams [a 1 cit]
91. panacea [2, 1590, Spenser *FQ*] Kiv^{r} See **serapion**, unrec.
92. paracelsist [B, 1625, Hart *Anat Ur.*] Cii^{r} great harme ... dayly is committed by the Paracellistes [*sic*] [a 1 cit]
93. particularity [1b, 1593, Shakespeare *2H6*] Cii^{r} For sithens experie[n]ce is but the observation or remembrance of the successe had in particuler things ... and ... neither art nor science consisted in particularities: it must needs folow [tha]t naked experience maketh no art

94. pastil [1, 1616, Jonson, B. *Devil*] Iiii^{r} See **andronis**, unrec. [a 1 cit]
95. peculiar [A, 3, 1590, Smyth, Sir. J. *Disc. Weapons*] Ciii^{r} places whiche require a peculter [*sic*] & distinct method & order of cure [a 1 cit]
96. periosteum [*a*, 1597, A. M. *Guill.*] Miii^{v} And so it is with the *Periosten, pericranium* and membranes [a 1 cit]
97. pneumatocele [1693, *Blancard's Phys. Dict.*] Qii^{r} See **hydrocele**, anted. [a 1 cit]
98. pompholyx [1, 1678, Phillips (ed. 4)] Liiii ^{r} *Pompholigoes* washed [a 1 cit]
99. quadrant [3, 1601, Holland *Pliny*] Rii^{v} *Quadrans* is the 4. parte of a pound
100. quenched [II, 6c, 1814, Byron *Lara*] Hiiii^{v} (margin) Quenched lime [a 1 cit]
101. radix [7, 1727–41, Chambers's *Cycl.*] Oii^{v} the *Radix chini* beeing a root very deer [a 1 cit]
102. raphanus [1730–6, Bailey] Kiiii^{v} if it be in *Alexandria*, you shall take *Oleum Recinum* and *Raphaninum* [a 1 cit]
103. reduce [17a, 1605, Timme *Q.*] Iiii^{r} others may be beaten and redused into poulder
104. relaxation [3, 1626, Bacon *Sylva*] Piv^{r} Hernies in childre[n] which came by the relaxasion … of *Peretoneu[m]*
105. resolute [14, 1607, Topsell *Ff. B.*] Liiii^{r} it is conuenient to vse medicines whiche haue a mene astrictio[n] with resolute vertue and without biting
106. revulsive [B, 1661, Fell, J. *Life Hammond*] Piii^{r} vse *Hebetonice Reuolsiue* or according to the cause of the greef [a 1 cit]
107. rhagades [1601, Holland *Pliny*] Mii^{v} for *Rhagadies*, for Tumours [a 1 cit]
108. ruptor [1656, Blount] Piii^{v} cutters for the stone and Ruptors [a 1 cit]
109. ruta [1800 Turk] Ri^{r} See **agnicasty**, unrec. [a 1 cit]
110. sagapenum [1579, Langham *Gard. Health*] Fiiii^{r} *Sagapenum* of the East [a 1 cit]
111. sapa [1624, Middleton *Game Ch.*] Gii^{v} he vsed *Trosis* dissolued in *Sapa* [a 1 cit]
112. sarcocele [1742, *Heister's Surg.*] Qii^{r} See **hydrocele**, anted. [a 1 cit]
113. scrotum [1597, A. M. *Guill.*] Qii^{r} no other then a certain descending down of the *Intestines* in *Scrotum* [a 1 cit]
114. slicked [1594, O. B. *Quest. P. C.*] Ri^{r} glistereth like vnto a slikt paper
115. solutive [B, 1, 1605, Timme *Q.*] Oii^{r} the solutiues may the better work vpon the aforesaid humors
116. spectacle [II, 5c, 1581, Wilkinson W. *Confut. Fam. L.*] Aii^{v} yea was not Grecia the Theatre, Spectacle and light of the whole world?
117. spermatic vessel [6, 1690, Maidment *Bk. Sc. Pasq.*] Qiv^{r} See **heritroides**, unrec.

118. state [7, 1607, Topsell *Ff. B.*] Gi^{r} See **declination,** ns.
119. straining [*vbl sb*, 4b, 1580, Blundevil, *Curing Horses*] Ei^{r} strain it, and to the strayning: put … good *Venice* Turpentine
120. succus [1719, Quincy *Lex. Physico-Med.*] Fiiii^{r} These medicens that are heer rehersed are of a thin suttle substance … as *Succus cerenæus, Succus medicus* [a 1 cit]
121. sulphur [1c, 1867, *Chambers's Encycl.*] Hiiii^{r} *Sulphur Viuum* is very good in these afore said compositio[n]s
122. tent [v^4, a, 1597, A. M. *Guill.*] Fi^{v} you shall tent bothe sides of the wound [a 1 cit]
123. terebinthine [*sb*, B, 2, 1578, Lyte *Dod.*] Iiv^{v} liquid Pich, whiche some merchants and Factors sel for *Terebenthine* [a 1 cit]
124. terrene [2, 1601, Holland *Pliny*] Iii^{v} all metalls are partly of groce and terrene substa[n]ce
125. tetrapharmacum [1727–41, *Chambers's Cycl.*] Hiiii^{r} mingled with *Tetrapharmacum* [a 1 cit]
126. theatre [6, 1581, *Confer II*] Aii^{v} See **spectacle,** anted.
127. tributory [*sb*, 1585, Washington, T. *Nict. Voy.*] Aiii^{r} the Spartanes consented not therto nor would become tributoryes [a 1 cit]
128. trigon [4, 1835, Kirby *Hab & Inst.*] Mii^{r} the venimouse fish called in Greek *Trigon Thalassia*
129. uncia [1, 1695, *Plut. Trans.*] Rii^{v} *Unsia* is to say an vnce [a 1 cit]
130. unclarified [*ppl a*, 1591, Percivall *Sp. Dict.*] Hiii^{r} that which is brought in erthen pots, which is vnclarified [a 1 cit]
131. unction [4, 1580, Hester *Fiori*] Gii^{v} applyed it in [th]e foresaid *Neruous* parte, & made particuler vnction
132. unequable [1692, Bentley *Boyle Lect.*] Qiv^{v} the signes are an vnequable hardenes, and inflation [a 1 cit]
133. unequal [3b, 1591, Fletcher, G. *Russe Com.*] Qiv^{v} with pain beeing vnequall and not euen
134. venerean [2b, 1612, Chapman *Wid. T.*] Oi^{r} The errors which be vsed at this present (touching the *Venerian* dissease) are very great

2. *New senses*

1. abrogate Bi^{r} how pernitious a thing it is to abrogate good lawes
2. cedrine Fiiii^{r} See **succus laurinus**, unrec.
3. contusion Fi^{v} See **bruised**, anted.
4. croton Qiv^{r} we wil begin with the [Hernia] *Aquose*, whiche is no other thing then a certain watrish tumor of *Croton*
5. declination Gi^{r} The parfit knoweledge of Simples is in three thinges, that is to say, of plants, of metalles, and of liuing things, and it is not sufficient to see them once or twise: but you must marke and beholde them often, as in their beginning, growing, state, and declination
6. denarius Rii^{v} *Denarius* or *Drachma* is the 8. parte of an vnce and is 3. Scrupples

7. denervation Miv^v The wounds of the ioynts are for the moste parte mortall by reason of their deneruations or Tendones and membranes
8. folium Liv^r medicines whiche haue a mene astrictio[n] with resolute vertue and without biting as ... *Folium Malabathri*
9. liquid *v*, Hii^v you shall take of the best wax, liquid it in Oile
10. must *sb*, Iiii^r *Sapa* is made of *Must*, that is to say sodden Wine
11. potential Nii^v although they be potentiall hot
12. quincunx Rii^v *Quincunx* is 5. vnces
13. renegate Piv^r these that bee Runnagates (for so may I wel terme them)
14. sextant Rii^v *Sextans* is the 6. part of a pound
15. urn Riii^r The *Vrne* is of wine & vinagre 40. l

3. Unrecorded

1. abiotina Hiii^r Turpentine wil remain moste liquid, the other dooth soon dry, as *Strobolina* and *Abiotina*
2. aeris squama Iii^v the abstersives, as *Aeris squama*
3. aggrestis Mi^v See **asarin**, anted.
4. agnicasty Ri^r there may be added to of Seeds and hearbes, as *Semen, anisi, Carui, Fœniculi, Agnicasti, Ruta*
5. amaricum Kiv^v they must be liquified with some kinde of Oil, or resolutiue Vnquent, namely *Amaricum* and *Oppobalsamum*
6. andronis Iiii^r The Pastils or *Trocis* of *Andronis Poluidas* and *Pacion*, be right excellent
7. asia petra Fiiii^r Like wise these are suttle, *Nitrum beronicum* and *Asia Petra* ... Of metalls *Lorpin* and *Sulphur* be both suttle and hot. After these *Misy, verdigrece* and *Chalcitis* ... be very hot
8. betonicum litrum Hiiii^r *Sulphur Viuum* ... may be vsed with Tetrapharmacu[m]. Also *Aphronitrum* may be vsed and *Beronictum litrum* [*sic*]
9. bis Qii^r *Bis* is 2. third partes which is 8. vnces and 240. Scrupples
10. carnificative *sb*, Ri^r This is to be cured with *Carnificatives* as *Oleum nucum, Oleum Anethinum, Costinum &c*
11. cataplasmus Fii^r they ... applyed *Cataplasmus* of whete meale
12. ceranium Qiii^r The *Ceranium* is of Wine and Vinagre 80. pound, and of Oile 72. pound, and of Hunny 120. pound
13. cerapion Kiiii^r There are also simples [tha]t wil aswel dissolue without fire as with fire, in most things as *Gutta Aminoniaci*, [th]e licour of *Sagapeni, Panacis, Cerapion* and *Oppoponax*
14. chalces Riii^r Scrupple is ... 2. *Obloes*, an *Obloes* is 2. *Siliques*, and a *Silique* 2. *Chalces*, & the *Chalces* is 8. graines
15. characias Fiiii^v The best of [th]e said *Tithimales* is [tha]t which the Greeks call *Characias*, which is the male & the greatest moouer
16. cheme Riii^v The *Cheme* is of Wine & Vinagre 3. Drams and one Scrupple and of Oile 3. Drams, and of Hunny 5. Drams
17. cicamini Mii^v then ye shall take the licour of *Cicamini*
18. cicatrasatise Giii^r consequently when *Galene* had thus vsed it [the med-

icine]: the[n] he came to *sicatrasatises* and for the outwarde parte he applyed *Euphorbium* mingled with Wax & *Rosin* in forme of an Emplaister

19. ciprinum Kiiii^v in sted of these *Susinum* and *Ciprinum*

20. ciroene Hii^v For to make Emplastrum Carotodes. That is to say a Cerat or Ciroene

21. comagenum Kiiii^v Then afterwards with Irinum and *Comagenum*, and in sted of these *Susinum* and *Ciprinum*

22. costinum Ri^r See **carnificative**, unrec.

23. cotile Qiii^v The *Cotile* is of Wine and Vinagre 18. Drams, of Oile 18 Drams, and of Hunny 27. Drams

24. deunx Rii^v *Deunx* is 11. vnces, which are .264. Scrupples

25. dextans Rii^v *Dextans* is the half and the third part of a pound, that is to say 10. vnces and 240. Scrupples

26. diaeuphorbium Kii^r The medicine which is called Dieuphorbium

27. diasteaton Kii^r the whiche *Cerot* shalbe proffitable for many purposes, and is called *Diasteaton*, that is to say made with Talow and greace

28. dodrans Rii^v *Dodrans* is the half and one quarter of a pound, which is 230. Scrupples

29. epigoni Gii^v the green Plaister of *Epigoni*, which the Greeks call *Isis*

30. erineon Fiiii^v a wilde Figge tree, whiche the *Greeks* call *Erineon*

31. ervus Fiii^v The Corne which the Greeks call *Sitera* that is to say Whete, and *Eruus* or *Orobus* is the moste suttelest

32. fæniculi Ri^r See **agnicasty**, unrec.

33. fricta Hii^v Of the dryest of these kindes [of Rosin] is that whiche some call *Fricta*, and others *Colophonia*

34. hebetonice Piii^r if the strength of the patient be good … vse *Hebetonice Reuolsiue*

35. heritroides Qiv^r a certain watrish tumor of *Croton* increased by little and little, & for the most part lies between *heritroides* and [th]e Spermatike vessels

36. hernia aquosa Piii^v vnder this cure of cutting the *Hernyes* they doo miserably take away the stone aswell in the *Hernia aquosa* or *ventosa* as in all the rest

37. hernia charneuse Qii^r See **hydrocele**, anted.

38. hernia humorale Qii^r See **hydrocele**, anted.

39. hernia inquinale Qii^r See **bubonocele**, anted.

40. hernia intestinale Piv^r he may see what kinde of *Hernies* they haue, and so … discerne the *Aquosa* or *Ventosa*, from *Intestinale* or *Omentales*

41. hernia omentale Piv^r See **hernia intestinale**, unrec.

42. hernia variquese Qii^r See **hydrocele**, anted.

43. hernia venteuse Qii^r See **hydrocele**, anted.

44. hernia ventosa Piii^v See **hernia aquosa**, unrec.

45. hernia zirbale Qii^r these are vii kind[es], that is *Enterocele* otherwise called *Hernie Intestinale, Epiplocele* or *Hernie Zirbale, Bubonocele* or *Hernie Inguinale*

46. homotribes Iiv^{r} Wherefore new Oil which the Greeks call *Homotribes*, is neither good nor conuenient
47. irinum Kiv^{v} See **comagenum**, unrec.
48. isis Gii^{v} See **epigoni**, unrec.
49. lorpin Fiiii^{r} See **asia petra**, unrec.
50. lues venerea Oi^{r} See **lues**, anted.
51. malus terrae Lii^{r} those herbes which were of a suttle substance, that is to wit of *Dictamus, Amaracus*, and *Malus terrae*, whiche is *Aristolochiae*
52. mirespice Liv^{r} the *Cerot* which the Greeks call *Mirespice*
53. nitrispuma Fiiii^{r} See **id est**, anted.
54. nitrum betonicum Fiiii^{r} See **asia petra**, unrec.
55. oleum Ri^{r} See **carnificative**, unrec.
56. oleum anethinum Ri^{r} See **carnificative**, unrec.
57. oleum costinum Ri^{r} See **carnificative**, unrec.
58. oleum magistrale (title page) the moste excellent and pretious Oil called *Oleum Magistrale*
59. oleum nucum Ri^{r} See **carnificative**, unrec.
60. oleum radicis Mi^{v} See **asarin**, anted.
61. oleum recinum Kiiii^{v} See **raphanus**, anted.
62. oleum sinapinum Kiiii^{v} But there is not to be found *Oleum sinapinum*
63. ossa pubis Ri^{v} which is called *Eiaculatores* ... the which goes vp to *Osepubis*
64. pacion Iiii^{r} See **andronis**, unrec.
65. phuliatum Liv^{r} See **pompholigo**, unrec.
66. politeleis Lii^{v} Compositio[n]s for wou[n]ds of the *Nerues*, which the Greeks call *Politeleis*, that is to say sumpteous
67. polvidas Iiii^{r} See **andronis**, unrec.
68. pompholigo Liv^{r} the Vnguents whiche the *Romains* call *Vnguentum spicatum*, and *Phuliatum*, in adding to the xij. part of *Pompholigoes* washed, which must be prepared with *Terrhenique*, Wax, and burnt *Nardus*
69. præcipitatum Oiii^{r} pledgets with *Basilicon* and *Præcipitatum* mingled together
70. preparans Ri^{v} The Spermatike vessels, as well they whiche bring the substance where with the Sperme is made which are named *Preparans*
71. psoicum Fiiii^{r} See **chrysocolla**, anted.
72. pultasis Giiii^{v} The Floures that are to be vsed to make *Pultasi*
73. resolutive Nii^{v} filled with some resolutive medicin
74. sanguis draconis Ei^{r} Sanguis draconis, one vnce
75. selibra Rii^{v} *Selibra* is half a pound or *Semis*, and 144. Scrupples
76. semis Rii^{v} See **selibra**, unrec.
77. sextunx Rii^{v} *Sextunx* is 1. half and 1. twelf parte that is 7. vnces and 168. Scrupples
78. silique Riii^{r} An Oboles is 2 Siliques
79. sinope Miii^{r} accident[es] ... as pain, vehement fluxion, inflamation, Feuer, losse of reason, *Sinope*

80. **siriphian** Bi^v no barbarous Siriphian may vpbraid your honor
81. **sitera** Fiiii^v See **ervus**, unrec.
82. **stacta** Fiiii^v licour or water of *Lixiuii* whiche the Greeks call *Stacta*
83. **strobolina** Hiii^r See **abiotina**, unrec.
84. **succus cedrinus** Fiiii^r See **succus laurinus**, unrec.
85. **succus cerenæus** Fiiii^r These medicens ... are of a thin suttle substance [*sic*] ... as *Succus cerenæus, Succus medicus*
86. **succus laurinus** Fiiii^r And of the like qualities are *Succus laurinus* and *Cedrinus*
87. **succus medicus** Fiiii^r See **succus cerenæus**, unrec.
88. **susinum** Kiv^v See **comagenum**, unrec.
89. **trosis** Gii^v See **sapa**, anted.
90. **tyrrhenique** Liii^v *Tryrrhenique Wax*
91. **zirbus** Qii^r The Intestines or *Zirbus*

4. Postdatings

1. **bursting** [*sb*, 2, 1544, Phaer] Qi^v I wil write all the kindes of *Ruptures* or burstings and how to knowe euery one of them
2. **conge** [1420, *Pallad on Husb.*] Riii^v The *Conge* is of Wine and Vinagre 10. pound, of Oil 9. pound, and of Hunny 15. pound
3. **mitigative** [B, 1530, *Remedy of Love*] Diii^r an approoued *Mitigatiue* or appeaser of pain
4. **zirbale** [1547, Borde] Qii^r See **bubonocele**, anted.

BANISTER, JOHN, *The historie of man*, 1578

1. Antedatings

1. **abdomen** [2, 1615, Crooke] Siii^v begynyng first somewhat further of with the partes of *abdomen*
2. **abort** [1621, Burton] Fii^r See **extract**, *v*, 3a, anted. [a 1 cit]
3. **abrase** [1593, Nashe] Ci^v which Membrane ... once abraced, or taken off fro[m] the bone [a 1 cit]
4. **acetable** [2, 1648, *Bonet*'s] Cii^v (margin) What is the *Acetable*
5. **acetabulum** [2b, 1709, Blair] Cii^v A deepe hole, or cauitie therfore, you shall call after the Latins, *Acetabulum*
6. **action** [6c, 1845, *Lond. Univ. Col.*] Ciii^v the more manifest motio[n] in *Arthrodia*, shalbe attributed for a kynde of *Diarthrosis*, & the obscure action, to *Synarthrosis*
7. **active** [5, 1597, Shakespeare] Li^v so doth it serue as the turne of a Ligament, and much auayle to the actiue mouyng of the ioynte
8. **acuminate** [1, 1646, Browne] Dii^r So *Pericles* ... his head ... being more long, and accuminate [a 1 cit]
9. **acuminated** [*ppl a*, 1, 1611, Coryat] Dii^r a sharpe or accuminated figure of the head [a 1 cit]

10. adherent [A, 1, 1615, Sandys] Diiii^{r} And for that these bones do represent scales, to the sides of other bones (to make vp the inclosure) adherent, they haue no other nomination than, *Ossa Squammosa*
11. admission [1, 1622, Bacon] Xiii^{r} whiche was necessary there to be deuided for the admission of the vmbellicall veyne
12. admit [4, 1661, Dryden] Eiiii^{r} The fourth bone of the upper iawe ... occupyeng no small scope, admitteth the distinction of that Suture, which we haue named to cut the Palate ouerthwartly
13. admit [II, 3, 1703, Maundrell] Fiii^{v} the whiche hole is produced into two sharpe corners, admittyng together with a *Veyne* and *Arterie*, a portion of the fourth co[n]iugation of Nerues
14. adnate [2, 1661, Lovell] Ffiii^{r} to speake of the manifold Membranes of the eyes ... The first ... hath many names, as all these, *Adnata, alba, Adhærens, and coniunctiua* [a 1 cit]
15. aegilops [1, 1601, Holland] Eiii^{v} where the disease called *Aegilopa* chaunceth [a 1 cit]
16. affect [v^{2}, 1, 1606, Shakespeare] Xi^{v} Somewhiles in deede it so affecteth the ventricle, as that the patient oft falleth into defect of mynde [a 1 cit]
17. affect [*v*, 5, 1605, Shakespeare] Aii^{v} For if so we be affected, that euery one may catch vnto himself, and hide from others, there is loue broken, then is humane societie buried
18. affected [III, 1, 1619, Donne] Aiiii^{r} meanes to cure the affected partes of the bodie
19. affirmation [4, 1593, H. Smith] Ui^{v} *Galen* before him also made the like affirmation
20. affixed [*ppl a*, 1651, *Life of F. Sarpi*] Hii^{v} At the sides ... are affixed and knit the prominent partes of *Os Ilium*
21. afore-going [afore, D, 1b, 1592, Junius] Qii^{v} It is not obscurely proued by this afore goyng, that the noblenes, and worthy nature of this Muscle may euill be spared in mans bodie [fpl]
22. aforenamed [afore, D, 1b, 1603, Knolles] Eiii^{r} as saith the aforenamed Authour [fpl]
23. agglutination [4, 1615, Crooke] Ei^{r} the bones of the temples, which, in their vpper part ... are equally circumscribed with scalie *Agglutinations*
24. alienate [*ppl a*, 2, 1599, A. M. *Gab.*] Hiiii^{v} much alienate from the naturall construction of the same in mankynd
25. alligate [*v*, 1626, Cockeram] Hiiii^{r} the *Ligamentes* wherby they are alligated to the *Vertebres* [a 1 cit]
26. allure [3, 1612, Drayton] Aai^{v} and this the splene allureth, and draweth vnto him by the trunke of *Vena Porta*
27. alterative [*a*, 1, 1605, Bacon] Uiii^{r} engendryng in it selfe the alterative facultie [a 1 cit]
28. ammission [1623, Ailesbury] Hhi^{v} in that parte shall neither continue ammision of sense, nor mouyng [a 1 cit]

29. ample [2, 1596, Spenser] Giii^{r} nature hath insculped the large and ample hole for the descense ... of the *Spinall* marey
30. amplify [2, 1580, North] Yii^{r} beyng amplified and cut into braunches
31. amplitude [1, 1599, Nashe] Gi^{r} two *Processes* which nature decreed to ... shut the amplitude of *Larinx*, and way of the rough *Arterie*, lest any thyng ... should slippe into the inner capacitie therof
32. anastomosis [1615, Crooke] Bbii^{r} The right veyne, and arterie ... being together, after a space, so contingent, and mutually growing together, as that most elegantly this word of the *Grecians Anastomosis* may be to them applyed [a 1 cit]
33. anatomical [1, 1585, T. B.] Dii^{v} the Assertio[n]s of *Realdus Collumbus* ... in matters *Anathomicall*, not meanly experienced [a 1 cit]
34. anatomist [B, 1594, T. B. *La Prim*] tp The Historie of Man, sucked from the sappe of the most approued Anathomistes, in this present age
35. ancyroid [1706, Phillips] Ii^{v} One of them compared to a Crowes beke, or anker, is therefore called *Ancryoides* or *Coracoides* [a 1 cit]
36. anfractuous [1621, Burton] Ei^{v} See **stonylike**, unrec. [a 1 cit]
37. anfractuouse [1, 1691, Ray] Uiiii^{r} such anfractuous foldes
38. angina [1, 1590, *Pasquils Apol.*] Yi^{v} This veyne the Phisitions commaund to be opened in the disease called *Angina* [a 1 cit]
39. angular [1, 1598, Florio] Ki^{r} fastened to the angular bosome of the *Postbrachiall* bones [a 1 cit]
40. angular [2, 1597, J. King] Gii^{r} the *Spinall* marey could not endure euery angular flexion [a 1 cit]
41. annex [*v*, II, 2, 1605, Bacon] Cii^{r} And those *Particles* so annexed to the bones, are called *Appendances*
42. annular [2, 1691, Ray] Pii^{r} Of these ix. muscles the ij first go forth from the *Anular* bone
43. answerable [3b, 1580, Lyly] Liii^{r} the first part, which immediately succeedeth the legge and Fibula, beyng called Tarsus, is aunswerable to the wrest of the hand
44. answerable [4b, 1617, J. Taylor] Cii^{v} as the fashion of the heades of the Processes, are diuersified accordyng to the places, so the hollowes that receiue them, must of necessitie also be diuers and different, euer answerable to their proportio[n]s
45. anterior [1, 1611, Cotgrave] Ciii^{r} the bone may not be suffered to moue: as appereth by the *Cauities* of the arme, that is, the *Anterior* corner admitting th[e] first *process* of the *Cubite* [a 1 cit]
46. aorta [1594, T. B.] Ii^{r} about the rootes of *Arteria aorta* [a 1 cit]
47. appellation [II, 3, 1581, Campion] Hiiii^{v} a *Cartilage*, which hath to name by propper appellation from the Latins, *mucronata Cartilago*
48. application [2, 1601, Shakespeare] Hhiii^{r} (margin) A *caveat* for the applicatio[n] of cauterie to the legge
49. application [6, 1605, Bacon] Sii^{v} the good successe of such cures, pur-

chased more by the benefit of nature, then their rare experience, or singular application

50. **apposition** [4, 1606, Carleton] Ciiii^{v} Either els the vnion, is made, by the apposition of fleshe, therfore by the Greeke name, *Syssarcosis*

51. **apprehension** [I, 1, 1646, Browne] Kiii^{r} Generall differences of Apprehension are v

52. **appropinquate** [1, 1623, Cockeram] Kii^{v} it behoveth vs now to appropinquate, and touch the effect [a 1 cit]

53. **aptly** [1, 1597, Morley] Ciiii^{r} Much more aptly is the obscure *Arthrodia* expressed, by the three bones of Tarsus, ioyned with the shiplike bone, & the bone *Cyboides*

54. **aqueous** [1b, 1643, Herle] Ffiiii^{r} that humour ... which is called *Aqueous* or watrishe, of *Galen Alluginius* [a 1 cit]

55. **arabia** [1711, Pope] Yiiii^{v} others of that *Arabia* sect [a 1 cit]

56. **arachnoides** [B, *sb*, 1751, *Chamb. Cycl.*] Ffiii^{v} The first Membran, called /S/αϱαξυοειδησ/S/ [a 1 cit]

57. **arbitrarious** [1642, H. More] Ggiii^{r} all the partes of the body vnder the head ... should haue bene destitute of arbitrarious mouiynge [a 1 cit]

58. **arterious** [1634, T. Johnson] Ddi^{v} The same *Vena caua*, not consistyng of any strong or arterious body, should greatly haue bene dangered [a 1 cit]

59. **arthrodia** [1634, T. Johnson] Ciii^{v} See **enarthrosis**, anted. [a 1 cit]

60. **articulate** [*a*, A, 1, 1610, Healey] Giii^{r} *Occiput* is *Articulate* vnto the ij. first *Vertebres*

61. **articulate** [*v*, 3, 1832, Lyell] Iii^{v} and be neuer the fitter to *Articulate* with their places

62. **articulate** [*v*, 1, 1616, Surflet and Markham] Ciii^{v} th[e] bone of the thighe, *Articulated* to the hippe

63. **articulation** [1, 1597, Lowe] Ciii^{v} See **explicate**, 6, anted. [a 1 cit]

64. **articulus** [1877, Huxley] Ciii^{v} *Hipocrates* esteemed simply the rou[n]d part of that bone, that entred into th[e] hollow of another, to be *Articulus* & so called it [a 1 cit]

65. **artificer** [3b, 1659, Pearson] Miii^{r} most sapiently hath the diuine artificer decreed this part

66. **artificially** [2b, 1708, Chamberlayne] Ggiii^{r} The first payre, therfore of these Nerues is sent forth betwene the bone of the hinder part of the head, and the first *Vertebre* of the necke, so priuely, and artificially

67. **artist** [I, 3a, 1592, Chettle] Bi^{r} honest Artistes, and professours of Chirurgerie [a 1 cit]

68. **arytenoid** [B, 1691, Ray] Pii^{r} the fourth muscles ... are entred into the sayd bones, which construe, and make *Aritenoides* [a 1 cit]

69. **ascendent** [A, 1a, 1591, Greene] Dii^{v} since to the brayne many vapors and excrementes are continually ascendent

70. **ascendent** [A, 1b, 1611, Cotgrave] Giii^{r} propper cauities of the first

Vertebre, made in the vpper part & middle seate of the ascendent *Processes* therof
71. aspect [*v*, 2, 1610, Gwillim] Giii^{v} ascendent *Processes* ... directly aspectyng the laterall *Processes*, haue through them flowyng the distinct number of coniugated *Nerues* from the same *Spinall* marey produced
72. aspect [*v*, 5, 1635, Person] Iii^{v} the same bones, inwardly aspectyng
73. assident [B, 1753, *Chamb. Cycl.*] Ti^{v} two litle thicke *Glandules* called *Parastates* and *Assidentes* [a 1 cit]
74. assimulate [1630, J. Taylor] Eiiii^{r} part of the bone that assimulateth a searse [a 1 cit]
75. attenuated [1, 1677, Plot] Kiiii^{r} beyng thinner both aboue and beneth ... the nearer towardes their middest, are the more also attenuated [a 1 cit]
76. attical [1660, Hammond] Dii^{r} the Atticall Poetes [a 1 cit]
77. attractive [4, 1603, Holland] Ui^{v} naturall vertues ... as attractiue, retentiue, concoctiue, and expulsiue
78. auditor [4, 1640, Bp. Reynolds] Aiiii^{r} the testimonie of a cleare conscience, before the highest Auditor
79. auricle [3, 1664 Power] Cci^{r} the coronall Veyne, neare adioyning to the right auricle [a 1 cit]
80. auricula [1, 1691, Ray] Ffi^{v} The eares ... of which the outward partes are called *Auricula* [a 1 cit]
81. axillary [1, 1615, Crooke] Ti^{v} Vena caua is deuided into two, that is, *Axillarie* and *Iugulare* [a 1 cit]
82. basilica [3, 1625, Hart] Yi^{r} Wherof one is called *Basilica*, or *Hepatica*, the inner veynes (after *Hypocrates*) of the cubitte
83. basis [4, 1615 Crooke] Ciii^{r} /S/*Βαθμιδεζ*/S/ or *basis* are certain corners, after the order of a firmament, or ground
84. bastard [B, 5d, 1625, Hart] Li^{r} their opinions, are accompted vayne, which, iudging this ioynt neuer plainly luxated, do terme it onely a bastard, or false and counterfaited luxation
85. bear [*v*, 38, 1601, Holland] Kiii^{v} These bearyng outward, likewise in the fore part, do meete and ioyne together
86. beating [*ppl a*, 3, 1702, Rowe] Ddiiii^{v} other partes of mans body are endewed with beatyng Arteries [a 1 cit]
87. belly [II, 11, 1591, Spenser] Riii^{r} the posteriour bellye of the legge called *Sura*
88. blasted [*ppl a*, 2, 1742, Collins] Pi^{v} the vnhappy husbandman ... reapeth a sorte of blasted cares mingled with that cursed coccle
89. blind gut [1594, T. B.] Xi^{r} *Cæcum*, that is the blynde gutte [a 1 cit]
90. boll [*sb*, 1, 4, 1600, *Turk & G*] Iiii^{r} the head of *Radius* standeth vpon the toppe or hinder part of this bole or turne
91. bottle [3, 1609, C. Butler] Aiii^{v} to flow through the Vrinarie passage to the bleddar as a bottell to that humor
92. brachial [1b, 1859, Todd] Iiiii^{v} *Brachiale*, which we call the wrest of the hand

93. branching [*ppl a*, 2, 1720, Pope] Oi^{r} store of braunching sinews
94. caecum [1, 1721, Bailey] Uiii^{v} That is to say *Duodenum, Denne, Cæcum, Colum* and *Rectum* [a 1 cit]
95. capable [2, 1594, T. B.] Ui^{r} all round thynges are more capable, and lesse subiect to iniuries
96. capacious [2, 1634, Brereton] Uiii^{v} [the intestines] ... are created round in fourme, to be the more capacious [a 1 cit]
97. capacity [3, 1649, Blithe] Gi^{r} See **amplitude**, anted.
98. capsule [2, 1693, Urquhart] Cciii^{v} The membran enuoluyng the whole hart ... is called of the Greekes *Pericardion*, in Latin, *Cordus inuolucrum*: some *Casula cordis*, for that it is as a certaine house vnto the hart: the barbarous number, by the addition of one letter pronounce it *Capsula* [a 1 cit]
99. cardia [1782, Heberden] Ui^{r} The auncient Greekes do call this /S/χαϱδια/S/, but we (after the Latins) name it the vpper mouth of the Ventricle [a 1 cit]
100. cardiac [A, 1, 1601, Holland] Ggii^{r} this disease is called *Cardiacus dolor* [a 1 cit]
101. caros [1678, Phillips] Eii^{r} See **convulsion**, anted. [a 1 cit]
102. cast [*v*, XIII, 70, 1591, Ralegh] Hhii^{v} it [the nerve] casteth about through the hinder partes of the thighe
103. catch [*v*, 22, 1597, J. King.] Aii^{v} See **affect**, *v*, 5, anted.
104. cava [1681, tr. *Willis*] Tiii^{v} The veynes enfloded in *Omentum* ... are onely the braunches of *Vena porta*, but none from *caua* commeth to *Omentum* [a 1 cit]
105. cave [2, 1605, Bacon] Ciii^{v} a deepe and profou[n]d caue, or case, which we haue called *Acetabulum*
106. cavernous [2, 1597, Lowe] Diii^{r} And therfore be the bones of the head, betwene the outmost, and the inner scales, cauernous
107. cele [1708–15, Kersey] Cii^{v} See **supercilium**, unrec. [a 1 cit]
108. cephalic [A, 1, 1599, A. M. *Gabel.*] Iii^{v} *Vena axillaris* and *Cephalica* [a 1 cit]
109. cerebrum [1615, Crooke] Ggii^{v} the nerues of the Spinall marey, called also *Cerebrum elongatum* [a 1 cit]
110. challenge [2b, 1796, Southey] Fiii^{r} In the bone of the hinder part of the head, nere to the hole of all other, within the scull the greatest, we finde one not uery large, where through the vii. coniugation seeketh way: chalenged partly of the toung, partly of *Larynx*, and partly of the temporall *Muscles*
111. charybdis [1597, Bacon] Bi^{v} I haue wholly abstained my pen[n]e: least, shunning *Charibdis* I should fall into *Scylla* headlong [a 1 cit]
112. chorion [4, 1650, Bulwer] Ffiii^{r} the fourth Membran of the eye which is called *Vuea* and *Chorion, Secundina* and *Choriformes*
113. choroid [2, 1696, Phillips] Eiiii^{v} all the foldes *Choroides*, that are in the anteriour ventricles of the brayne [a 1 cit]

114. clavicle [1, 1615, Crooke] Iii^{r} the *Clavicles* or Cannell bones [a 1 cit]
115. coagmentation [2, 1678, Cudworth] Eii^{r} placyng the temporall *Muscle* vnder this *Iugall* coagmentation
116. coarticulation [1615, Crooke] Cii^{r} where no *Coarticulation* is made also: as in Ilium [a 1 cit]
117. cobweblike [1663, Gerbier] Ffiii^{v} the copweblike Membran [fpl]
118. coccyx [1615, Crooke] Gii^{v} the v. partes wherinto the backe is deuided … are … the Necke, the Brest, the Loynes, *Os Sacrum*, and *Coccix* [a 1 cit]
119. columella [1, 1585, Lloyd] Ccii^{r} a round, long, and litle thicke Pendule, called by diuers names: as *Vna, Vuula, Columella, Gargareon* [a 1 cit]
120. combination [1, 1613, R. C. *Table Alph.*] Lii^{v} ech structure, and combynation therof [the legge], being by *Arthrodia* and *Synarthrosis*
121. commit [10a, 1770, *Junius letters*] Diii^{r} by breaking one place, you shall commit the rest also to peeces
122. communicate [10, 1731, Arbuthnot] Uii^{v} sinews … haue poured out Nerues and braunches to the involucre of the hart, and by the like also communicatyng with lunges
123. community [2, 1587, Golding] Hhii^{v} the fourth with the fift hath such communitie, that of them both but one payre can be described
124. complicate [1, 1631, Donne] Fii^{r} Which three vessels, penetrate and pearse into th[e] little cauities and foundations of the teeth, where they are complicate [a 1 cit]
125. comprehend [1, 1584, Cecil] Kiii^{r} when we comprehend anythyng within the compasse of them, or hold any substaunce within the palme of the hand
126. comprehension [III, 8, 1656, More] Kiii^{r} (margin) When comprehension is made the fingers are all of one length
127. compressed [*ppl a*, 2, 1668, Wilkins] Diiii^{r} the two skales, that keepe the compressed sides of the head
128. compression [2, 1603, Florio] Miii^{v} the false ribbes yeld an excellent effect vnto the body … since all do know what great incommodities to the body, compression at that instant might inferre
129. conarium [1656, H. More] Ti^{v} The first [glandule] … betwene the [brayne] and *Cerebellum*, which is called *Conarion pineale* [a 1 cit]
130. concaved [*v*, 1652, Benlowes] Gi^{v} beyng also together mutually concaued [a 1 cit]
131. concreted [*a*, 1, 1634, Holland] Aai^{r} much blacke concreted bloud [a 1 cit]
132. concupiscible faculty [2b, 1594, Carew] Xiii^{r} the liuer, the retainer of all concupiscible facultie
133. conducted [1646, Crashaw] Ci^{r} the splendant sparke of reason, which shall light ech mans iudgement into the right conducted way of truth [a 1 cit]
134. confused [3b, 1776, Withering] Biiii^{r} To prætermitte those whiche

Vesalius obserued, because they are confused, let vs come to the most notable, by others descriued and set in order

135. confused [*ppl a*, 5, 1611, Bp. Hall] Pi^{r} a confused muscle of flesh, fat, and glandulous matter together

136. conjugated [*ppl a*, 1690, Norris] Giii^{v} See **aspect**, *v*, 2, anted. [a 1 cit]

137. connect [*v*, 1, 1691, Boyle] Diiii^{v} a *Cartilage*, which, after the maner of a *Ligament*, connecteth the head to the first and second *Vertebre*

138. connectively [1745 Swift] Ciii^{v} See **glene**, anted. [a 1 cit]

139. consistence [1b, 1613, Overbury] Fi^{v} the bones ther ceasse to enlarge after the consistence of yeares [a 1 cit]

140. consistence [4, 1626, Bacon] Bii^{v} they kept the compressed heades of their children, swathed so, till some consistence of yeares grew on them [a 1 cit]

141. constituting [*vbl sb* 1642, Milton] Diiii^{v} for the better constituting of the head his articulation [a 1 cit]

142. constituting [*vbl sb* 1642, Milton] Dii^{r} See **construction**, anted. [a 1 cit]

143. constringe [1, 1606, Shakespeare] Ciii^{v} Who are both co[n]stringed, & also dilated [a 1 cit]

144. constringe [2, 1604, T. Wright] Yi^{v} the *Muscle* constringing and pulling together the eye lidde [a 1 cit]

145. construction [2, 1707, *Curios. in Husb.*] Dii^{r} Bones ... which to the brayne, in their construction, are so safe a muniment, as it is small thankes to say nature was most carefull in constitutyng of it

146. construction [I, 4, 1796, Morse] Eiii^{r} the *Ligamentes* produced from his *Sutures* might enter the construction of the *Muscles*

147. contendent [A, 1, 1641, Bp. Mountagu] Aaii^{v} the posteriour part of the same body ... is digested into braunches, to the outside of the kidney contendaunt [a 1 cit]

148. contexture [2a, 1605, Bacon] Hhiiii^{r} the mervailous workemanshyp, and subtill contexture of the members [a 1 cit]

149. contract [III, 7, 1626, Bacon] Bbi^{r} *Cuti*, which ... is not fat, lest it should not extend, and contract

150. contract [III, 8, 1602, Shakespeare] Oi^{r} the forehead, where we contract and wrinckle the skinne

151. contraction [5b, 1871, T. Holmes] Eiii^{r} no commoditie (but in ridiculous manner to defourme the face of man) might ensue by contraction [a 1 cit]

152. contraction [5a, 1589, Nashe] Ciii^{v} all kynde of motions, and turnings: as *Extension*, *Contraction*, *Circumaction* [a 1 cit]

153. contraction [II, 8a, 1706, Phillips ed. Kersey] Fiiii^{r} it is called /S/υψιλοειδιζ/S/, but with more contractio[n] of speach *Hyoides* [a 1 cit]

154. contractive [1624, Bargrave] Uii^{v} melancolie iuyce ... which is ... of necessitie contractiue, & astringent [a 1 cit]

155. contusion [1b, 1626, Bacon] Hi^{r} (margin) The tranuerse Processe of

the 12 Vertebre appeareth in somme as though the head therof were deuided with some vigorous contusio[n]
156. convexity [1, 1605, Bacon] Hiii^{r} bones, which are extended with such ample scope and conuexitie [a 1 cit]
157. convict [*v*, 1b, 1609 Holland] Aiii^{v} he shall be reiected, when he is conuicted to haue done all for the cause of his owne vtilitie
158. convulsion [2a, 1585, Lloyd] Eii^{r} For among all other *Muscles* ... chiefly this ... causeth ... co[n]uulsions, feuers, caros, & dotage [a 1 cit]
159. coracoid [1, 1706, Phillips] Ii^{v} See **ancryoid**, ns [a 1 cit]
160. corona [6, 1712, Arbuthnot] Cii^{v} Others also beyng sharpe but not so slender, as the knagge of a hartes horne, that is to say thicke and pointyng, such as are to be found in the nether iawe: *Galena* calleth such *Corona Processus*
161. coronal [2c, 1656, Blount] Xiiii^{v} a veyne, whiche ... embraceth the hart like vnto a crowne, wherefore it is accordingly called *Coronalis Vena*
162. coronal suture [2a, 1615, Crooke] Diii^{v} (margin) The names, description, and vse of the Coronall Suture
163. corpulent [3, 1619, Fotherby] Giii^{v} (margin) The bodie of the Vertebre is the corpulent and grosse parte therof
164. corpus [2, 1706, Phillips] Bbii^{v} this same *Varicosum corpus*
165. correspondent [2c, 1656, Ussher] Ii^{v} a hole agreeyng, or correspondent to the greatness of the head of the shoulder
166. coursing [*ppl a*, 1599, Shakespeare] Tii^{v} it [*Peritonæum*] ... deuideth from the outer coursing *Muscles* [a 1 cit]
167. coxendix [1615, Crooke] Ri^{v} And from Coxendix amplecteth the lesser *Trochanter* [a 1 cit]
168. cremaster [1678, Phillips] Qiiii^{v} The auncient writers haue called these *Muscles Cremasteres* [a 1 cit]
169. crus [2a, 1727–51 *Chamb. Cycl.*] Li^{v} that therfore possesseth the hole name of *Tibia*, or *Crus* [a 1 cit]
170. crystalloid [A, 1862, H. Spenser] Ffiii^{v} The second humor of the eye is *Christalloides* or *Christallinus* [a 1 cit]
171. cubiform [1730-6, Bailey] Liiii^{r} The fourth is *Cyboide*, or after the Latins *Cubeforme os*, as it were squared lyke a dye [a 1 cit]
172. cuticula [1, 1621, Burton] Siii^{v} The outmost skinne therfore which is in Greeke called *Epidermis*, in Latin *Cuticulus* [a 1 cit]
173. cutis [1603, Jonson] Siiii^{r} (margin) The trew skinne called *Derma*, and *Cutis* [a 1 cit]
174. cyst [1, 1720, W. Gibson] Yiiii^{r} The bleddar ... called of some *Cistis Fellis* [a 1 cit]
175. damp [1b, 1869, Martineau] Ii^{r} so truth (like vnto the flames of fire) beyng neuer so couered & damped for a space
176. dartos [1634, T. Johnson] Qiiii^{v} Euery of the testicles retaynyng one Muscle ... situated in the Membran called in Greeke *Dartos* [a 1 cit]

177. decency [1c, 1610 Guillim] Hhiiii^{r} heares are made also ... for decencie of fourme

178. decipher [3a, 1605, Daniel] Eii^{v} Which three [bones] orderly to decyffer

179. deciphered [*ppl a*, 1845, Graves] Ciii^{r} those fewe decyffered names [fpl]

180. decorum [1c, 1586, T. B.] Bbiiii^{v} I shall [not] commit more indecencie agaynst the office of *Decorum*

181. deduction [2, 1615, Chapman] Diiii^{v} by benefite of which transuerse deductio[n] of the same Suture

182. defect [*v*, 1, 1586, Hooker] Oiiii^{r} they happen transuersly to separate his *Fibres*: which beyng done ... the life defecteth [a 1 cit]

183. defer [v^{2}, 1, 1626, Bacon] Kiiii^{v} those that be deferred downe to the thigh

184. deferent [A, 1626, Bacon] Qiii^{v} the vessels bringing seede called *Deferentia vasa*

185. deferent [B, 1, 1626, Bacon] Kiiii^{v} a certaine litle hollow gutter ... by the whiche couertly runne, as well *Deferentia* as *Preparantia vasa*

186. deglution [1657, Tomlinson] Pi^{v} the deglution and swallowyng of meate and drinke [a 1 cit] [fpl]

187. delay [*sb*, 1b, 1748, F. Smith] Uiiii^{r} with longer delay the excrementes tary

188. delineation [4, 1603, Daniel] Eiiii^{v} I haue ... in the delineation of these bones, imitated somewhat narrowly the iudgement of *Collumbus*

189. deliver [IV, 9, 1597, T. J.] Xi^{r} into many partes broken, and deliuered to the intrels

190. deltoid [B, 1, 1681, tr. *Willis*] Piii^{r} The second muscle of the shoulder is ... called by Anathomists /S/επωμιξ/S/ and /S/δελτοειδισ/S/, and *Humeralis* [a 1 cit]

191. dental [A, 1, 1599, A. M. *Guill.*] Giii^{r} the *Dental Process* of the second *Vertebre* [a 1 cit]

192. dentition [1, 1615, Crooke] Fii^{r} the first *Dentition* of children bryngeth forth *Appendances* [a 1 cit]

193. depraved [*ppl a*, 1, 1610, Guillim] Eii^{r} *Fuchsius* coniecture, in explicating this hard and depraued place [a 1 cit]

194. depressed [*ppl a*, 3, 1753, *Chambers's Cycl.*] Giiii^{v} they (the vertebrae of the breast) are neither so flatte ... nor yet so depressed as those we haue spoken of

195. depression [1, 1656, Blount] Hiiii^{v} the elation and depression of the ribbes

196. derivation [sb^{1},1a, 1607, Topsell] Gi^{v} th[e] vppermost deriuations [of nerves] seeke not out the nether partes

197. derive [3b, 1597, Harington] Giii^{v} From the sides likewise of the first *Vertebre* are stretched two *Processes* ... deriuyng braunches from themselues

198. derma [1706, Phillips] Siiii^{r} See **cutis**, anted. [a 1 cit]
199. descendent [A, 1, 1644, Digby] Diii^{v} from the extremitie of the discendent *Coronalis*
200. descendent [B, 1, 1600, E. Blount] Kiiii^{v} the insertion of the oblique descendentes of the bellye
201. difficult [1, 1586, T. B.] Fiii^{r} penetratyng the laberinthe with a blind and difficult conduict
202. difficulty [2a, 1619, Daniel] Mi^{v} hard to be rightly restored but by a skilful Artist who knoweth the reason of such difficultie
203. diffuse [I, 2, 1590, Spenser] Uiii^{r} the vessels which therin are diffused
204. digit [1, 1644, Bulwer] Iiiii^{v} *Digitis*, or the fingers [a 1 cit]
205. dike [I, 2b, 1616, Surflet & Markham] Xiiii^{v} This veyne is rightly compared vnto a great river. For from thence as there be many dikes issuyng, so very many braunches are deriued from this veyne
206. direct [6, 1596, Shakespeare] Rii^{v} this muscle being taken away: direct flexion can in no wise be brought to passe
207. disjoin [4b, 1592, Shakespeare] Diiii^{r} *Os cuneale* disioyneth it selfe from *Os frontis*
208. disjoined [*ppl a*, 1594, Southwell] Piiii^{r} they go somewhat disioyned [a 1 cit]
209. dislocate [*v*, 2b, 1605, Shakespeare] Gii^{r} the small number of Bones, should offer ouer readyly occasion, vpon euery light motion to be dislocated, or rather *Luxated* [a 1 cit]
210. dissect [1, 1607, Topsell] Gi^{v} (margin) That Vesalius dissected commo[n]ly the *Larinx* in beastes
211. dissect [2, 1611, Florio] Biiii^{r} amongest those very few bodies ... I haue dissected, I haue found some of Galens Sceletons in sundry pointes [a 1 cit]
212. dissected [*ppl a*, 1, 1634, Sir T. Herbert] Dii^{v} the due obseruation of the *Dissected* parts [a 1 cit]
213. dissecting [*vbl sb*, 1888, *Daily Tel.*] Hi^{v} a labourer in the Arte of dissecting [a 1 cit]
214. dissection [1, 1611, Cotgrave] Dii^{v} Who ... found by *Dissection*, that through out his head, scarse the tract of one *Suture* could be obserued [a 1 cit]
215. dissection [2, 1605, Bacon] Biiii^{r} Much mervailous shall it be to him that vseth dissection, to see such sundry and often varieties: yea the Anathomist shall see ... sundry notes of new shapes in nature [a 1 cit]
216. disseminate [1b, 1664, Power] Hii^{v} strowed diuersly in the haunches, & disseminated amo[n]g the *Muscles* of the thighes [a 1 cit]
217. disseminate [1c, 1677, Grew] Ci^{r} no portio[n] of sinewes ... is in their substance disseminated [a 1 cit]
218. dissimilar [a, 1621, Burton] Ci^{r} *Dissimilar*, or *instrumentall* [a 1 cit]
219. dissipate [3c, 1626, Bacon] Eiiii^{r} the vj. *Suture* ... departeth into a large cauitie, where it is dissipated and wasted

220. distend [3, 1650, Bulwer] Tiiii^{r} the stomach filled with meate, if very long it should be distended

221. distention [1, 1607, Topsell] Aaiii^{r} lest … *Rectum intestinum*, beyng stretched … should ouermuch bynde or hold in the diste[n]tion therof [a 1 cit]

222. distinct [1b, 1674, Clarendon] Giii^{v} See **aspect**, *v*, anted.

223. distinguish [*v*, I, i, 1609, (Douay) Bible] Diiii^{v} as this bone in the hinder part of the head, in persons of strengthned yeares, is all one, and undeuided: so in young chidre[n], into foure or fiue partes, yea sometime into vij. distinguished

224. distraction [1d, 1720, W. Gibson] Gii^{r} many *Vertebres* beyng luxated … inciteth a great distraction

225. distribute [4, 1664, Evelyn] Ffiiii^{r} the fiue Muscles seruing to the eye … the vj. Membrans … all which I haue sufficiently in this discourse distributed

226. distribution [2, 1589, Puttenham] Siiii^{r} among all the partes of of th[e] skinne is not alike distribution of Nerues

227. distribution [2, 1659, *Vulg. Errors*] Ffiiii^{v} Their distribution is diuers, but their originall is from the seate or foundation of the brayne

228. divinely [1, 1594, Spenser] Hhiii^{v} how deuinely the incomprehensible creator hath made the body of ma[n] [a 1 cit]

229. doctrine [3, 1594, West] Ci^{r} The doctrine of this History is most obscure, vnless the Bones be first learned

230. dodeca- [1879, Sir G. Scott] Uiiii^{r} that parte of the gutte … wheras the gutte first begynneth to be infolded … is called of the Greekes /S/*δοδεχαδαχτψλοσ*/S/ [a 1 cit]

231. dorsum [1a, 1840, G. V. Ellis] Gi^{v} thou shalt note to be … nominated of the … Latins *Dorsum*, or *Spina*, which our English phrase termeth the backe [a 1 cit]

232. double [C, 1, 1767, *Byron's Voy.*] Diiii^{v} See **eminent**, anted.

233. dura [1882, Wilder & Gage] Ffiii^{r} called … in Latin *Cornea*, and of some *Dura* [a 1 cit]

234. earthy [2a, 1626, Bacon] Siii^{v} the Splene [receives] that which is more earthy and thick

235. edged [*ppl a*, 1, 1591, Shakespeare] Liiii^{v} the inferiour part … is most narrow, and as it were edged [a 1 cit]

236. educe [2, 1613, Bayne] Aaiii^{v} (margin) The way educing Vrine from the infant as yet in the Wombe

237. ejaculation [2, 1603, Holland] Aaiiii^{r} the eiaculation of sperme [a 1 cit]

238. elaboration [1a, 1612, Woodall] Bbii^{v} the same matter of seede, whiche first is red, should begin by litle and litle to be prepared, altered and made white. By which elaboration … a great part of labour to the Testicles is diminished

239. elegant [2, 1658, W. Burton] Diii^{v} diligence shal finde it [the head of a dog] most directly distinguished with Sutures: and those, more elegant than in men
240. elevate [II, 2d, 1607, Walkington] Hhiiii^{r} fuliginous vapours which are eleuated in the thyrd co[n]coctio[n] of nourishment
241. elongate [1828, Stark] Ggii^{v} the Spinall marey, called the *Cerebrum elongatum* [a 1 cit]
242. elongated [*ppl a*, 1, 1751, R. Cambridge] Ggii^{v} the outmost end of this elongated body [a 1 cit]
243. eminence [2a, 1615, Crooke] Dii^{r} both eminences of the head [a 1 cit]
244. eminent [3, 1612, T. Taylor] Diiii^{v} as the partes incident to small daunger, haue litle wherewith to defend them selues, so such as are sited in most eminent perilles, and as it were in the forefront of irrepugnable damages, those commonly are armed with double shielded defenses
245. emission [1, 1607, Topsell] Ddii^{v} wickettes ... of the hollow veyne and veniall arterie ... seruing to the emission of bloud [a 1 cit]
246. emission [4, 1619, Donne] Bbiiii^{r} for the emission of Vrine [a 1 cit]
247. empyema [1, 1615, Crooke] Hiiii^{r} the disease called of the Greekes *Empyema* [a 1 cit]
248. emulgent [B, 1612, S. H.] Yii^{r} a large veyne ... called *Emulgens*
249. enarthrosis [1634, T. Johnson] Ciii^{v} both [motions] are publikly deuided agayne in tripple wise ... as *Enarthrosis*, *Arthrodia*, and *Gynglyman* [*sic*] [a 1 cit]
250. enclasp [1596, Fitz-Geffray] Xiii^{r} the apter to enclapse [*sic*] the ventricle, as with the fingers of ones hand [a 1 cit]
251. enclosure [3b, 1594, Plat] Biiii^{r} It was straunge to behold pericardium, the enclosure of the hart, wantyng
252. enclosure [4, 1580, Hollyband] Hiii^{r} the brest ... a certayne strong enclosure
253. enfold [4, 1605, Bacon] Uiiii^{r} the gutte first begynneth to be infolded [a 1 cit]
254. enfolding [*vbl sb*, 1586, W. Webbe] Oi^{r} the skinne ... by replication and enfoldyng therof [a 1 cit]
255. engraving [2, 1611, Bible] Giii^{v} it was made thinner and weaker, by the engrauyng on the inside of the aforesayd cauitie [a 1 cit]
256. engross [10, 1611, Chapman] Li^{r} the more it descendeth the more also it engrosseth and enlargeth
257. entertain [14, 1586, A. Day] Bi^{r} Let these my simple labours, what soeuer they are, be entertained in the handes of thee [*sic*] true, vertuous, and honest Artistes, and Professours of Chirurgerie
258. entire [5, 1590, Spenser] Dii^{v} as the head had bene of one *Solid*, & entier Bone
259. epidermis [1, 1626, Bacon] Siii^{v} The outmost skinne ... in Greeke called *Epidermis* [a 1 cit]

260. epididymus [1610, Jonson] Bbi[v] the first professours of Anathomie, which named the Testicles *Didimos*, haue called it (sayth *Vesalius*) *Epididymos* [a 1 cit]
261. epiglottis [1615, Crooke] Fiiii[v] a door or gate seruiceable to *Larinx* ... called of the Greekes *Epiglottis* [a 1 cit]
262. equal [2c, 1677, Yarranton] Hi[r] which thing shall truly be proued in the xij. *Vertebre* of ma[n], which purchaseth one [sic] ether syde an equall kinde of *Articulation*: that is, both aboue & beneth it hath *Processes* puttyng forth, th[at] it might be on both sides receiued
263. equal [4, 1661, Morgan] Siiii[v] very neare approchyng to the waight with equall temperature
264. equally [1, 1615, Sir T. Herbert] Ki[r] The seuenth endeth at the first, second, sixt, and viij. but not equally, or in like order committed to one, as to an other
265. equally [5, 1664 Evelyn] Ui[r] In the Anterior part it is equally euery where Gibbous
266. erect [1, 1609, *Man in the Moone*] Giiii[v] Neither are the transuerse *Processes*, biforked and guttured, but lo[n]g and great, endyng with round and thicke heades; whiche rising also from the sides of the *Vertebres*, do erect their exorture vpwardes
267. erect [II, 4, 1626, Bacon] Bbiii[v] the yard ... should, beyng filled with spirite, be erected, produced and notably swelled
268. erected [*ppl a*, 3a, 1603, Jonson] Bbiii[v] the yard ... in the time of carnal societie, ought to be swelled, stiffe, and erected [a 1 cit]
269. erection [3, 1622, Sparrow] Gii[v] the erection of the same Necke could not be made firme and stedfast, without the supportable ground and frameworke of Bones
270. erection [4, 1594, Plat] Bbiiii[r] the necessary erection in coiture
271. erythroid [1847, Craig] Bbi[v] that coate called *Erithrocides* [a 1 cit]
272. ethmoid [B, 1842, Col. H. Smith] Eeiiii[r] the Bone named *Sphenoides*, towardes *Ethmoides* [a 1 cit]
273. european [B, 1632, Massinger] Biii[v] The Europæans co[n]trariwise are in magnitude much different amo[n]g them selves [a 1 cit]
274. exact [I, 1, 1633, Herbert] Pi[r] So exacte therfor is the makyng therof, and with such commoderation is it measured
275. exactly [2, 1612, Brinsley] Ci[r] For if you doe not first exactely examine ... this History of Bones
276. exactly [5, 1662, Stillingfleet] Xiii[r] It is not in figure exactly round
277. excluding [*sb*, 1581, J. Bell] Qii[r] (margin) How *Septum* auayleth to the excludyng of excrementes [a 1 cit]
278. exclusion [4, 1646, Browne] Qii[r] a most strong, and certaine exclusion of the superfluous dregges of the thyrd digestion [a 1 cit]
279. excremental [3, 1599, A. M. *Gabel.*] Eiii[v] the excrementall purgyngs of the brayne

280. exist [4, 1790, Burns] Qi^{r} the life it selfe by no means could exist, or stand [a 1 cit]
281. expiration [1, 1642, *Preparative*] Eii^{r} neither could be auoyded through the holes, neither any vapor of smel ascend, vnlesse nature did puruey the same, both by inspiration, and expiration
282. expired [*ppl a*, 1, 1794, Hutton] Miii^{v} to transport the ayre inspired and expired [a 1 cit]
283. expiring [*ppl a*, 1612, R. Sheldon] Miii^{r} mouynge which is caused by continuall expiryng and inspiryng [a 1 cit]
284. expiring [*vbl sb*, 1612, R. Sheldon] Miii^{r} caused by continuall expiryng and inspiryng
285. explicate [1, 1620, Bp. King] Ddiiii^{r} others [arteries] enter into the Scull ... and lyke a tree through the sides of the hard Membran ... are explicated
286. explicate [6, 1622-62, Heylin] Ciii^{v} These examples do explicate the maner of *Enarthrosis Articulation*, under the name of *Diarthrosis*
287. expressed [*ppl a*, 1, 1599, A. M. *Gabel.*] Di^{v} See **lightly**, anted.
288. exquisite [7, 1643, Prynne] Riiii^{r} (margin) The broad tendo[n] of th[e] foote of most exquisite sense
289. extend [5, 1673, Evelyn] Hi^{v} (margin) Why ribbes were not exte[n]ded ouer the region of the belly
290. extension [3, 1674, Betterton] Ciii^{r} when *Extension* is made neither can any of the *Processes* passe further in their *Celles*, then the utmost seat, to them by nature limited
291. extension [9a, 1796–7 *Instr. & Reg.*] Hi^{v} the iust length, and magnitude of the ribbes [whose] extension ouer the region of the bellye had not bene conuenient
292. extract [*v*, 2b, 1607, Topsell] Aiiii^{v} I saw *Fuchsius* to haue extract a notable Epitome out of *Vesalius*
293. extract [*v*, 3a, 1628, Wither] Fii^{r} he had occasion to search in childre[n] that neuer were extract, or brought to light, as also in *Abortes*
294. extraordinary [5, 1649, Blithe] Hiii^{r} We must note, that by the extraordinarie number of *Vertebres*, may grow the like effect in accompt of the ribbes
295. extrinsical [1, 1594, Blundevil] Ki^{v} they [the tendons] of the extrinsecall region of the wrest
296. extrinsical [2, 1608, D. T.] Diii^{r} See **involution**, anted.
297. extrusion [1, 1638, W. Rowley?] Yiiii^{v} a small extrusion of the excrementes
298. fabricate [*v*, 1598, Yong] Miii^{r} had the nostrels bene otherwise made, or of the substaunce of bones fabricated [a 1 cit]
299. face [12, 1632, Lithgow] Li^{r} their endes, or extreme faces be smooth
300. false rib [**false**, 15, 1594, T. B.] Giiii^{v} comprehendyng but the false ribbes

301. fibre [2, 1607, Topsell] Ci^{r} *Ligamentes, Fibres, Membrans, Flesh*
302. fibrous [1a, 1657, Purchas] Niiii^{r} A *Muscle* … is construct and made of *Fibrous* flesh [a 1 cit]
303. fibula [2, 1706, Phillips (Kersey)] Cii^{v} See **tarsus**, anted.
304. figure [IV, 18, 1597, Morley] Iii^{v} their makyng is not vnlike this figure .S
305. filament [1, 1594, T. B.] Oii^{v} Sinewy Filamentes [a 1 cit]
306. fixedly [1598, Sylvester] Ciiii^{r} the bones: whiche are otherwise so fixedly compact together [a 1 cit]
307. flat [v^2, 14a, 1670, Cotton] Yiiii^{r} it might flat or shrinke in [a 1 cit]
308. flat [v^2, 3a, 1613, Ridley] Eiiii^{v} the heades of other beastes are more depressed, and flatted [a 1 cit]
309. flatness [2, 1683, Ray] Giiii^{r} a certaine kind of flatnes in the foreface of them, not improvidently ordained
310. flexion [1b, 1615, Crooke] Gii^{r} See **angular**, anted. [a 1 cit]
311. foreguard [1588, Greene] Tii^{v} that, which foregardeth, and circumplecteth all the subiect vessels and bowels [a 1 cit]
312. formal [2b, 1691, Ray] Ggi^{v} the formall instrument of voyce, named /S/γλοττιζ/S/
313. fornix [a, 1681, tr. *Willis Rem. Med.*] Eeiiii^{v} an other portion named *Fornix* and *Psalloides*, in figure of a halfe circle [a 1 cit]
314. foundation [7, 1874, Knight] Ii^{r} in the foundation of the hart, (about the rootes of *Arteria aorta*
315. fracture [1, 1803, M. Cutler] Diii^{r} the head, beyng thus of bonye substaunce, whiche by the violence of some stroke might be fractured, or contused [a 1 cit]
316. fragile [1a, 1607, Shakespeare] Iii^{r} their hollones maketh them more fragill, and britle [a 1 cit]
317. framework [1a, 1644, Milton] Fi^{v} no otherwise then the frame worke of a house, do supporte [a 1 cit]
318. frequentation [1, 1585, Washington] Ffii^{r} *Collumbus* reproued such as haue hitherto made description of the eyes, by frequentation of brutish Anathomies
319. frons [1856–8, W. Clark] Oiiii^{r} It springeth therfore … from *Frons* and *Sinciput* [a 1 cit]
320. function [3a, 1590, Shakespeare] Uii^{v} all the functions therof [the splene], which co[n]sist in a certaine kynd of embracyng
321. furcula [B, 1859, Darwin] Iii^{r} in Latin *Furcula, Clavicula*, or *Iugula* [a 1 cit]
322. fused [a, 1699, Salmon] Ffiiii^{r} it representeth fused or moulten glasse [a 1 cit]
323. futility [1, 1623, Cockeram] Aaiiii^{r} the futilitie of their subtill inuention [a 1 cit]
324. gargareon [1653, Urquhart] Ccii^{r} See **columella**, anted. [a 1 cit]

325. ginglymos [1657, *Phys. Dict.*] Ciiii^{r} The thyrd kynde of *Articulation* hath to name *Gynglymos*, and that is a mutuall *Congresse*, or *Coarticulation* of the bones, whe[n] as in either of the endes that mete, perminent partes appeare, as also cauities or little hollowes [a 1 cit]
326. glans [1, 1650, Bulwer] Bbiiii^{r} *Glans* is harder than the other partes of the yard [a 1 cit]
327. glene [1706, Phillips (Kersey)] Ciii^{v} *Arthrodia* is a coniunctio[n] of bones, wherof the one hath a head depressed, the other a shallow or playne cauitie, called *Glene* ... aunsweryng the head of the other so conuectiuely [*sic*], as it is hard to know the head, from the hollow [a 1 cit]
328. godly-minded [4, 1856, R. A. Vaughan] Aiii^{r} There is one thing also, which ought to be a great comfort vnto the godly minded, that is, that none do persecute vertuous proceedynges, saue only the enemies of vertue [a 1 cit] [fpl]
329. gracile [1623, Cockeram] Xi^{r} The thyrd intestine succeedyng *Ieieunum* is called *Ileon*, of some *Tenue*, or *Gracile* [a 1 cit]
330. grave [6, 1609, Douland] Pii^{r} by their office, ech graue or bace voyce is vttered
331. great artery [6d, 1715, Burnet] Ti^{r} the braunches of the great *Arterie* [fpl]
332. hairlike [1656, Blount] Aaiii^{v} small twistes and hearelike surcles [a 1 cit]
333. hammer [2d, 1615, Crooke] Eii^{v} See **mallet**, anted.
334. harmonia [1657, *Phys. Dict.*] Ciiii^{r} Of these [symphyses] are three differences, thus called by proper names, *Sutura*, *Gomphosis*, & *Harmonia* [a 1 cit]
335. hepatic [A, 1, 1599, A. M. *Gabel.*] Yi^{r} Wherof one is called *Basilica* or *Hepatica*, the inner veynes (after *Hypocrates*) of the cubitte
336. historiographer [3, 1579-80, North] Bii^{v} Aristotle, Plinie, and others [*sic*] most famous Historiographers
337. holloing [1596, Shakespeare] Qii^{v} the vse of hollowyng, crying, blowynges of trumpets [fpl]
338. hollow vein [A, 7, 1591, Sylvester] Xiiii^{v} the hollow veyne ascendeth [fpl]
339. hollowed [4, 1613, Purchas] Kiiii^{r} neare to the seate ... of *Coxendix*, there is an other hollowed corner [a 1 cit] [fpl]
340. hoodlike [8, 1861, J. R. Greene] Pii^{v} a hoodlike *Muscle*, or more seemely in Latin *Cucullaris Musculus* [fpl]
341. hopper [4, 1763, Lewis] Ffi^{r} this cauitie is called *Pelvis*, or *Infundibulum*, which is to be Englished a tunnell or hopper made to receiue the excrementes
342. humeral [A, 1, 1615, Crooke] Xiiii^{v} the humerall veyne called also *Capitalis* [a 1 cit]
343. humeral [B, 1641, Trapp] Piii^{r} The second muscle of the shoulder ... called ... *Humeralis* [a 1 cit]

344. **hyoid** [B, *sb*, 1, 1706, Phillips] Oiiii[v] The muscles therfore that make the mouynge of *Hyoides* are in number viij [a 1 cit]
345. **hypsiloid** [1886, *Syd. Soc. Lex.*] Fiiii[r] (margin) It is more rightly called *Ypsiloides* then *Lamdoides* [a 1 cit]
346. **ilium** [2, 1590, Barrough] Xii[r] in the region of the right *Ilium*
347. **ilium** [3, 1706, Phillips] Cii[r] See **coarticulation**, anted.
348. **imagine** [9, 1586, A. Day] Aiiii[r] the partes themselues beyng altogether vnknowen, or falsely imagined of
349. **imbecility** [2, 1624, Capt. Smith] Uiiii[v] It happeneth rather through imbecillitie of his interpretour *Tho. Linacre*
350. **impel** [2, 1611, Florio] Pi[r] The vij. and viij. [*Muscles*] haue propertie now hether now thether to impell and moue the tongue
351. **impend** [4, 1652, Gaule] Diiii[v] For so nature carefully impended her study [a 1 cit]
352. **impose** [1a, 1597, A. M. *Guill.*] Kiiii[r] tendons ... hidde in their *Muscle* as as if they were in a purse imposed
353. **improvidently** [1, 1607, Donne] Giiii[r] See **flatness**, anted. [a 1 cit]
354. **inarticulate** [1713, Derham] Iiiii[r] wherein, the two vppermost bones of the wrest, are inarticulated and knit [a 1 cit]
355. **incisor** [a, 1672, T. Browne] Fi[r] the formost foure are named *Incisorij* [a 1 cit]
356. **incisory** [1, 1594, T. B.] Eiii[v] See **recurrent**, anted.
357. **incrust** [1663, Beale] Iiii[r] deeply incrusted with a *Cartilage* [a 1 cit]
358. **incursion** [2b, 1640, Bp. Reynolds] Fi[v] such cruciable torments of Rheumaticke incursions
359. **indagation** [1589, Nashe] Ei[r] *Realdus Collumbus*, a famous man to be remembered, who, in these matters *Anathomicall* by his exploratiue indagation seemeth to haue sifted a mite, and clouen a heare [a 1 cit]
360. **indecency** [1, 1589 Puttenham] Bbiiii[v] I shall commit more indecencie agaynst the office of *Decorum* [a 1 cit]
361. **indented** [*ppl a*, 1635, Braithwait] Eiiii[v] (margin) The xi. bone is likened to a plow share without a handle, and with an inde[n]ted or vnequall edge [a 1 cit]
362. **indurated** [*ppl a*, 1677, Plot] Ciiii[v] which flesh is made so callons [*sic*], and indurated, as that the teeth therby are not a little delited, and bowlstered [a 1 cit]
363. **inequality** [3a, 1607, Topsell] Iii[r] (margin) The inequalitie of th[e] scaple bones in thicknes and thinnes
364. **infection** [9, 1616, R. C.] Pi[v] from these my simple labors I may clearely wipe the blotte of errour, least by such meanes or [*sic*] infection, they become odious to the hearers
365. **inferior** [2, 1589, Puttenham] Hiiii[r] The first superiours, and last inferiours beyng farre shorter then the middlemost
366. **influx** [1a, 1626, Bacon] Uiiii[v] the influxe of choler stimulatyng and styring by the force of the guttes [a 1 cit]

367. infundibulum [2, 1706, Phillips] Ffi^r See **hopper**, anted. [a 1 cit]
368. injuriously [6b, 1809–10, Coleridge] Diii^r Therfore not injuriously, or vaynly, is the healthfull head distinct with *Sutures*
369. innest [*v*, 1611, Florio] Siiii^r That which innesteth the inside of the hand [a 1 cit]
370. insert [2, 1601, Holland] Di^v a rounde or long head is inserted within some cauitie answerable to it
371. insinuate [1, 1647, H. More] Yiiii^r nor ouermuch insinuated in the liuer
372. insinuate [1b, 1598, Hakluyt] Ggi^v insinuatyng it selfe into the cauitie of *Larinx*
373. inter [1641, Bp. Montagu] Di^v See **lightly**, anted. [a 1 cit]
374. interceptive [1819, Foster] Eiii^v See **recurrent**, anted. [a 1 cit]
375. intercostal [A, 1597, A. M. *Guill.*] Pii^r (margin) *Collumbus* demeth them to be like th[e] intercostall Muscles [a 1 cit]
376. intercostal [B, 1681, Willis] Pii^r the muscles callled *Intercostales* [a 1 cit]
377. intercourse [5, 1626, Bacon] Siiii^v Whiche happeneth by the intercourse of Veynes and Arteries
378. interjacent [1594, Rowland] Ffiii^v no other Membran interiacent or lyeng betwene [a 1 cit]
379. interjected [*ppl a*, 1619, Cooper] Kiii^r betweene them all are interiected *Cartilages* [a 1 cit] [fpl]
380. interlay [2, 1613, Purchas] Kiii^r (margin) Why their ioynts are interlayd with Cartilages [a 1 cit]
381. intersect [*v*, 1a, 1615, Crooke] Oii^r a circle intersected with diuerse Fibres [a 1 cit]
382. interseptum [1753, Chambers] Ffi^v a seuerall diuision, or hedge: called therfore *Narium interseptum*, or *Interseptum Cartilaginosum* [a 1 cit] [fpl]
383. intestinal [1, 1599, A. M. *Gabel.*] Bbii^r that kinde of rupture called *Intestinalis* [a 1 cit]
384. intestine [1a, 1597, A. M. *Guill.*] Tii^v the Ventricle, intestines, the kell
385. intestine [b, 1651, Ralegh] Xi^v [this gutte] finishyng his course at *Kellum intestinum* in the toppe of *Os Sacrum*
386. intrench [1, 1754, P. H.] Lii^r a *Veyne, Arterie*, and Sinew, which that way downewardes are intrenched [a 1 cit]
387. inverse [*v*, 1611, Florio] Ffiii^v where it is made double and inuersed
388. invert [*v*, I, 1a, 1613, Beau. & Fl.] Iiiii^r (margin) How the hand is inuerted both vpward and downward
389. invest [2b, 1632, Lithgow] Tii^v *Septum transuersum* as is aforesayd, clothed, it inuesteth the liuer
390. involution [1b, 1646, Browne] Diii^r on the outside of the scalpe, an

other *Membran*, which involutio[n] is ordained, for the *Extrinsecall Obduction* of the capitall Bones [a 1 cit]

391. involution [2, 1661, Cotgrave] Bbiii^{r} that body groweth to the inner coate of the Testicle, and is on the outside, the impressions of those inuolutions beyng taken away, smooth [a 1 cit]

392. involvement [2, 1630, H. R.] Eeiii^{v} the hard Membran is ... to the brayne an involvement [a 1 cit]

393. irrigate [1, 1615, Crooke] Tiiii^{v} these do irrigate, and moysten the way of Urine [a 1 cit]

394. ischium [1646, Browne, and ns] Yiii^{v} that veyne ... called *Vena Scia. Iscij*, or *Coxendicis* [a 1 cit]

395. janitor [2, 1584, *Grant Burgh Sch. Scot.*] Ui^{r} the Grecians call it /S/πυλωϱοσ/S/; the Latins *Ianitor* [a 1 cit]

396. jugal [2, 1598, Florio] Ei^{r} The thyrd Processe of the temporall bone ... maketh somewhat a slender reflection, the more aptly to mete with the iugall bone [a 1 cit]

397. jugal [B, 1854, Owen] Eii^{r} the bone called ... in Latin *Iugula* [a 1 cit]

398. jugular [A, 1, 1597, A. M. *Guill.*] Fiii^{r} No lesse seruiceable seemeth this hole to th[e] Iugular Veyne, suffryng the ascense therof [a 1 cit]

399. jugulum [1706, Phillips] Iii^{r} in Latin *Furcula*, *Clavicula*, or *Iugulum* [a 1 cit]

400. junior [2, 1766, B. Peirce] Eiiii^{r} the which seat of the eye, because it is exculped round, the Iunior sort do call a *Roundell*

401. just age [11, 1668, Culpepper and Cole] Bii^{r} matrimonie is ouer liberally & before the iust age, permitted

402. labrum [1816, T. Brown] Cii^{v} See **supercilium**, anted. [a 1 cit]

403. labyrinth [3a, 1696, Phillips] Ei^{v} that noble Labyrinthe, resonant to the reflectyng ayre of euery noyse

404. lambdoides [1597, A. M. *Guill.*] Ciiii^{v} The seame called *Lambdoides* in the hinder part of the head [a 1 cit]

405. lateral [A, 1, 1600, Jonson] Pii^{r} the posteriour and laterall part of th[e] *Anular* bone [a 1 cit]

406. lateral [3a, 1722, Quincey] Giii^{v} (margin) the vse of th[e] hole of th[e] laterall Processes [a 1 cit]

407. lateral [3c, 1724, Bailey] Gi^{v} the true ambulatiue motion of the body is obteyned, forewardes, backwardes, rounde, or laterall reflection admitted [a 1 cit]

408. lateral [B, 1, 1635, Swan] Hi^{r} ij. tranuerse or laterals [a 1 cit]

409. latitant [a, 1646, Browne] Piiii^{r} *Muscles* whiche are called *Latitantes sub Æsophago* [a 1 cit]

410. lawful [1b, 1599, Shakespeare] Iiiii^{r} it is not onely lawfull for the hand, to turne both vpward and downward

411. lengthways [b, 1702, *Providence rec.*] Qiii^{r} the rectitude, and length wayes of the body [a 1 cit]

412. levigate [2, 1694, Salmon] Fi^{r} consideryng that their [th[e] hindmost Grinders] vse and labour is lesse, in Leuigatyng the meate [a 1 cit]
413. lightly [2b, 1594, Shakespeare] Di^{v} *Arthrodia* is, where a place beyng lightly hollow, & that in the enter part, admitteth a litle expressed head
414. limit [*v*, 2b, 1582, Stanyhurst] Ciii^{r} See **extension**, anted.
415. lithoid [1841, Spalding, and ns] Ei^{v} (margin) Why th[e] Greekes call these Bones *Lithoide* [a 1 cit]
416. lumbal [B, 1708, Keill] Hhii^{r} the fift *Muscle* of the thighe, called by his proper name *Lumbalis* [a 1 cit]
417. luxate [1623, Cockeram] Gii^{r} dislocated, or rather *Luxated* [a 1 cit]
418. macrocephaly [1889, NSSL and ns] Bii^{v} In Asia are a people named Macrocephali, hauing very long heades [a 1 cit] [fpl]
419. mallet [5, 1796, Nemnich] Eii^{v} The other part, which is thicker, and endewed with a head ... after th[e] manner of a *Timpan* ... is called a *Mallet* or *Hammer*
420. mamilla [1, 1693, Blancard] Diii^{v} two seames ... are caried aboue the eares ... and in some reache downe to the lowest seat of *Labdoides*, in others agayne, not passing *Mamillares* [a 1 cit]
421. mamillar [1648, J. Beaumont] Ei^{r} The first of which, are the *Mamillar Processes* [a 1 cit]
422. manus [1, 1826, Kirby & Sp.] Iiiii^{v} *Hipocrates* vnderstode the like that we do by the name of *Manus*
423. march [3a, 1604, Grimstone] Piii^{r} The first [Muscle] marcheth forwardes from the middest of the Cannell bone
424. marking [*vbl sb*, 2, 1585, T. Washington] Ciii^{v} hard to be iudged, without diligent heed and markyng
425. masseter [1666, J. Smith] Fii^{v} The originall of the muscle called masseter or *Mansoria* [a 1 cit]
426. mastoid [A, a, 1732, Monro] Ei^{r} representyng the fashion of *Tetes* in a Cowes vdder, called therfore of the *Grecians* /S/*μαστοιδισ*/S/
427. maxillary [B, 1836, Todd] Fi^{r} Now of the Grinders, called *Maxillares*, or *Molares* [a 1 cit]
428. meadowy [1598, Florio] Biii^{r} places more meadowy, or grou[n]des flowing with herbes [a 1 cit]
429. mediate [*v*, c, 1592, Marlowe] Aiiii^{v} before you take any occasion to accuse me of temeritie, whiche crime I had worthely incurred if zeale should not mediate my cause
430. medulla [1a, 1651, *Ralegh's Ghost*] Eeiiii^{r} the Nerues of *Spinalis Medula* [a 1 cit]
431. melancholy [1b, 1646, T. Wright] Uii^{v} the splene might poure forth vnto the ventricle melancholie iuyce
432. membrane [1a, 1615, Crooke] Ci^{r} All the partes of mans body are either *Similar* or *Simple*, with sence, as are *Ligamentes*, *Fibres*, *Membrans*, *Flesh*, and *Fatte*: or els *Dissimilar* or *Instrumentall*, as the *Veine*, *Artery*,

Sinewe, *Muscle*, *Finger*, and other *Organs* of the whole body

433. membraneous [1633, Fletcher] Fiiii^{v} with *Membraneous* bandes, are tyed to the lower sides of the bones [a 1 cit]

434. meninx [a, 1616, Bullokar] Ddiii^{v} they reach to *Dura* and *Tenuis meninx* [a 1 cit]

435. menstruous [2, 1599, Moufet] Yiii^{r} out of whiche place their menstruous purgations flowe

436. mesaræum [1594, T. B.] Xii^{r} those veynes which happe to be called *Mesaraica* or *Mesaraea* [a 1 cit]

437. mucous [1, 1646, Browne] Liii^{v} a certaine mucous, or slimie substance [a 1 cit]

438. mucronate [1776, J. Lee] Miiii^{r} the shieldlyke *Cartilage* … *Mucronatum* [a 1 cit]

439. mysterious [1, 1622, Massinger and Dekker] Ci^{r} in searchyng the true Secresie of this Misterious Science [a 1 cit]

440. narrowly [1708, Swift] See **delineation**, anted.

441. nates [2, 1681, tr. *Willis*] Ggii^{r} *Processes* of the brayne called *Nates, Penes, Testes* [a 1 cit]

442. naviform [1816, Faber] Liiii^{r} (margin) The bone of the foote called *Scaphoides* and *Naviforme* [a 1 cit]

443. neb [3b, 1611, Cotgrave] Liiii^{r} a *Processe* like the neb of a shyppe or boate

444. neck [14b, 1726, Munro] Cii^{v} we call the slender part therof, from the body of the bone, vnto the head of the *Processe*, a necke

445. nerve [II, 8, 1606, Shakespeare] Ci^{v} the Nerues, whiche are the organs of sence

446. nomad [1, 1587, Golding] Biii^{r} True it is also that the Scythia[n]s, named Nomades, are very corpule[n]t [a 1 cit]

447. nominate [1b, 1597, Hooker] Gi^{v} thou shalt note to be of the *Grecians* nominated /S/*βαχιξ*/S/ and /S/*υοτυμ*/S/

448. nominate [2, 1593, G. Harvey] Hii^{v} The fift and last portion of the backe which heartofore we haue nominated, called *Coccix*

449. notum [1877, Huxley] Gi^{v} See **nominate**, 1b, anted. [a 1 cit]

450. nutrition [1, 1615, Crooke] Siii^{v} instruments seruyng to nutrition

451. nutrition [2, 1603, Holland] Ffiiii^{r} by meanes of renewyng these nutricions, that humour is also ingendred

452. obelion [1878, Bartley] Ciiii^{v} (margin) The seame called *Obelaia*, or *Sagitalis* [a 1 cit]

453. obligate [*v*, 1, 1600 Shakespeare] Diiii^{v} a *Cartilage* … connecteth the head to the first and second *Veterbre*, whereby the same … might more firmely be bound and obligated to those smal bones

454. oblique [2c, 1615, Crooke] Eii^{r} knit together by an oblique Suture

455. obliterate [1a, 1611, Speed] Bii^{v} let vs … wholy obliterate their writyngs [a 1 cit]

456. obnoxious [1a, 1597, Hooker] Biii^{r} they would not be able to hold their bowes, or cast their darts, for losenes of their ioints, through slippery humours so obnoxious to luxation [a 1 cit]
457. obscurity [2, 1619, Drayton] Giiii^{r} neither the hollownes of the one, nor the head of the other are (for their obscuritie) to be so termed playnly
458. observed [*ppl a*, 1602, Shakespeare] Biiii^{r} the obserued stones in the lunges [fpl]
459. obstriction [1671, Milton, and ns] Ii^{r} Brayne ... the obstriction and dilatation therof [a 1 cit]
460. obstruct [*v*, 1, 1611, Cotgrave] Xi^{v} it is obstruct, and stopped [a 1 cit]
461. obtuse [1, 1589, Puttenham] Tiiii^{v} with an obtuse or blunt corner
462. odontoides [B, 1706, Phillips] Giii^{r} (margin) What is the process called *Odontoides* [a 1 cit]
463. olecranon [a, 1727-41 *Chamb. Cycl.*] Sii^{r} the superior part of the cubit called *Olecranon* [a 1 cit]
464. operation [6, 1597, A. M. *Guill.*] Ci^{v} the good Artiste ... after he passeth (in his operation) *Periosteon*
465. opposite [2, 1594, R. Ashley] Uiii^{r} the straight *Fibres* of the stomach moue in opposite order to natures first decree
466. oppressive [1, 1627–77, Feltham] Dii^{v} the other ouer heauy, and to much (more then nature would) oppressiue [a 1 cit]
467. orbicular [A, 1b, 1615, Crooke] Eiiii^{v} The fashion of the neither iawe is *Orbicular* like a halfe long *Circle*, the vtmost endes wherof are ascendently reflected
468. os hyoides [1842, F. Wilson] Fiiii^{v} For by these *Processes*, is *Os Hyoides* fast knit with the *Stiliformed Processes* [fpl]
469. os ilium [1611, Cotgrave] Hii^{r} yeldyng on ech side from *Os Ilium* in tyme of bringyng forth Child [a 1 cit] [fpl]
470. os pubis [1754-64, Smellie] Kiii^{v} an other part [of *Os sacrum*] ... is called *Os pubis* [fpl]
471. os sacrum [1741, Monro] Biiii^{v} And first (touchyng the Sceleton) in the number of Vertebres; as ... fiue in Os sacrum [fpl]
472. outgoing [1633, Struther] Giii^{r} ii. *Processes*, or outgoyng portions [a 1 cit]
473. outstretching [1654, Gataker] Dii^{r} the fore part and the hinder part be eminent, or out stretching
474. over-liberally [1601, Holland] Bii^{r} wheras matrimonie is ouer liberally, & before the iust age, permitted [a 1 cit] [fpl]
475. overspreading [1610, Willet] Liii^{r} without the ouerspreadyng, or deffensive clothyng of a *Cartilage* [a 1 cit] [fpl]
476. overtake [*v*, 8, 1581, W. Charke] Xi^{r} others ... were greatly ouertaken with errour
477. parastatic [a^{2}, 1693, Urquhart's *Rab.*] Qiii^{v} the *Glandules* called *Parastata* [a 1 cit]

478. parenchyma [1a, 1657, Purchas] Aai^{r} the small twigges or *Fibres* of the vessels ... are couered with much thicke and feaculent bloud, which *Eristratus* called *Parenchina* [a 1 cit]
479. parotid [B, 2, 1747, Astruc] Tii^{r} those abcesses, called of the Greekes *Parotides* [a 1 cit]
480. patella [1, 1693, tr. Blancard] Lii^{v} called of the latins diuersly: as *Patella, genu mola, scutiforme os*, and *Rotula genu*, in English the *Patell* ... the eye of the knee
481. pectus [1693, tr. Blancard and ns] Hiiii^{v} The brestbone ... in Latin *Pectus* [a 1 cit]
482. pelvis [2, 1678, Tyson] Ffi^{r} See **hopper**, anted. [a 1 cit]
483. penis [1693, tr. Blancard] Kiiii^{v} *Penis*, and the *Testicles* [a 1 cit]
484. perfector [1587, Golding] Cciiii^{r} the fountaine of vitall heate, and perfector of vitall spirites
485. perforated [*ppl a*, 1e, 1886, Cassell's *Enc.*] Fii^{r} the Holes of the head, and such Perforated places as yeld no lesse pleasure to the passage of *Veynes, Nerues*, and *Arteries*
486. perforating [*ppl a*, 1661, K. W.] Riiii^{r} the tendons of the perforatyng *Muscle* [a 1 cit]
487. periosteum [1597, A. M. *Guill.*] *i^{r} To these I haue added a ninth, least (otherwise) the marey, Periosteon, and the heares should haue bene sought in vayne in the History of Man [a 1 cit]
488. perpetual [2b, 1658, Earl Monm.] Siiii^{v} the skinne is not left perpetuall
489. perspicuity [3, 1609, B. Jonson] Diiii^{r} both *Sistole*, and *Diastole* of the brayne, most euident, and with pleasaunt perspicuitie ... is to be discerned
490. pertinacious [1b, 1646, Lawrence] Kiii^{v} their composition is made more strong, and pertinatious [a 1 cit]
491. phrase [2b, 1597, Shakespeare] Iii^{v} *Humerus*, whiche in English phrase is interpreted the shoulder
492. phrenes [1706, Phillips] Qi^{v} *Grecians* called it *Phrenes* whiche is by interpretation the mynde. [a 1 cit]
493. piety [3, 1579, Lyly] Aii^{r} With no lesse pietie haue abandoned themselues, lest, by their own prosperitie, the state of the com[m]ons might be impaired
494. pineal [a, 1681, Willis] Ti^{v} the first [Glandule] in the Scull ... is called *Conarion Pineale* [a 1 cit]
495. pituitous [a, 1607, Topsell] Eiii^{v} the pituitous excrements expurged fro[m] the head vnto the eyes [a 1 cit]
496. plectrum [2, 1826, Kirby & Sp.] Ei^{r} See **belonoides**, unrec. [a 1 cit]
497. pleura [1a, 1664, Power] Hiiii^{r} a most Tensible *Membran* called *Pleura* [a 1 cit]
498. plexus [1, 1682, T. Gibson] Eeiiii^{r} (margin) *Plexus coriformes*. The vse [a 1 cit]

499. podium [2, 1858, Mayne] Liii[r] The second, called *Podium*, is co[m]parable to the *Postbrachial* bones
500. pointing [a, 1630, Milton] Cii[v] Others also beyng sharpe but not so slender, as the knagge of a hartes horne, that is to say thicke and poynting [a 1 cit]
501. postbrachial [B, 2, 1852, and ncit] Iiiii[v] *Postbrachiale*, which is the space betwene the wrest, and the first ioynt of the fingers [fpl]
502. posterior [a, A, 3, 1632, Lithgow] Ciii[r] the *Posterior Processe* of the *Cubite*
503. præcordia [1601, Holland] Qi[v] *Plinie*, and others after him, named it *Præcordia*
504. predicate [2b, 1882–3, *Schaff's Enc.*] Ii i[r] the Reader is forewarned that euery Prædicate is to be sought vnder his subiect
505. prepared [1b, 1663, Boyle] Ddii[v] the hart ... receiueth ... prepared bloud and spirite into the left ventricle
506. pretend [*v*, I, 1, 1596, Spenser] Li[r] The head [of *Tibia*] is thicke, round and ouercrusted with a *Cartilage*, hauyng the necke therof, which is lo[n]g, much inwardly prete[n]ded
507. processus [1651, H. More] Ffi[v] /S/*Αποφυλισ*/S/ which the Latin interpretours call *Processus* is thus: when a bone in any part, stretcheth forth his substance in an excreasing manner [a 1 cit]
508. procrastination [1, 1632, Lithgow] Gii[r] the necessarie, and healthfull procrastination of lyfe [a 1 cit]
509. produced [*ppl a*, 1644, Bulwer] Hi[r] *Processes* or produced portio[n]s [fpl]
510. progress [3a, 1595, Shakespeare] Iii[v] vnder that regio[n] lyeth the progresse of principall vessels
511. prominence [2, 1598, Florio] Diiii[v] Neither not elegantly hath nature erected a *Prominence*, fro[m] that hole, wherby th[e] brayne is deriued into the spinall marey
512. promptitude [1b, 1660, Jer. Taylor] Yiii[v] I prayse the promptitude of his mynde
513. prone [*a*, 6b, 1607, Horden] Lii[v] prone to be luxated forward
514. protuberated [*ppl a*, 1683, Snape] Kiiii[r] their protuberated or swelled portions [fpl]
515. protuberating [*ppl a*, 1615, Crooke] Iiii[v] these Protuberatyng *Processes* [fpl]
516. psalloid [1756, Douglas] Eeiiii[v] See **fornix**, anted. [a 1 cit]
517. psoas [1681, Willis] Piiii[v] The three *Muscles* are of the loynes, which the *Grecians* call /S/*Πψοασ*/S/ [a 1 cit]
518. pterigoid [1a, 1722, Quincy *Lex Physico-med.*] Ei[v] (margin) The processes of the *Cuneall* bone called *Pterigoides* [a 1 cit]
519. pubis [1, 1597, A. M. *Guill.*] Ciiii[v] *Synchondrosis*, is to be noted by the bones of the brest, and *Pubis*, the *Vertebres* themselues [a 1 cit]

520. puff [*v*, 4b, 1725, Bradley] Hi^{r} the Loynes, ... whose turnyng Ioyntes we acco[m]pt in number, fiue, greater than all we haue hitherto described, but most in substaunce puffed, and of lesse soliditie
521. pylorus [a, 1615, Crooke] Ui^{r} the Grecians call it /S/πυλοϱοσ/S/, the Latins *Ianitor*[a 1 cit]
522. quadrangular [1592, G. Harvey] Diiii^{v} a quadra[n]gular, or four square maner [a 1 cit]
523. quote [*v*, I, 4, 1680, Butler] Hi^{v} *Collumbus*, who without all maner of indifferent excusation coateth *Vesalius*
524. radius [1c, 1615, Crooke] Cii^{r} Likewise the bone of the shoulder, with the scaple bone: and that which in like sort is tyed to *Radius*, and *Vlna*
525. ramex [1608-9, Middleton] Tiii^{r} in Latin *Ramex* and in English a rupture [a 1 cit]
526. ready [7c, 1730, *Coll. Rec. Pennslyv.*] Eiiii^{v} this neither iawe ... retayneth not such Solliditie, as might be an impediment to the light and ready motio[n] therof
527. recited [*ppl a*, 1630, Prynne] Ii^{v} the two last recited *Processes* [a 1 cit]
528. recrement [2a, 1615, Crooke] Diii^{r} the fuliginous recrements, inwardly ascending without any transpirative vent [a 1 cit]
529. rectus [a, 1704, J. Harris] Diii^{v} The thyrd *Suture* ... or *Recta Sutura*
530. recurrent [1, 1611, Florio] Eiii^{v} as though betweene the *Incissorie*, and Dogge teeth, were some interceptive Seame recurre[n]t [a 1 cit]
531. reduce [14a, 1605, Timme] Siii^{v} And so alway to the old estate we maintaine and reduce them both
532. reduplication [1b, 1698, Tyson] Tiii^{r} a simple membran, but from the nauell downwardes doubled, the vse of which reduplication is [a 1 cit]
533. refer [8, B, 1605, Shakespeare] Ciii^{v} for familiar exa[m]ple sake, I referre you to the beholdyng of the *Articulation* of *Talus*, with the botelike bone
534. reflected [*ppl a*, 1, 1611, Speed] Fiiii^{r} a very *Obtuse* or blunt corner: but the hinder part therof, which is more inward ... is hollow in reflected or bowed manner
535. reflecting [*ppl a*, 1, 1591, *Troub. Reign K. John*, and ns] Ei^{v} See **resonant**, anted. [a 1 cit]
536. regurgitate [1a, 1653, H. More] Yiiii^{r} neither admittyng ... any of the choler to regurgitate backe agayne [a 1 cit]
537. regurgitate [2, 1753, Torrland] Dii^{v} findyng no passage to regurgitate the superfluities [a 1 cit]
538. relax [11b, 1620, Venner] Li^{r} this *Ligament* ... is relaxed, & slacked
539. resistance [3b, 1656, Boyle] Lii^{r} these ii. make strong resistaunce
540. resistant [A, 1620, Guillim] Ciii^{r} hauyng the offices also of *Propugnacles*, or resistant defences [a 1 cit]
541. resonant [2, 1685, tr. Hobbes] Ei^{v} that noble Laberinthe, resonant to the reflectyng ayre of euery noyse [a 1 cit]

542. respect [6c, 1583, Stubbes] Ciiii^{r} Somme adde an exa[m]ple of the *Commissures* like the nayles, not for that they mutually respect one another, but do occupy and stoppe the vacant places reside[n]t betwene the nayles of the fingers
543. respect [II, 8b, 1581, J. Bell] Dii^{r} *Realdus Collumbus*: who denyeth not *Galens* opinion in this respect
544. reticular [1a, 1597, Lowe] Eeiiii^{r} the reticular or net like foldes [a 1 cit]
545. rite [1b, 1581, Pettie] Niiii^{v} Neither doe the *Muscles* obserue one rite or order their exorture
546. rotator [1, 1676 Wiseman, and ns] Cii^{v} See **trochanter**, anted.
547. rotatory [A, 1b, 1812, H. & J. Smith] Eii^{v} those which in the thighe we call the *Rotatorie Processes*
548. rotundity [1a, 1597, A. M. *Guill.*] Kii^{v} with their magnitude; and rotunditie, fulfill the flattenes so on that side [a 1 cit]
549. rounded [*ppl a*, 5, 1796, Withering] Iiii^{v} the hollow or rounded gutter in the lower end and shoulder bone
550. runged [1694, *Phil. Trans.* XVIII] Ciiii^{v} some where concurryng euen, & in other places ronged: being therfore a mixed vnio[n] [a 1 cit] [fpl]
551. sacrum [1753, *Cham. Cycl. Supp.*] Hii^{r} the two last partes or diuisions of the backe ... called ... of the Latins *Sacrum* [a 1 cit]
552. sagged [*ppl a*, 1647, Staplyton] Bbiiii^{r} they incontinent become slacke, narrow together, sagde, and shorter [a 1 cit]
553. scaphoid [A, 1741, Monro] Liii^{r} The first of all therefore is named *Talus*, the second *Calx*, the thyrd *Scaphoides* [a 1 cit]
554. scope [6a, 1600, Shakespeare] Aiiii^{v} I perceiued I might both more playnly describe the partes to the iudgement of the Reader, as also vse sufficient scope vpon the dissention of Authours in the most notable causes
555. scope [6b, 1830, Herschel] Aiiii^{r} as men not retayning the whole summe and scope of Arte to them selues ... their wordes are not as Gospel in all thynges
556. scope [9, 1590, Spenser] Ei^{v} the *Palate* and nostrels, the wayes of which one, haue sufficie[n]t scope into the other
557. scrotum [1597, A. M. *Guill.*] Bbi^{r} to dissect *Scrotum*, for the sight, and administration of the Testicles [a 1 cit]
558. scrupulous [5, 1638, Junius] Eiiii^{v} needless to contend vpon such scrupulous and sharpe poynted diuision
559. scutiform [1656, Blount] Fiiii^{v} See **scutalem**, unrec. [a 1 cit]
560. seam [v^{2}, 2b, 1695, Blackmore] Eiii^{v} *Os malæ*, is greater the[n] the rest, but of strau[n]ge fourme, and diuersly seamed [a 1 cit]
561. seamy [2, Mickle 1776] Dii^{v} vaporous fumosities (which otherwise by the seamy *Commisures*, would transpirately evaporate) [a 1 cit]
562. seat [9a, 1607, Topsell] Xii^{r} the fundament or seat, in men vnder the bleddar

563. secure [II, 3e, 1841, T. R. Jones] Xii^{v} it [*Mesenterium*] ... might safely gather together, and shield the secure course of the veynes from *Porta*
564. securely [2, 1615, Braithwait] Uiii^{v} the Membrans of *Peritoneum* securely carrying the vessels to the intestines [a 1 cit] [fpl]
565. seed vein [1615, Crooke] Yii^{v} a veyne called *Seminalis*, or a seede veyne [a 1 cit]
566. semicircled [1586, Marlowe] Gii^{r} a blunt bowyng, and *Semicircled* corner [a 1 cit]
567. seminary [1, 1592, Nashe] Biiii^{v} a woman who had outwardly a perfect shape, & no matrice, seminarie vessels, or Testicles at all [a 1 cit]
568. sensible [IV, 14, 1584, Scot] Ci^{r} you shall finde the rest of this booke, not onely in reading vnsauery, but also to your sensible vnderstandyng very obscure
569. sensibly [4, 1755, Johnson] Oiii^{r} thou hast to consider of the Muscles of the eyes, abstract sensibly from *Galen*
570. separation [6, 1615, Crooke] Diiii^{v} In which hole, appeareth foure seperations, or diuisions, so that it seemeth to be deuided into foure partes
571. septum [1b, 1726, Monro] Hiii^{r} stayed and bound to *Septum transversum* [a 1 cit]
572. serous [1a, 1594, T. B.] Yii^{r} the bloud, which together with the serous matter is deduced to the reynes [a 1 cit]
573. sesaminae [B, 1607, Topsell] Ci^{v} the bones of the nose, and *Sesaminae*
574. sesamine [A, 1608, Topsell] Mi^{v} They are called *Sesamina Ossicula* for their litlenes, and likenes to the *Sesamine* seede
575. sharp [3b, 1580, Spenser] Dii^{r} (margin) A sharpe reason, in that the eyes of Cankers are hard
576. sharp [B, 3, 1633, *Verney Mem.*] Gi^{r} the thyrd vnnamed bone ... in the posteriour part towardes the stomacke, it is broader, & is exte[n]ded into a sharpe
577. sharp-bellied [C, 1, 1804, Shaw] Giiii^{r} Euery turnyng ioynt hath his body, besides the first & vppermost, which hath onely a light compassyng proportion, beyng sharpe bellied towardes the forepartes [fpl]
578. shiplike [8d, 1842, Faber] Ciiii^{r} ioyned with the shiplike bone [fpl]
579. sideway [A, 1612, Peacham] Iiii^{v} the head of *Radius* is admitted sideway [a 1 cit]
580. sifting [*ppl a*, 1642, H. More] Fiii^{r} as it were the small siftyng holes of a searse [a 1 cit]
581. sigmoid [A, 1, 1670, *Phil. Trans.*] Iiii^{v} the whiche cauitie ... represe[n]teth the figure of a C in Latin ... and for that cause *Galen* named it *Sigmoides* [a 1 cit]
582. similar [A, 1, 1626, Bacon] Tii^{v} the simple bodyes, called *similar* partes [a 1 cit]
583. sinuate [1848, *Blackwood's Mag.*] Li^{r} the outer side of *Talus* is largely sinuated [a 1 cit]

584. site [*v*², 2, 1630, *R. Johnson's Kingd.*] Eiii^v the excrementall purgyngs of the brayne, are receiued by this peece of flesh in this angle sited [a 1 cit]
585. situation [3a, 1600, Shakespeare] Bii^r how ... do our bodies testifie, how sondry of the inner partes both in magnitude, number, figure, and situation, do differ from those in others of other regions?
586. slope [*sb*², 2a, 1611, Cotgrave] Piii^v their race is a slope, or oblique
587. society [1b, 1588, Shakespeare] Aii^r Nothing ioyeth without societie of other
588. solid [II, 7, *Reg. Privy Council Scot.*] Aii^r See **procrastinate**, ns.
589. solidity [2a, 1603, Holland] Ci^v *Andreas Vesalius* also supposed that neither the bones of the nose, and *Sesaminae*, neither the little *Ossicles* that constitute the organ of hearyng, should be other wise then made of massive *Soliditie*
590. soporiferous [2b, 1601, Holland] Ddiiii^v so many distributions of the *Soporiferous* Arteries aboue the sell of the Cuneall bone [a 1 cit]
591. spinal [1b, 1725, Pope] Gi^v Construed of *Vertebres* or *Spondilles* most exquisitely: Which beyng also together mutually concaued, make in them selues by strict *Coarticualation* the closse [*sic*] Cloysture and safe Gallery for the *Spinall* marey
592. spinal process [1b, 1726, Monro] Ii^v next to the *Spinall Processes* of the pectorall *Vertebres* [fpl]
593. spine [3, 1706, Phillips] Piiii^v fastened to all the Spines of the *Vertebres* of the brest
594. spriggy [1597, Gerarde] Diii^r See **tendring**, unrec.
595. spur [II, 5b, 1681, Grew] Liii^v heele bone, or ... the Spurre of the foote
596. spur-like [1829, T. Castle] Ei^r And these stiliforme, or spurrelike processes are prominent next vnder *Mamillares* [a 1 cit]
597. steady [2b, 1885, Horner] Eii^v the second Ossicle, called by the name of a stedy or an anueld [a 1 cit]
598. stephanion [1878, Bartley] Ciiii^v (margin) The seame called *Stephaneia* in the fore parte of the head [a 1 cit]
599. sternon [1597, A. M. *Guill.*] Hiiii^v (margin) *Sternon* ... the brest bone [a 1 cit]
600. stethos [1876, Ransom] Hiiii^v Stethos is rather the region of the brest [a 1 cit]
601. stimulate [3a, 1707, Floyer] Uiiii^v See **influx**, anted.
602. stock [3a, 1616, Beau. & Fl.] Oi^r the *Fibres* of that Musculous stocke
603. straight [1h, 1585, Higins] Xii^r *Rectum Intestinu[m]*, in English the straight gutte
604. strainer [1b, 1626, Bacon] Aaii^v they haue ... written, this fatnes of the Urinarie way to be a certaine worke to be made in the reynes to the excretion ... of Urine: and therfore to be as a certaine strayner
605. straitening [1598, Stow] Qi^v straitening of the brest [fpl]

606. strengthened [*ppl a*, 1586, Sidney] Diiii^{v} See **distinguish**, anted. [a 1 cit] [fpl]
607. structure [3b, 1615, Crooke] Ciiii^{v} For by *Harmonia* is vndersta[n]ded, that kynde of *structure* in the Bones, made by a simple meetyng
608. styloid [1615, Crooke] Cii^{v} like the fashion of a sharpe bodkin: wherfore the *Grecians* call such *Processes*, *Slyloides* [a 1 cit]
609. subduction [3, 1612, Woodall] Kiiii^{r} open on eche side ... for the subduction of uery many, and large surcles [a 1 cit]
610. sublevate [1597, A. M. *Guill.*] Oiiii^{v} the waight beyng subleuated by the attraction of these *Muscles* [a 1 cit]
611. subsisting [*vbl sb*, 1a, 1592, Hooker] Kiiii^{v} a voyde, and empty corner, for the subsistyng of *Penis* [a 1 cit]
612. supercilium [3, 1706, Phillips] Cii^{v} there are certaine *Circular Processes* which augme[n]t the profundities of such *Celes* ... called *Labra*, or *Supercilia*, as it were the lippes or browes ... to those caues [a 1 cit]
613. superior [4, 1634, Ford] Hi^{v} we finde not these holes so round as there [*sic*] superiors
614. superjacent [1611, Guillim] Diiii^{r} These are the lineall coagmentatio[n]s of the two skales, that keepe the compressed sides of the head, bordryng vpon the other bones, or on their endes Superiacent [a 1 cit]
615. supernaturally [2, 1597, A. M. *Guill.*] Bbiiii^{v} without fatnes altogether ... lest supernaturally therewith encreasing, it might be greuous to the matrice
616. suppress [*v*, 7, 1621, Burton] Bii^{v} some of them beyng a while frutefull, but after widowes, and for that suppressed of naturall course, put on virilitie, being then bearded, hearie, and chau[n]ged in voyce
617. suspensor [1746, tr. Le Cat, and ns] Qiiii^{v} The auncient writers haue called these *Muscles Cremasteres*, as it were, *Suspensores* or hangers vp [a 1 cit]
618. suspensory [B, *sb*, 1699, de la Vauguion] Niii^{r} The right of these two *Ligamentes* is called a *Suspensory*
619. swallowed [1600, Shakespeare] Ui^{r} auoyde great swallowed bones [a 1 cit]
620. sweating [3, 1586, Day] Iiii^{v} *Collumbus*, (whose sweatyng labours could neuer appale the indefatigable courage of this searchyng skill)
621. synchondrosis [1615, Crooke] Ciiii^{v} a *Cartilage* goeth betwene, and this vnion the Grecians call *Synchondrosis* [a 1 cit]
622. syndesmo- [1848, Dunglison] Ni^{r} A Ligament is called of the Greekes /S/συνδισμοσ/S/, the Latins *Vinculum* [a 1 cit]
623. syndesmosis [1720, Monro] Ciiii^{v} See **syndesmos**, unrec. [a 1 cit] [fpl]
624. synneurosis [1676 Wiseman] Ciiii^{v} by the helpe of a *Nerue* or *Ligament* they are conioyned, and that they call Synneurosis [a 1 cit]
625. syssarcosis [1, 1676, Wiseman] Ciiii^{v} Either els the vnion, is made, by the apposition of fleshe, therfore by the Greeke name *Syssarcosis*

626. table [II, 16, 1612, Woodall] Diii[v] some haue sayd, the scull to be condited and made of two walles, which they call tables: meanyng those .ii. crustes, or scales, which beyng hard, and therewith a little thicke, do shut in on eche side that sayd *Spongious* & medullous substaunce
627. talus [*sb*², 1, 1693, Blancard] Ciii[v] to set … the bone of the heele, to that under the ancle called *Talus* [a 1 cit]
628. tarsus [1a, 1676, Wiseman] Cii[v] the insteppe, meeting with the Bones of *Tarsus* and *Fibula* [a 1 cit]
629. temporal [*a*², A, 1597, A. M. *Guill.*] Diiii[v] *Galen* hath named them … temporall *Sutures*
630. tend [*v*², 1c, 1641, Wilkins] Giiii[r] neither altogether so much forwardly tendyng
631. tenderly [1b, 1604, Grimstone] Eiiii[r] a uery large cauitie, tenderly walled on ech side with thinne scally bones
632. tendinous [1658, Rowland] Hiiii[v] in that place is much of sinewye, or tendinous substaunce [a 1 cit]
633. terrestrial [2b, 1658, Rowland] Ci[r] they are not accou[n]ted voyde of feeling, because they are most of th[e] terrestrial element
634. testis [2, 1681, *Willis Rem. Med.*] Eeiiii[v] called therfore of Anathomists *Testes* [a 1 cit]
635. theatre [5, 1613, Purchas] Gi[v] *Col.* writeth that *Vesa.* neglected the bodie of ma[n], for this part *Larinx*, & dissected it of custome in beastes: yea, and i[n] publicke Theaters
636. thymus [1, 1693, Blancard] Ti[v] other *Glandules* slender in vs, but thicker in beastes, called *Lacies* and *Thymus* [a 1 cit]
637. thyroid [1a, 1693, *Blancard*] Fiiii[v] the *Anathomistes* … call it, for the liknes of the thyng, *Scutalem* … the Grecians /S/*θυρoειδισ*/S/ [a 1 cit]
638. tibia [1, 1726-41, Munro] Cii[v] the bone of the cubite called *Vlna*, and the inferior part of *Tibia*
639. tonsil [1, 1601, Holland] Tiiii[v] The Latins terme them *Tonsilla* [a 1 cit]
640. tooth [II, 3b, 1694, Salmon] Di[r] that *Ligament*, wherewith, the tooth of the second *Verterbre* of the necke, is knitte to the hinder part of the head
641. topic [II, 2b, 1601, Holland] Xiii[r] (margin) *Topic Medicinis* are rashly applied vppon the sharpe cartilage
642. topic medicinis [II, 2b, 1601, Holland] Xiii[r] See **topic**, anted.
643. torcular [*sb*, 1, 1657, *Phys. Dict.*] Ddiiii[r] (margin) *Torcular* is the forth cauitie of *Dura Mater* [a 1 cit]
644. track [*sb*, 4b, 1807–26, S. Cooper] Eiiii[r] the tra[n]suerse *Suture* in the *Palate* … is in elder persons quite abolished, so that the tracke therof may not be found
645. tract [*sb*³, III, 11, 1583, Golding] Dii[v] See **dissection**, 1, anted.
646. transmission [1a, 1611, Florio] Hii[r] (margin) th[e] transmission of Nerues [a 1 cit]

647. transmitting [1681, Fleming] Siii[v] seruyng to the transmittyng of these excretions [fpl]
648. transporter [2, 1893, *Westm. Gaz.*] Hi[v] the transporters of sense produced from the Spinall marey
649. transversely [1650, Bulwer] Diiii[r] The ... last *Suture* ... creeping through the middle regio[n] of the lesser corner of the eye ... thence transversly spedeth to the toppe of the nose [a 1 cit]
650. triangle [*v*, 1, 1595, *Aberdeen Regr.*] Lii[v] it is in like sorte triangled [a 1 cit]
651. triple-formed [1606, Sylvester] Fi[v] And thus much of the triple-formed difference
652. trochanter [1, 1615, Crooke] Cii[v] the processes of the thighe called *Trochanteres* or *Rotatores* [a 1 cit]
653. turning [7, 1734, *Rollins Anc. Hist.*] Ggiii[r] the first *Vertebre*, or turnyng ioynt of the necke
654. twig [3, 1683, Snape] Fi[r] departyng from the sensible Surcles of twigges of the Sinowe aforesayd
655. type [5, 1843, Mill] Fii[r] *Vesalius* ... concluded with my selfe, to imitate the type of their Assertio[n]s
656. ulceration [2, 1580, T. Newton] Aaiii[v] subiect to vlcerations
657. umbilical [A, 1b, 1615, Crooke] Ti[r] the *Umbelical* Veyne
658. umbilical [B, 1774, Cooper] Tiii[r] the arteries called *Vmbelicales*
659. umbilicus [1a, 1615, Crooke] Ti[r] a line, and round pitte, called the nauell, of the Latins *Vmbelicus* [a 1 cit]
660. unequal [*a*, 3c, 1613, Purchas] Eiiii[v] See **indented**, anted.
661. union [1c, 1631, H. Crooke] Ciiii[v] wherefore doubtlesse the true unio[n] of such Bones, is rather to be attributed to that kynde of *Symphysis* called *Harmonia*, then *Sutura*
662. unite [1b, 1597, Shakespeare] Eiiii[r] where both these bones are vnited with the common line, they cleave to that diuision
663. unnamed [2a, 1611, Donne] Fiiii[v] See **unnamed**, 2b, anted.
664. unnamed [2b, 1845, *Encyc. Metrop.*] Fiiii[v] other *Anathomistes* do call the seco[n]d vnnamed *Cartilage*, but *Collumbus* maketh it the thyrd vnnamed bone
665. urge [III, 6a, 1594, Kyd] Gii[r] the dayly motion of such few bones, so outragiously urged
666. vas [1a, 1651, Biggs] Bbii[v] the seminall veynes, and arteries, which also are named *Vasa præparantia* [a 1 cit]
667. vault [1d, 1594, T. B.] Ki[r] the vault on th[e] inside of th[e] wrest[1]
668. vena axillaris [1598, Florio] Iii[v] principall vessels, caryeng the Animall, Vitall, and Naturall Faculties that is to saye *Vena axillaris* and *Cephalica* [a 1 cit] [fpl]
669. vena porta [1626, Jonson] Biiii[r] he obserued stones in the lunges, liuer, Vena Porta, vrinarie wayes [a 1 cit] [fpl]

670. vestigium [a, 1637, Nabbes and ns] Mi^{r} the second part of the foote, called of the Latins *Planta*, or *Vestigium*, as it were the footesteppe [a 1 cit]
671. vicinity [1b, 1651, Baxter] Mii^{v} bycause of their vicinitie which [*sic*] the temporall bone
672. vigorous [3a, 1599, Hakluyt] Hi^{r} (margin) deuided with some vigorous contusio[n]
673. vinculum [3, 1859, Mayne] Ni^{r} A Ligament is called of ... the Latins *Vinculum*, which we translate a Bond [a 1 cit]
674. violate [4b, 1595, Daniel] Tiii^{r} the continuitie hereof beyng violated and broken
675. virility [1c, 1890, *Am. Naturalist]* Bii^{v} See **suppress**, anted. [a 1 cit]
676. vitreous [2b, 1663, Boyle] Ffiiii^{r} (margin) Situation of the vitreous humor [a 1 cit]
677. vocal [6, 1644, Digby] Pii^{v} the vocall organ
678. vomiting [*sb*, 1b, 1601, Holland] Yiiii^{v} the vomityng forth of choler from his vessicle: as one to the intrels, an other to the ventricle
679. waterish [2a, 1583, Stubbes] Aai^{v} serous and watrish humiditie
680. watery [4c, 1615, Crooke] Ffiii^{v} betwene the glassie and watrie humor
681. welter [*v*, 2c, 1629, J. Cole] Hhi^{v} in whiche absurditie many are weltred, whose names on earth resounde as ecchoes from the rockes
682. wheeling [a, 1628, Milton] Iii^{r} the circumaction and round, or wheelyng motion of the shoulder [a 1 cit]
683. white line [1, 1598, Florio] Ti^{r} the lyne or hollow tyeng from it [the nauell] for the whitenes therof, *Linea Alba*, the white line [a 1 cit]
684. who [11c, 1588, Shakespeare] Ciii^{v} the *Vertebres* & their *Processes*, Who are both co[n]stringed, & also dilated
685. wing [10, 1650, Bulwer] Miii^{r} the extreme partes of the nose, wherof two constitute the sides called the wynges
686. writhing [2, 1798, R. Bloomfield] Yiiii^{r} they haue into the intrell not onely a writhyng entrance [a 1 cit]
687. xiphoid [1746, Glass] Hiiii^{v} some also call it *Ensiformis* and *Gladialis*, other, for that it ha[n]geth like a shield, say *Clypealis*, some agayne, *Malum granatu[m]* but the Greekes, *Xiphoides* [a 1 cit]

2. *New senses*

1. addict Riiii^{r} to euery toe ii. *Muscles* are addicted
2. ancyroid [not as *sb*] Ii^{v} One of them compared to a Crowes beke, or anker, is therefore called *Ancryoides*, or *Coracoides*
3. appurtinent [not as *adv.*] Bii^{v} But, to speake more appertine[n]t to the bodie of man
4. arabia Yiiii^{v} See **arabia**, anted.
5. ascendent [*sb*, cf *a*, 1b] Giiii^{r} the ascendentes cut obliquely or slopwise backwardes
6. assistant Aaiiii^{r} *Glandules* called *Parastatæ*, or *Assistentes*

7. author [*sb*] Oiiii^r This muscle … is therfore the Author, of mouyng th[e] nether iawe
8. axillary [not as *sb*.] Ti^v See **axillary**, anted.
9. bond [*sb*] Ni^r See **vinculum**, anted.
10. brine [*sb*] Aai^v the serous humour, which we call brine
11. bringing Bbiii^r See **bringing vessels**, unrec.
12. calx Liii^r See **scaphoid**, anted.
13. caryatid Ddiii^r arteries called *Cariatidas*, or *Soporarias*
14. caulis (?) [= **cole**, *sb1* ?] Bbiii^v for the apt acte of generation, the omnipotent maker hath giuen a member (called in Latin *Coles, penis, mentula, virga*, or *Pudendu[m] virile*, in English the yard)
15. cele Cii^v See **circular process**, unrec.
16. contendent Aaii^v See **contendent,** *a*, anted.
17. cutter [*sb*] Qiiii^v (margin) The errour which our cunning cutters for the most part commit in taking away the stone
18. descendent Giiii^r the desce[n]dentes therfore … cut obliquely forwardes
19. dura Ffiii^r See **dura**, anted.
20. enter [*a*] Di^v See **lightly**, anted.
21. exile [*v*] Hhi^r from these whiche we sayd to go forward to the thombe, are exiled very small surcles, or twigges[2]
22. frons Oiiii^r It springeth from the Cannell bone … from *Frons*, from *Sinciput*
23. gallery Gi^v See **spinal**, anted.
24. gracile Xi^r See **gracile**, anted.
25. humeralis [not as *sb* in this sense] Piii^r See **deltoid**, anted.
26. intestinal Bbii^r that kinde of rupture called *Intestinalis*
27. ischium Yiii^v that veyne … called *Vena Sci. Ischeum*, or *Coxendicis*
28. janitor Ui^r See **pylorus**, anted.
29. labrum Cii^v *Labra*, or *Supercilia*, as it were the lippes, or browes, or as we may terme them, the brinkes to those caues
30. lambdoid Fiiii^r It is more rightly called *Ypsiloides* then *Lambdoides*
31. lithoid Ei^v See **lithoid**; anted.
32. macrocephaly Bii^v See **macrocephaly**, anted.
33. maxillary Fi^r See **maxillary**, anted.
34. mutation Tiiii^r the Ventricle … into whiche liuynge creatures receiue their meate … concoctyng & makyng the first mutation
35. notum Gi^v See **nominate**, 1b, anted.
36. obstriction Ii^r See **obstriction**, anted.
37. obstruct [not as *pp*.] Xi^v it is obstruct, and stopped
38. oppressive Dii^v ouer heauy, and to much (more then nature would) oppressiue
39. palate Gi^r Pypes and Shalmes, wherein are put certaine litle tongues, made of two *Palates* of reed

40. pectus [1693, Blancard] Hiiii^{v} the brestbone … in Latin *Pectus* [a 1 cit]
41. pin Oi^{v} the pinnes or wynges of the nostrels
42. pineal [not as *sb.*] Eeiiii^{v} This *Glandule* is called *Pinealis*, or *Conarium*, fitly representyng the shape of the yard
43. pretensed [*ppl a*] Uiiii^{r} The creatures in whiche none of those foldes or turnyng, spoken of, are founde, but haue one simple intrell, or gutte from the ventricle to the fundament straight pretensed, we see to be rauenous
44. prick Eeiii^{r} as one should say to the centre, pricke, or half way of any rounde fashion or fourme
45. prickle [= prick?] Oiiii^{r} the *Fibres* of it runne from the outer borders to the centre or middle prickle therof
46. procrastinate Aii^{r} If … a solid commonwealth is most prosperous … we that are the partes, [ought] to vse, inuent, and communicate that … amongest our selues, which may procrastinate the continuance of the healthfull state of our body, that is, the common wealth
47. reflecting [also anted] Ei^{v} See **resonant**, anted.
48. rising [cf. II, 6a] Iii^{v} the placyng, knittyng, and rising of the *Muscles*
49. rotator Cii^{v} See **trochanter**, anted.
50. secundine Ffiii^{r} the fourth Membran of the eye, which is called *Vuea* and *Chorion, Secundine* and *Choriformes*
51. secundine Eeiii^{v} *Tenuis meninx* with which indument the brayne [is] clad … beyng of some called *Chorion*, that is to saye *Secundina*
52. soporiferous Ddiiii^{v} See **soporiferous**, anted.
53. squared Ii^{v} Their fashion is after a *Triangular* manner, although not equally sided, or squared
54. steady Eii^{v} the bone called the *Stedie*
55. styloid [not as *vbl sb*] Cii^{v} like the fashion of a sharpe bodkin: wherfore the Grecians call such processes styloides
56. suspensor Qiiii^{v} See **suspensor**, anted.
57. tenuis Ddiii^{v} they reach to *Dura* and *Tenuis meninx*
58. testicle [cf. **testis,** 2] Eeiiii^{v} In the forepart of these Testicles (as we call them) stretchyng to the thyrd ventricle, an other part of the brayne appeareth
59. underset Bbiii^{v} an underset, or proppe
60. vestigium Mi^{r} See **vestigium**, anted.
61. visible Fii^{v} the Opticke Sinew … which like vnto a roote, is implanted into the middle of the eye, for the transportyng of the visible vertue thereunto
62. wicket Ddii^{v} See **emission**, 1, anted.

3. Unrecorded

1. abortures Fii^{r} (margin) *Collumbus* tried it in newe borne and in such Abortures as come vij or viij. monethes ere due tyme

2. **adhærens** Ffiii^{r} See **alba**, unrec.
3. **affusio** Ti^{v} The name therof is *Panchreas*, that is, *Affusio*, lying flat or prostrate
4. **alba** Ffiii^{r} The first of them [the Membranes of the eyes] is the outmost, and has many names, as all these, *Adnata, alba, adhærens*, and *coniunctiua*
5. **alluginius** Ffiiii^{r} See **aqueous**, anted.
6. **amigdala** Ccii^{v} On both sides of the iawe are two *Glandules* ... they haue to name *Paristhimia, tonsillæ, amigdala, fauces*
7. **amphiblistroides** Ffii^{r} (margin) What doth constitute the membran called *Amphiblistroides* or *Retina*
8. **annular bone** Pii^{r} See **annular**, anted.
9. **aplant** Bbii^{v} See **varicosum corpus**, unrec.
10. **apophilis** Cii^{r} /S/*Αποφιλισ*/S/ which the Latin interpretours call *Processus*
11. **applantation** Bbiii^{v} the applantation of this vessel to the testicle
12. **approbable** Pi^{v} his opinion herein is scarce approbable
13. **approprimate** [misspelling for approximate?] Giii^{v} the vpper turnyng Joynt altogether receiueth the insertion, both of the superior, and inferior Bones therto approprimate
14. **aranea** [cf. **araneous**] Ffiii^{v} the first Membran, called /S/*αϱαχνοειζ*/S/, in Latin *Aranea*, for that it seemeth to represent a Spider's webb
15. **arteria cephalica** Iii^{v} (margin) *Vena* and *Arteria Cephalica*
16. **arteria magna** Gii^{v} the *Vertebres*, and *Processes* beneth are wonderfull safegardes to *Vena concaua*, and *Arteria Magna*
17. **arterialis** Yiii^{v} The thyrd from the right ventricle of the hart is spread into the lunges, onely that veyne maketh this peculiar challenge, because it consisteth of the body of Arteries to be called *Arterialis*
18. **ascendently** Eiiii^{v} See **orbicular**, anted.
19. **ascense** Eiiii^{v} of one bone is made the neither iawe, without distinction, or dissolution: except in Children onely, who by hauing in the vtmost part of the chinne a lineall ascense, perhaps incited the other opinion
20. **ascygon** Xiiii^{v} (margin) the rising of the veyne without a felow(?) called *Ascygon*
21. **aspera arteria** Fiiii^{v} *Larinx* is the toppe of *Aspera arteria*
22. **assimule** [*v*, cf **assimile**] Ii^{v} the last of the three *Processes* ... we assimuled and likened to the ridge, or rising of a hill
23. **athenian** Aiii^{r} For therefore sayth the renowmed Athenian Oratour
24. **auditory cavity** Eii^{v} within the Auditorie cauitie
25. **auditory organ** Eiii^{v} the small Ossicles, or little Bones of the Auditorie Organ
26. **auditory passage** Eii^{v} The way vnto them [these ossicles] is by the Auditorie passage
27. **bathmidas** Iiii^{r} Wherfore *Hypocrates* calleth these holes /S/*Βαθμιδασ*/S/, beyng the seates, and groundes, of the cubittes motion

28. belonoides Ei^{r} (margin) This Process hath diuers names, as *Belonoides*, *Graphoides*, *Styloides* and *Plectron*
29. black coloured muscle Hhii^{v} See **leady coloured muscle**, unrec.
30. blind hole [cf. **blind**, 16] Fiii^{r} the extreme region of the eare: beyng called the blynd hole, in consideration of the obscure passage
31. boatlike Ciii^{v} the *Articulation* of *Talus*, with the botelike bone
32. boatlike bone Ciii^{v} See **boatlike**, unrec.
33. bringing vessels Bbiii^{r} (margin) Where the bringing vessels do meete
34. caecum intestinum Xi^{v} they come to this *Cæcum Intestinum*
35. calicreas Tiii^{v} the *Grecians* therfore call it *Calicreas* and *Panchreas*
36. callosum corpus Eeiiii^{v} Aboue the thyrd ventricle of the brayne, you may behold a portion supereminent, or appearyng ouer it sufficiently white, whiche is called *Callosum corpus*, a Callous body
37. callous body Eeiiii^{v} See **callosum corpus**, unrec.
38. cardiacus dolor Ggii^{r} this disease is called *Cardiacus dolor*
39. casula cordis Cciii^{v} the Membran enuoluyng the whole hart … like a certaine casket … is called of the Greekes *Percardion*, in Latin, *Cordis inuolucrum*: some *Casula cordis* … the barbarous number, by the addition of one letter pronounce it *Capsula*
40. cauda Biiii^{v} the number of Vertebres … sometyme one in Cauda
41. ceratoides Ffiii^{r} The thyrd Membran is called in Greeke /S/*κερα-⋆τοιδεσ*/S/ (margin *Ceratoides*)
42. cercis Iiiii^{v} The other and vppermost bone, called of the *Grecia[n]s* /S/*χερχισ*/S/ (margin *Cercis*)
43. cerebrum elongatum Ggii^{v} See **cerebrum**, anted.
44. choriformes Ffiii^{r} See **secundine**, ns.
45. cinna Aiii^{r} such Cinnaes, as perpetually laugh at the meruailous pietie of Aelius
46. circular process Cii^{v} Nothwithstanding there are certaine *Circular Processes*, which augment the profundities of such *Celes* as are largely excaued
47. clavicula Iii^{r} the Canell bones therfore, called in Greke /S/*χλειδεσ*/S/, in Latin *Furcula*, *Clavicula*, or *Iugula*
48. cleides Iii^{r} See **clavicula**, unrec.
49. clunes Eeiiii^{v} *Testes*: neare vnto which, two other particles yet somewhat greater are to be discerned, called according to their figure clunes, the haunches or buttockes
50. clypealis [cf. **clypeal]** Hiiii^{v} See **xiphoid**, anted.
51. colona torquendo Xi^{v} The first portion is called *Colona torquendo*, that is to say of writhyng
52. concava Xiiii^{r} a veyne called *Concaua*, *Chilis*, or *Magna*, beyng the mother of all other veynes in our body
53. connit[3] Eiii^{v} See **cuneiformed**, unrec.
54. contrahere Hhi^{r} in that place where it should *Retrahere*, and *Contrahere*

55. **cordis involucrum** Cciii^{v} See **casula cordis**, unrec.
56. **coriza** Eii^{r}(margin) The reason why in th[e] disease called Coriza the sense of smellyng is lost
57. **coronon** Oiiii^{r} the sharpe Processe of the nether iawe called *Coronon*
58. **coxendicis os** Kiii^{v} a large caue, is called *Coxendicis os*
59. **crassa** Eeii^{v} The vttermost of these inner Pannicles ... next vnto the scull ... in Latin *Crassa*
60. **crassa meninx** Diii^{r} the *Membran* of the brayne called *Crassa Meninx*, or Dura mater, which, as shalbe sayd hereafter more largely, beyng effused by *Fiberlike* tyeng through the same seames
61. **cubitus** Iiii^{v} (margin) The inferiour part of *Cubitus*
62. **cucullaris** Ggiii^{v} The Muscle called *Cucullaris*
63. **cucullaris musculus** Pii^{v} likened to a monkes hoode, and ... therfore ... called *Cucullaris Musc*
64. **cuneal cell** Ti^{v} What is ment by the Cuneall cell thou hast learned that in the Hystorie of bones
65. **cuneal process** Eiiii^{r} the Cuneall Processes which we haue compared to the wyngs of Battes
66. **cuneiformed** Eiii^{v} by the benefite of the *Cuneiformed* or *Cuneall* bone, it is connitted to the vj. *Suture*
67. **cyboides** Ciiii^{r} See **aptly**, anted.
68. **deferentia vasa** Qiii^{v} the vessels bringng seede called *Deferentia vasa*
69. **dodecadactylos** [See **dodec-**] Uiiii^{r} called of the Greekes /S/δωδεχα-δαχτυλοσ/S/, and of the Latins *Duodenum*
70. **dura membrana** Eii^{r} *Dura Membrana* is also accordyngly perforated
71. **eating muscle** Eii^{v} the mansorious, or eatyng *Muscle*
72. **enstrew**[4] Ggiiii^{r} Sondry others [nerves] to the cauitie of the shoulder blade, where there [*sic*] are enstrewed to the *Muscle t*here lurkyng
73. **epomida** Ggiiii^{r} the *Muscles* called /S/επωμιδα/S/ & *Cucullares*
74. **exsanguis** [cf. **exsanguine**] Tii^{r} it be lawfull to call the propper [flesh] *Sanguinea*, and the impropper *Exanguis*. As that to be the propper or *Sanguinea* which is engendred of bloud ... *Exsanguis* which conteineth not bloud
75. **extrahed** Kiiii^{v} these same bones, should in women bryngyng forth, be losed, and departed ... that more easely, the byrth might be extrahed
76. **fanwind** Ddii^{r} The opinion of other Anathomists is, that the vse of these diuisions of this vessel into the lunges, is to cary vnto the lunges the altered ayre, which are as a fanwynde to the hart, to coole the same
77. **faseoli** Aaii^{r} a litle pulse or grayne, called of the Herbarians *Faseoli*
78. **fibrelike** Diii^{r} See **crassa meninx**, unrec.
79. **focile minus** Li^{v} The lesser hath sundry names as *Sura*, *Fibula*, and of the barbarous sort, *Focile minus*
80. **gladialis** Qii^{r} the *Cartilage*, called *Gladialis*, or commonly, *Mucronata*
81. **glandula pinealis** Ddiiii^{r} these two arteries ... passe into the substaunce

of the brayne, in that place, whiche is called *Conarium*, or *Glandula Pinealis*

82. glouton [cf. **glutæus]** Li^{r} (margin) The description of the Processes o[f] the thigh. *Glouton* what

83. graphoides Ei^{r} See **belonoides**, unrec.

84. half circle like Sii^{v} their begynnyng is half circle lyke

85. hanger up Qiiii^{v} See **suspensor**, anted.

86. hill of venus Sii^{r} a litle transuerse muscle, placed vpon the hill of *Venus*

87. hioloida Ffiiii^{r} the thyrd humor [of the eye] called *Hioloida*, of all sortes of Anathomistes *Vitreum* because it representeth fused or moulten glasse

88. hipogunder Qiii^{v} Their duety is to compresse the belly, and bynd together the *Hipogunder*

89. incrase Ei^{v} nere to th[e] auditorie passage, is a cauitie, deepely incrased with a Cartilage

90. innitted Kii^{r} a cauitie ... whereunto, the head of the ioynt, after a certaine manner long, and forward protensed, or stretched, is innitted

91. inserp Iii^{v} slender surcles, and twigges of *Veynes*, which inserpyng their substaunce here and there

92. insited [cf **insite** *v*] Siii^{v} the whole mass of man for the insited heate therin

93. interseminum Bbiiii^{v} the part betwene the involucre of the testicles ... and the fundament ... [t]hat is *Intersæminum*

94. interseptum cartilaginos Ffi^{v} a seuerall diuision, or hedge: called therfore *Narium septum*, or *Interseptum Cartilaginosum*

95. inwards-looking Gi^{r} the toppe of the thyrd bone inwardes lookyng

96. inventing Qiiii^{r} (margin) *Collumbus* against the inuentyng of mo Muscles to *Abdomen*

97. kellum intestinum Xi^{v} at length finishyng his course at *Kellum Intestinum* in the toppe of *Os sacrum*

98. labdall Diiii^{v} The third bone is called Occiput, endyng at the Labdall Suture: besides that in the fou[n]dation of the head, it is disioyned from Os Sphenoides

99. lacies Ti^{v} other *Glandules* slender in vs, but thicker in beastes, called *Lacies* and *Thymus*

100. lapidoid Oiiii^{r} the bone of the temples called *Lapidoides*

101. latitans [cf, **latitant]** Ggii^{r} Nerues ... called therfore of *Galen Latitans*

102. leady coloured muscle Hhii^{v} the black or leady coulored Muscle, growyng ... from the greater *Trochanter*

103. linea alba Ti^{r} See **white line**, anted.

104. magna Xiiii^{r} See **concava**, unrec.

105. malum granatum Hiiii^{v} See **xiphoid**, anted.

106. mamillar process Ei^{r} The first of which are the *Mamillar Processes*

107. mansoria Fii^{v} See **masseter**, anted.

108. manus pectus Ki^{v} some of *Galens* interpretours haue called it *Palma*, others *Manus Pectus*

109. marvellous net Ddiiii^{r} from the Arterie *Carotides*, the meruailous net is effourmed

110. membrana carnea Siiii^{v} a Membran called fleshy, in Latin *Panniculus Carnosus*, or *Membrana Carnea*

111. mentula Bbiii^{v} See **caulis**, ns.

112. meserical[5] Qiiii^{r} dreined by the *mesericall* veynes

113. monoculus Xi^{r} the blinde gutte ... is endewed with one onely mouth. Hence ... some ... haue named it *Orbus*, or *Monoculus*

114. mucronata cartilago Miiii^{r} (margin) The vse of *Mucronata Cartilage*

115. musculus Niiii^{r} *Muscle* which the *Grecians call μυζ*, the Latins *Musculus*

116. narium septum Ffi^{v} See **interseptum cartilaginos**, unrec.

117. ocium Aiii^{v} Whereupon also if your worship, sometyme in Ciceroes ocium ... shall chaunce to looke

118. oirachos Ti^{r} a fourth vessel called *Oirachos*, which beginneth at the bottome of the bleddar

119. olfactilis Ffi^{v} in the forepart of the brayne ... the rising of two organs are playne to be discerned, which the *Grecians* call *Olfactilis*, but other Anathomistes *Processus Mamillares*

120. orbus Xi^{r} See **monoculus**, unrec.

121. os coccix Hii^{r} (margin) *Os Coccix*

122. os cubeforme Liiii^{r} The fourth is *Cyboides*, or after the Latins *Cubeforme os*

123. os cuneale [fpl; see **os**] Diiii^{r} See **disjoin**, *v*, anted.

124. os cuneiforme [fpl; see **os**] Ei^{v} *Os Cuneiforme*, or *Cuneale*

125. os frontis [fpl; see **os**] Diiii^{r} See **disjoin**, anted.

126. os iugale [fpl; see **os**] Ei^{r} The thyrd Process of the temporall bone maketh a portion of *Os iugale*

127. os malae Eiii^{v} The thyrd, which *Galen* calleth *Os malæ*, is greater the[n] the rest

128. os pectoris Iii^{v} the begynnyng at *Os Pectoris*

129. os scutiforme Lii^{v} See **patella**, anted.

130. os sphenoides Diiii^{v} See **labdall**, unrec.

131. ossa squamosa Diiii^{r} See **adherent**, anted.

132. os sternon Biiii^{r} Os Sternon Galen with the elders, obserued perpetually to consist of seuen Bones

133. over-corrective Ggiii^{r} we will consume no tyme to aunswere, and reply vpon euery selfe opinion, for seemyng ouer correctiue

134. over-readily Gii^{r} the small number of Bones, should often ouer readyly occasion ... to be dislocated

135. palma Ki^{v} See **manus pectus**, unrec.

136. parastatæ Qiiii^{v} At the end or necke of the bleddar, in man groweth two *Glandules* or kernels called *Parastatæ*

137. parenchyma affusio Ccii^{v} The substaunce of the lunges is rare, light,

and porie ... which kynde of substaunce the elders haue named *Parenchyma Affusio*
138. paristhimia Ti^{v} See **amigdala**, unrec.
139. pedium Liii^{r} The second, called *Pedium*, is co[m]parable to the *Postbrachial* bones
140. peltalem [cf. **peltate**] Fiiii^{v} See **scutalem**, unrec.
141. planta Liiii^{v} the second part of the foote, called of the Latins *Planta*
142. polymorphon [cf. **polymorph**] Liiii^{r} Why *Cyboides* is called *Polimorphon*
143. poplaris Yiii^{v} The braunche that is borne under the knee is named *Vena poplaris*
144. praeparantia vasa Kiiii^{v} by the whiche couertly runne, as well *Deferentia*, as *Preparantia vasa*
145. processus mamillaris Ffi^{v} See **olfactilis**, unrec.
146. pudendum virile Bbiii^{v} See **caulis**, ns.
147. reclude Hii^{r} Neyther doth *Os sacrum* obscurely reclude, but playne, and largely open and discouer the passages on eche syde
148. recta Diii^{v} it is nominated of the *Grecia[n]s* /S/*Oβιλαια*/S/, the Latins Sagittalis or *Recta Sutura*
149. rectum intestinum Xii^{r} See **straight**, anted.
150. retrahere Hhi^{r} See **contrahere**, unrec.
151. reversive nerve Ggi^{v} the right recurrent, or reuersiue Nerue
152. rotatory process Eii^{v} See **rotatory**, anted.
153. rotula genu Lii^{v} See **patella**, anted.
154. rough-forged Aii^{v} and fashion these my rough forged labours
155. sagittalis [but cf. **sagittal**] Ciiii^{v} the third is straight in the middest of the top, in like sort (of the *Grecians*) called *obeliaia*, as we should say, *Sagittalis*
156. sanguinea Tii^{r} See **exsanguis**, unrec.
157. scutalem Fiiii^{v} the *Anathomistes* ... call it, for the likenes of the thyng, *Scutalem*, or *Scutiformem Cartilaginem*, or *Peltalem*
158. seminal artery Xi^{r} the going forth of the seminall Arteries
159. seminal passage Yii^{v} the left Seminall passage
160. seminal vein Yii^{v} one of these Seminall veynes
161. seminary vein Yii^{v} the Seminarie veyne
162. septum transversum Miiii^{r} it gardeth the hart, & defendeth *Septum transuersum*
163. sharp cartilage Xiii^{r} (margin) *Topic medicinis* are rashly applied vppon the sharpe cartilage
164. sharp gristle Xiii^{r} ungue[n]tes, which some men minister vpon the sharpe Gristell
165. shieldlike cartilage Miiii^{r} Some therfore haue called it a litle sword, others the shieldlyke *Cartilage*
166. sight side Xii^{r} he more endeuoureth to decke the toppe and sight side

of his house, then hath care to set firme his foundation

167. sleepy artery Fiii^{r} the progress of the slepy *Arterie*

168. soporarias [cf. **soporal**] Ddiii^{r} ii. arteries called *Cariatidis* and *Soporarias*

169. spinalis medulla Eeiiii^{r} the nerues of *Spinalis Medula*

170. stoides Oiiii^{r} the *Processe* called *Stoides*

171. stomachus Tiiii^{r} called by all these names as *Æsophagus, Stomachus, Gula* and after the *Arabians, Meri*

172. stonylike Ei^{v} Which bones are ... anfractuous, rough, and stony like

173. subenter Ei^{v} the thyrd processe ... crooketh vp, toward the iugall bone, in *Circular* sorte, not vnlike the arche of a Bridge, vnder which, subentreth, the hollow of the temples

174. substrewed Xii^{v} *Panchreas* ... so substrewed, and circumposed to the singular scissions of the vesselles euery where

175. succingens Cci^{v} named in Latin *Succingens*, and commonly called *Pleara* [*sic*]

176. sura Li^{v} See **focile minus**, unrec.

177. surceade Hiii^{v} no otherwise then as it surceadeth all others in bredth

178. sutura Ciiii^{r} First *Sutura*, whiche the Grecians call *ϱαφη*, is a coniunction of the bones

179. sutura coronalis Di^{v} *Sutura* is that maner of co[m]position sene in the head, wherein the bones are committed together & lyke the teeth of a sawe, as is *Sutura Coronalis* [,] *Sagittalis* [,] *Labdoides*

180. sutura labdoides See **sutura coronalis**, anted.

181. sutura sagittalis See **sutura coronalis**, anted.

182. syndesmos [cf. **syndesmo-**] Ciiii^{v} we shall call it more rightly a *Ligament*, which the Greekes nominate *Syndesmos*: therefore this knittyng, after that rate, *Syndesmosis*

183. tendring [*sb*] Diii^{r} the little *Tendringes* or *Spriggie* braunches of veines, and *Arteries*

184. tenue Xi^{r} See **gracile**, anted.

185. tenuis meninx Ddiii^{v} See **meninx**, anted.

186. trifulca Ddii^{v} at the seate of the hart, xi. Membra[n]s do stand, called *Trifulca* or iij. edged

187. turning joint Diiii^{r} the first *Vertebre* or turning ioynt

188. two horned muscle Sii^{r} the two horned Muscle, springeth ... from the inferiour part of the shoulder

189. una Ccii^{r} See **columella**, anted.

190. unnamed cartilage Fiiii^{v} See **unnamed**, anted.

191. urinarius Yii^{v} a vessel called *Vreter*, that is *Vrinarius*

192. uvea membrana Ffiii^{r} *Iris* is that circle in the eye [whose] varietie of colours, proceedeth not through the humor therin closed, but through *Vuea membrana*

193. vale of abdomen Ti^{v} in the vale of *Abdomen*

194. varicosum corpus Bbii^v this same *Varicosum corpus*, where it is to the Testicles applanted.
195. vaulted place Eeiiii^v (margin) The vse of the callous body and vaulted place
196. vena chilia Qiiii^r the office of *Vena Chilia*
197. vena concava Gii^v wonderfull safegardes to *Vena concaua* and *Arteria magna*
198. vena coronalis Xiii^v an other [branch] embraceth aboue his Orifice is a crowne, and is therefore called *Vena Coronalis*
199. vena coxendicis Yiii^v See **ischium**, anted.
200. vena ischeum Yiii^v See **ischium**, anted.
201. vena iugularis Fiii^r no more stoppage is offred, to a branch of *Vena iugularis*
202. vena poplaris Yiii^v See **poplaris**, unrec.
203. vena sciatica Yiii^v See **ischium**, anted.
204. venial artery [cf. **venal**, 2] Cci^r drawne, by the veniall arterie, into the left Ventricle of the hart
205. virga Bbiii^v See **caulis**, ns.
206. visible nerve Oii^r the roundell at the visible Nerue
207. visible sinew Ffiiii^v the visible sinews, ... because they bryng the vertue visible vnto the eyes
208. vitreum Ffiiii^r See **hioloida**, unrec.

4. Postdatings

1. abstract [*ppl a*, A, 1, 1496, *Bk. St. Albans*] Oiii^r thou hast to consider the Muscles of the eyes, abstract sensibly from *Galen*, *Vesalius* and the rest
2. ancienty [3, 1556, Vernon] Oii^v yeld auncientie vnto the truth, whether the Author therof was first or last
3. boss [v^1, 1b, 1542, Udall] Liii^r in fourme bossyng out aboue like a rou[n]d heaued, or swelled thing
4. confusedly [3, 1530, Palsgrave] Oi^v They haue confusedly mingled them together with the Muscles of the vpper lippe
5. entrail [2b, 1483, *Cath. Angl.*] Uiiii^v this intrell alone doth not receiue the rehearsed vtilitie
6. exort [*v*, *c*.1400, *Cov. Myst.*] Hhiii^r nerues ... as well from the greater, as the lesser *Focile* exorted or sprong
7. eye of the knee [*c*.1400, Lanfranc] Lii^v See **patella**, anted.
8. meri [1547, Boorde] Tiiii^r See **stomachus**, unrec.
9. private [*v*, I, 1, 1548,] Giii^r the whole body of the sayd *Vertebre*, for the large compasse that by this meanes it is hollowed, should not be wholly priuated, nor the passage for the *Spinall* marey marred
10. prompt [1, *c*.1425, *Found. St. Bart.*] Yiii^v not in prompt to euery ruption
11. reversive [*c*.1400 Lanfranc] Ggi^v the right recurrent, or reuersiue nerue
12. supportable [1, 1533, Bellenden] Gii^v the supportable ground and framework of Bones

13. white [*v*², 1, 1471, Ripley] Hhiii^v doth white, & concrease till it become a substaunce fit to the nourishing of the bones

5. *Other*

1. postbrachial Iiiii^v ncit See **postbrachial**, anted.
2. prostrate [3b] Ti^v ncit See **affusio**, unrec.

BARROUGH, PHILLIP, *The method of physicke*, 1583

1. *Antedatings*

1. abdomen [2, 1615, Crooke] 154 When inflammation afflicteth the mouth of the matrice, there is paine in the *Abdomen*
2. abridgement [3b, 1609, Skene] *vi^v a breuiarie or abridgement of phisicke
3. abruptly [1, 1590, Greene] *vii^v And thus (good Reader) I will abruptly ende
4. abscession [1, 1599, A. M. *Gabel.*] 211 two thinges are speciallie required: vidz. the perfect generation of the matter, and also his abscession into some space by it selfe [a 1 cit]
5. abscession [2, 1610, Barrough] 200 the abscessions are those tumours which the Latines call *Abscessus* [a 1 cit]
6. absinth [1, 1612, Benvenuto] 215 oyle of *chammomil*, absynthium, horehound, *nux cupressi* [a 1 cit]
7. absolute [12, 1625–49, Ch. I *Works*] 38 For mine own part I will not promise any absolute worke, but as learned Physitians haue thought of it and (as I my self have by experience learned) so will I frame and fashion my Treatise
8. absolutely [7, 1644, Quarles] 234 But melancholy we neuer absolutely do tearme choler
9. acanth [1662, Gerbier] 249 branke vrsine, or hircina, which is called *Achanthus* and *achanta*
10. acceptation *[*sb*, 2b, 1611, *Bible*] *ii^r the acceptation of my labour
11. accomplisher [1611, Cotgrave] *v^v the true and sincere accomplisher
12. achanthus [1, 1616, Surflet & Markham] 249 branke vrsine, or hircina, which is called *Acanthus* and *achanta*
13. achor [1585, Lloyd] 276 vlcers appearing in the head, which the Greekes call *achoræ* [a 1 cit]
14. acorus [1714, French *Bk. Rates*] 153 frankensence, squinant, *acorus*, nutmegs [a 1 cit]
15. acrochordon [1720, Shadwell] 202 To this kinde also may be referred *myrmeciæ*, as if one should call them *formiculæ*, and *acrochordones*, which of our countriemen are termed *pensiles verruca* and *clauus* also [a 1 cit]
16. acute [2, 1667, *Phil. Trans.*] 154 The companions to inflammation of the matrice be these: an acute feuer

17. adduce [*v*, 1616, Brent] *ii^{r} these causes meeting thus together did especially adduce me … to rush into your presence
18. aden [1653, Urquhart] 220 recourse of matter from the kernells (which the Greekes call *Adenæ*, and commonly they be called *Emunctoria*) [a 1 cit]
19. adiantum [1, 1706, Phillips] 283 Rx. … maidenhaire, *adiantum* [a 1 cit]
20. adjuvant [B, 1609, Yelverton] 46 an adiuuant and aide to all medicines [a 1 cit]
21. admire [*v*, 1590, Greene] *v^{v} he sitteth still, and admireth himselfe
22. aerugo [1753, *Chambers's Cycl.*] 262 Rx. … of *ærugo rasa* z.8 [a 1 cit]
23. affect [v^2 1, 1606, Shakespeare] 145 the whole bodie being euill affected [a 1 cit]
24. affectation *[2, 1607, Topsell] *ii^{v} the affectation of any popular praise
25. affected [III, 1, 1619, Donne] 200 There be many and sundrie differences of tumours … [proceeding] from the affected partes
26. affinity [II, 8, 1616, Suflet & Markham] *ii^{r} the affinitie betweene the matter of the worke … and the minde of him to whom it is presented
27. affluxion [1646, Browne] 247 But *oxyrhodinum* with salt, doth partly digest & drie up, and partly restraine and stop the affluxion of humours
28. aggrieved [*ppl a*, 3, 1725, Bradley *Fam. Dict.*] 59 when the aggreaued place is weake through the nature of the impostume
29. alcanna [1625, Hart *Anat. Ur.*] 271 oyle of *alchanna* which they call *cyprinum* [a 1 cit]
30. alkermes [1, 1621, Burton] Rx. … graines of Alkermes [a 1 cit]
31. alphos [1706, Phillips, ed. Kersey] 203 *alphon*, in which disease the whole flesh is not affected, but onely the externall partes … as though … it were set about with certaine scales … comprehended vnder the name of *vitiligo* [a 1 cit]
32. althea [1669, W[orlidge] 38 other simple medicines … (that is) *Castoreum*, roote of Althea [a 1 cit]
33. alum-water [5, 1656, Du Gard] 122 After this they must be washed with alommewater, or sulphure water [a 1 cit]
34. amplitude [1, 1599, Nashe] 125 it is caused through the amplitude of the reines
35. anabatic [1811, Hooper *Med. Dict.*] 169 Some [feuers] alwaies encrease and augment by little and litle, those the Greekes do call, *anabaticos*, & *epacmaticos*, (that is) encreasing and augmenting more and more [a 1 cit]
36. anatomist [B, 1594, T. B. *La Prim.*] 39 See **evict**, anted.
37. angina [1, 1590, *Pasquil's Apol.*] 61 Angina in latin, squinancie in englishe … is properly an inflamacion which is in the throte, or in the iawes [a 1 cit]
38. antecedent [1, 1612, Taylor, T.] 259 The cure … is … to appoint such an ordinarie and conuenient diet to the sicke, as that the matter, which causeth such abscessions be not heaped vp together in the body, and by all meanes to preuent and turne away the antecedent matter

39. antecedent [*sb*, 1, 1612, Taylor, T] 207 causes antecedent, which we name *antecedentes*
40. antevert [*v*, 1, 1649, Bp. Hall] 212 it will expell and thrust foorth the conceaued humour without anie forreine aide, unlesse a man by making incision will anteuert and preuent his voluntarie opening [a 1 cit]
41. anthos [1585, Lloyd] 37 conserues of Borage, endyue, violettes, roses, anthos [a 1 cit]
42. apertion [1, 1615, Crooke] 212 that opening or apertion which is made by nature [a 1 cit]
43. aphtha [1657, *Phys. Dict.*] 55 The ulcers which are bredde, in the overmost parte of the mouth and have a certaine burning heat, in greek they ar called *Apthæ* and of the barbarous sort *alcola* [a 1 cit]
44. apnœa [1719, *Glossogr. Nova*] 294 diseases of the breast & the lounges, (as is) *Dispneas*, *Apneas* [a 1 cit]
45. apophlegmatic [B, 1727, Swift] 302 Apophlegmatismvs is a medicine which causeth one to vomit vp fleume [a 1 cit]
46. apozem [1603, Jonson, B.] 285 make a long syrupe, that is as it were in the forme of an *Apozema* (which is a decoction so called of the Greekes [a 1 cit]
47. appositively [1881, Whitney] 199 this cannot appositiuely be sayd to be besides nature [a 1 cit]
48. appropriate [3, 1635, Austin] *iiii^{v} kinges haue appropriated it to themselues, and haue thought themselues honoured by the profession of the same
49. arrest [*v*, 14, 1814, Byron] *v^{r} this excessiue pride, which hath arested as it were the mindes of many Phisitions
50. assumption [II, 5b, 1871, *Atheneum*] 213 we will rehearse out of Galene certaine thinges concerning the order of curing, which haue their assumption from the partes which are affected
51. asthmatic [*sb*, B, 1610, Barrough] 65 Therefore then you must giue vnto the Astmatickes ... Antidotes
52. atheroma [1706, Phillips] 202 such kindes of *abscessus* ... those be *atheromata steatomata*, *melicerides* [a 1 cit]
53. attenuation [1, 1631, Donne] 247 sixe unnaturall thinges, which ... shall decline vnto heate and drinesse with a certaine attenuation or deminishing
54. augmentation [7, 1853, Mayne] 88 But if it chaunce in the beginning of the augmentacion or in the vigour and strength of the feauer
55. aversion [2, 1664, Evelyn] 126 it is better to parte the drawing out of the blood, that his pulling backe and auersion may be done by litle and litle [a 1 cit]
56. balaustine [1671, Salmon] 51 Rx ... balaustium [a 1 cit]
57. balneum [1, 1652, French] 295 Balneum is a baine
58. basilica [3, 1625, Hart] 194 you must cut the innermost veyne of the arme ... commonly called *basilica*

59. bastard rib [5c, 1594, T. B.] 113 paine and heauinesse all over the right side coming vp to the necke, and downe to the bastard ribs [a 1 cit]
60. bastardly [3, 1607, Topsell] 184 Against a bastardly tertain
61. bdellium [2, 1585, Lloyd] 51 mollifiers, as is ... *bdellium styrax*
62. beating [*sb*, 5, 1601, Shakespeare] 48 But if heauines, distension, and beating heate & paine be felt in the head[6]
63. belking [1650, *Balm Gil.*] 36 much windines, sharp belkings
64. blatta [1601, Holland] 215 hote repulsives are ... *blatta bizantia* [a 1 cit]
65. blind gut [1594, T. B.] 100 the stopping of harde dounge in the blinde gut [a 1 cit]
66. bole [*sb*², 2, 1601, Holland] 7 For them that are delicate, you may vse this bole
67. bolus [1603, Florio] 288 Bolus in English is called a morsell. It is a medicine laxatiue, in forme & fashion it is meanely whole, & it is swallowed by litle gobbets [a 1 cit]
68. border [10, 1728, Young] 199 for they have not yet passed the boundes of nature, neither are the actions and duities of their part maymed or anoyed, which is the border of those increments which are besides nature
69. brassica [1832, *Veg. Subst. Food*] 260 red coleworts (which of some are thought to be brassica marucina) [a 1 cit]
70. bronchocele [1657, *Phys. Dict.*] 255 Ganglia so called of Grecians, *Chœrades* (that is, *Strumæ* which they also call *Scrofule*, *Bronchocele*, which they name *Bocium*, and *Hernia gutturis* [a 1 cit]
71. burst [*v*, 8b, 1712, Arbuthnot] 68 naughtie bloud, gnawing asunder the vaines, & brusting open the heades of them
72. caked [1691, Boyle] 246 of caked fleame, there doe arise all those harde knottes [a 1 cit]
73. calastic [1621, Burton] 216 remedies that doe mitigate, which the Greekes call *chalastica* [a 1 cit]
74. calycle [1731, Bailey] 55 Rx. ... *calyculorum glandium* [a 1 cit]
75. cancer [3, 1601, Holland] 202 Celsus maketh a difference betweene *cancer*, and *carcinoma*
76. carcinoma [1, 1721, Bailey] 202 See **cancer**, anted. [a 1 cit]
77. carminative [B, 1671, Salmon] 280 If ventositie be present, adde carminatiues [a 1 cit]
78. carotid [B, 1741, Monro] 259 the greatest veines and arteries (which are called *Carotides*) [a 1 cit]
79. carus [1678, Phillips] 22 Carus ... is a disease, in which both sense & mouing is altogether taken awaie and yet ther breathing remaineth safe [a 1 cit]
80. castor [2, 1601, Holland] 50 put in the pouders of Comin and Castor
81. castor [*sb*, 1, 5, 1727-51, *Chamber's Cycl.*] 50 Rx oile of Castor
82. catheter [1601, Manningham] 30 you must get out the vrine by a fine pype made of siluer for that purpose called *Cathetera* [a 1 cit]

83. catholicon [1, 1611, Bible] 233 the medicine which is called *Catholicon* [a 1 cit]
84. catoche [1656, Ridgeley] 23 See **deprehension**, ns [a 1 cit]
85. caution [3, 1605, Shakespeare] 128 Neither may this caution be omitted
86. cecily [1597, Gerarde] 45 Rx … netles … or [of] Cecelian, of fennell [a 1 cit]
87. cele [1708–15, Kersey] 143 Cele in Greek, *ramex* and *hernia* in Latin, the barbarous writers call it *rupura* [a 1 cit]
88. cenchrine [1608, Topsell, and ns] 241 the other kinde of herpetes … we haue saide to be called in Greeke *miliaris* and cenchria [a 1 cit]
89. cerule [b, 1830, Phillips, W.] 260 *lapis lazuli*, which the Greekes call *Cyaneus*, the Romanes *Caruleus* [a 1 cit]
90. chalcite [1849, Murchison] 226 that resolution with oile of roses, which is made of the stone *chalcitis* [a 1 cit]
91. chive [*sb*^{2}, 1610, Barrough] 47 if any chyue, chippe or dust skippe into the eye
92. cholagogue [1671, Salmon] 23 medicine which can expell choler (called of the Greekes *cholagogon*) [a 1 cit]
93. cholerous [1610, Barrough] mitigate the cholerous heat [a 1 cit]
94. cicatrix [1, 1641, Prynne] 46 it will consume the wound, so that there shall appeare no Cicatrice [a 1 cit]
95. cimolia [1658, Rowland] 78 the earth called *cimolia* [a 1 cit]
96. circuit [2b, 1597, Payne, J.] *iiii^r there is nothing within this mortall circuite, that God hathe … kept to himselfe
97. clavus [1879, *Syd. Soc. Lex.*] 243 meane inflammation … turned into corrupted matter … called of Avicene *clavi*, but the Latines doe terme *claui, verrucæ albæ*
98. cocker [*v*, d, 1592, Harvey, G.] *vi^r The yong man … cockereth in himselfe a foolis[h] imaginatio[n]
99. colature [2, 1601, Holland] 286 water of the decoction of the common colature
100. colliquation [3a, 1662, Stubbe] 110 Hote diste[m]pure vexing the liuer, there are *colliquations*, first of the humours, and after that of the liuer it selfe [a 1 cit]
101. colliquation [3b, 1601, Holland] 131 these do further the colliquation and consuming of the bodie [a 1 cit]
102. collution [1, 1601, Holland] 30 Let him vse *Masticatoris*, and collusions of mustard seeds and such like [a 1 cit]
103. columella [1, 1585, Lloyd] 58 against the inflammation of this *Columella* apeareth a certaine fleshie peece, hanging in the vpper parte of the mouth [a 1 cit]
104. coma [*sb*^{1}, a, 1646, Browne] 24 Coma in Greeke, *sopor*, or *granis* & *profundus somnus* in Latin. It may be called in Englishe a dead sleepe [a 1 cit]
105. commixing [1610, Barrough] 84 the commixing of those thinges [a 1 cit]

106. compact [*ppl a*, 2, 1655, W. F.] 162 humours vehemently compact and thickened together

107. complicate [*a*, 1626, Bacon] 210 true apostemes ... are greatly complicate and folded together [a 1 cit]

108. complicate [*ppl a*, 2, 1638, Whitaker] 170 feauers ... are sometime complicate and ioyned togeather [a 1 cit]

109. complication [4, 1793, Beddoes and ns] 171 Complicatio[n] ... is when the feauers invade the patient at diuerse houres [a 1 cit]

110. compositum [1652, French and ns] 281 Practitioners doe put a double vnderstanding in syrupes ... *simplex*, which is called vsuall, and *compositum*, which is called magistrall [a 1 cit]

111. comprehend [III, 10b, 1631, Weever] 91 a great cupping glasse comprehending the nauell every where

112. conceivable [*a*, 1, 1586, T. B. and ns] *iiii^{r} he [God] had infused into man a conceauable mind [a 1 cit]

113. conceived [4, 1586, Marlowe] 212 it will expell and thrust foorth the conceaued humour [a 1 cit]

114. concoction [2b, 1685, Cooke, J.] 71 you must helpe the concoction of the impostume

115. concretion [6, 1646, Browne] 268 The third *species* of vnnaturall melancholie is that, which borroweth his originall of a certaine stonie concretion

116. condite [1586, Cogan] 9 You may commodiously minister inwardly cubebes, condite, or diambros, diamoscha [a 1 cit]

117. confidency [1600, Holland] *iii^{v} with such a bold confidency ... to rush into your presence [a 1 cit]

118. conflate [*v*, 1, 1610, Barrough] 210 the humours whereof they [tumours] be conflated or engendred [a 1 cit]

119. confusion [7b, 1612, Woodall] 171 confusion is, when they [fevers] begine at one time

120. congestion [2, 1634, Johnson, T.] 200 But the efficient causes ... are congestion and fluxe [a 1 cit]

121. conjunct [B, 1, 1650, Baxter] 120 The Coniunct or continent cause, is the bloud it selfe

122. connexion [1a, 1609, *Douay Bible*] 164 neither is there anie connexion or knitting of boanes [a 1 cit]

123. connexion [4, 1742, Young] 264 seperate it with the poynt of a penknyfe from the other partes therunto adioyned, and when you have drawen and loosed the connexion [a 1 cit]

124. consent [5, 1615, Crooke] 10 we intreate of paine in the head, which cometh by consent

125. consistence [2, 1606, Woodcocke] 23 But the lethargie hath a certaine peculiar consistence of him selfe [a 1 cit]

126. consistency [3a, 1661, Fuller] 208 all the humours are conteined in the

veynes and arteries, the which may appeare by their varietie of colour and consistencie [a 1 cit]
127. consolidate [4b, 1656, Ridgeley] 281 clysters be made of milcke verie well for his whey portion, which doth restraine and consolydate
128. consolidating [*ppl a*, 1707, Vulpone] 281 A clyster consolidating is made [a 1 cit]
129. constitution [4, 1601, Holland] *iv[r] constitution of mans bodie
130. construction [2, 1707, *Cur. in H. & G.*] 199 the difference of other ... like infirmities, which doe happen by the composition & construction of the instrumentes
131. continent [*a*, 6b, 1605, Bacon] 220 See **conjunct**, anted.
132. contraction [II, 51 b, 1871, Holmes. T.] 80 contraction & paine of the hammes [a 1 cit]
133. contractive [1624, Bargrave] 139 and the contractiue vertue of it should be hurt [a 1 cit]
134. convulsion [2a, 1585, Lloyd] 31 Epilepsia ... is a conuulsion, drawing, and stretching of all the whole partes of the body [a 1 cit]
135. core [*v*, 1a, 1597, *2nd pt. gd. H. Jewell*] 43 Take four crabbes ... and then ... being pilled and cored, incorporate them ... in maner of an ointment [a 1 cit]
136. corrosiving [1592, Chettle] 264 some of these corrosiuing medicines [a 1 cit]
137. cotton-wool [2, 1870, Emerson] 32 make a twilt with iij. sheetes of graie paper, & bast upon it cotton woll [a 1 cit]
138. cotyledon [2, 1601, Holland] 215 These things following do represse flux ... sengreene, lettuce, *psillium*, *cotyledon* ... (that is to say) *vmbilicus Veneris, lenticula palustris, caphura*
139. coxa [1, 1706 Phillips ed. Kersey] 162 *Coxa*, in English the huckle bone
140. crab [3, 1614, W. B. *Phil. Ban.*] 274 The euill called *crabro*
141. crudity [1b, 1626, Bacon] 132 let the sicke eschewe crudities, and sacietie or fulnesse
142. curd [*v*, 1b, 1601, Shakespeare] 133 Of bloud broken out of the bladder or curded in it
143. cyprine [1656, Blount] 271 oyle of *alchanna*, which they call *cyprinum* [a 1 cit]
144. dacryd [1846, Lindley] 237 *scammonium*, called of new Greece *dacrydion*
145. dark [13c, 1687, Burnet] 15 See **dark vertigo**, unrec.
146. dartre [1829, Bateman *Sun*] 205 The Frenchmen ... doe call both these kyndes ... *dartræ* [a 1 cit]
147. decorticate [*ppl a*, 1872, W. Blair] 18 Barley decorticate [a 1 cit]
148. defect [1, 1589, Nashe] Av[r] there hath not bene nor is, any such blocke or stay, which hath impeached so much their endeauours, as the defect of experience

149. defedation [1634, Johnson] 204 euilles and defedations of the skinne [a 1 cit]
150. defer [1, 1626, Bacon] 39 if it lye deepe within, it deferreth three visible colours
151. dejection [5, 1605, Timme] 147 Fat women must be cured with a dyet that can extenuate, and with swifte exercises, and with other medicines which can make the bodie slender and leane: as be continuall deiection and solution of the bellie
152. deligature [1610, Barrough] 144 he must vse apt and convenient deligatures and trusses [a 1 cit]
153. delineate [*v*, 1618] *iiii[v] to fashion out & as it were to delineat
154. demit [*v*, 1, 1646, Browne] 207 (vnnatural humours) are demitted and sent into certayne receptakles
155. depascent [1651, Biggs] 241 But those medicines, which besides their cooling are also apt by nature to moysten, *herpetes* especially *depascentes* doe in no wyse require, but they doe onelie admitte those refrigeratiues, which can also greatlie drie vp
156. derivation [1c, 1600, Vaughan] 213 The quantitie therefore which in a tumour aboue nature varieth the cure is either great or small. The qualitie is the fluxe, or (as some tearme it) the derivation and congestion
157. derive [*v*, 2, 1598, Stow] 35 it is deriued from other places, and ascendeth vp thither
158. desudation [1727–51, *Chambers's Cycl.*] 204 Auicene his desudations may well be the Greekes *hidroa* [a 1 cit]
159. detention [1b, 1650, Fuller] 23 Congelation ... is a sodaine detention & taking both of mind and body, both sense and mouing being lost
160. determination [6, 1677, Hale] 234 it followeth (after the determination of *phlegmone*, and of other tumoures consisting above nature, which proceed of bloude) that we now speake of those swellings, which are caused of choler
161. detersion [1607, Topsell] 233 detersion of the filthie corruption
162. diacalaminthe [1658, Eng. Dicts.] 138 the antidotes of *diacalaminthes, dialactia* [fpl]
163. diacapparis [1658, Phillips] 291 made of the powders of ... *Diacapparis*
164. diacorallion [2, 1741, *Compl. Fam.*] 293 To stoppe the fluxe take Trochiskes of *Diacorallus* [a 1 cit]
165. diacorum [1658, Eng. Dicts.] 9 diacorum, conserue of maiorum
166. diacyminon [1611, Cotgrave[7]] 91 See **dianisum**, anted.
167. dialacca [1658, English Dicts.] 154 powder of *dialacha* [a 1 cit]
168. dialthea [1658, English Dicts.] 249 boile them with *dialthea* [a 1 cit]
169. diamoschum [1658, English Dicts.] 9 See **condite**, anted. [a 1 cit]
170. dianisum [1658, English Dicts.] 10 eyther *Diacuminum*, or *Dianisum* [fpl]

171. dianthos [1849, *Florist*] 143 Rx *Dianthos, plirisarcoticon* [a 1 cit] [fpl]
172. diapalma [1646, Browne] 276 that which consisteth of *chalcites* commonly called *diapalma* [a 1 cit]
173. diapapaver [1658, English Dicts.] 190 *diapapauer* and such like [a 1 cit]
174. diaphœnicon [1625, Hart] 123 the Antidotes *diaphœnicon*, and *Electuarium nidum* be good
175. diapompholygos [1658, Phillips] 276 the ointment named diapompholygos, which is made of oyle of roses, of white waxe, ana 3. z. v. of the iuice of red pomegranates, and of nightshade [a 1 cit]
176. diaprune [1625, Hart] 7 *Diacatholicon*, or *Diaprunes solutiue*
177. diarrhodon [1789, *Archaeol.* IX] 123 you may well minister *diarrhodon abbatis, aromaticum rosarum, dialacca diacurcuma*
178. diary [*a*, 2, 1592, Unton] being ingendered as diary feuers be, either of sorrow, or anger
179. diary [*sb*, 3, 1639, Horn & Rob] 168 you must note, that there be feauers called *Diariæ*, which last untill the thirde daie
180. diasatyrion [1658, Eng. Dicts.] 143 Among compoundes it is good to vse this medicine Rx. *dianthos, plirisarcoticon, diagalangæ.* ana. z.iii. *diasatyrion* [a 1 cit]
181. diatragacanth [1657, *Phys. Dict.*] 289 with one lozenge of *Diatragacantum frigidum* [a 1 cit]
182. diduction [1640, Jackson *Creed*] 62 Take heed also that there be litle diduction of the veine [a 1 cit]
183. differentia [1827, Whateley] 199 it hath pleased some of the later sort to make *Apostemata* as the *species* or *differentia* of those tumours besides nature [a 1 cit]
184. digesting [*ppl a*, 1605, Timme] 223 both of them do cary with them a digesting qualitie [a 1 cit]
185. direction [5b, 1596, Spenser] *v[v] euery starre which he had hoped to haue vsed as guides and directions
186. discolorate [1850, *Recent dicts.* and ns] 39 the second they terme *discolorata* (that is, hauing no colour) [a 1 cit]
187. discussing [*ppl a*, 1607, Topsell] 116 frictions are most conuenient for this, which haue a discussing vertue [a 1 cit]
188. discussion [4, 1620, Venner] 222 it is requisite to euacuate by digestiues onely that which is compact together, if that *phlegmone* must be ended by resolution or discussion
189. discussive [3, B, 1612, *Enchir. Med.*] 59 you may safelie minister discussiues
190. disobedient [A, b, 1588, Read, J.] 276 for the most parte grosse and thicke and disobedient to resolution
191. dispersing [1604, Hieron] 141 all your whole cure must be turned to the dispersing and dissoluing of it [a 1 cit]

192. dissipation [2, 1615, Crooke] 86 it chaunceth thorough vnmeasurable dissipation and spreading abrode of the whole bodie
193. dissolver [2, 1651, Biggs] 297 In the declination, take and applie onely dissoluers, and looseners [a 1 cit]
194. dissolving [*ppl a*, a 1620, Venner] 160 she must vse releasing & dissoluing bathes [a 1 cit]
195. distend [*v*, 3, 1650, Bulwer] 199 as it were distended both in breadth and profunditie
196. distension [1, 1607, Topsell] 140 distention and stretching out of the synewes [a 1 cit]
197. distribute [*v*, 4, 1664, Evelyn] 39 it shall not be vnneccessarie also to distribute it into his parts
198. distribution [2, 1589, Puttenham] 76 it causeth swift distribution into other partes of the body
199. distribution [3, 1605, Bacon] 39 this Christalline humour begetteth the varietie of colours in sundrie eyes, which gaue our Anathomistes to deuise their distributio[n]s
200. diuretical [A, 1601, Holland] 258 Now these strumous tumours are greatly helped by vsing purging medicines, diureticall potions, & electuaries [a 1 cit]
201. doglike [1605, Timme] 86 A doglike appetite is contrarie to losse of appetite [a 1 cit]
202. dracunculus [1, 1706, Phillips ed. Kersey and ns] 202 this euill, which the grecians call *dracontion*, the Latines *dracunculus* [a 1 cit]
203. dropax [1621, Burton] 151 dropaces made of *Euphorbium*, pellitorie, pepper, and mustard seede [a 1 cit]
204. duplex [1, 1817, Peacock] 182 it is called *duplex tertiana*, a double tertian [a 1 cit]
205. eclegme [1605, Daniel] 31 this *Ecligma* is praised of many [a 1 cit]
206. ecthyma [1834, Good] 205 Those pushes, which grow in the skinne ... are termed *Ecthymata* [a 1 cit]
207. effectrix [1610, Barrough] 79 distempure of the effectrix and working qualities
208. effluxion [1, 1646, Sir T. Browne] 267 that slimie bloud ... is purged out neither by anie sensible nor secret effluxion [a 1 cit]
209. egestion [2c, 1633, Adams, T.] 126 And generallie egestion of the wombe, and much excretion of vrine do go before those paines
210. egestion [2d, 1607, Topsell] 19 their egestions be liquide
211. elevate [II, 2d, 1607, Walkington] 12 humours ... eleuate vp to the head
212. embrocation [*sb*, 2, 1610, Barrough] 3 Yt profitteth also to vse embrocations [a 1 cit]
213. embroch [1585, Lloyd] 4 make an embrocha [a 1 cit]

214. eminence [I, 2a, 1615, Crooke] 200 Little tumours are called of them little eminences or appearings [a 1 cit]
215. emissary [*sb*, 2b, 1657, Tomlinson] 212 if there be anie emissarie, or way made into the tumour either by nature or by Art [a 1 cit]
216. emission [1, 1607, Topsell] 214 through the emission of bloud we helpe and remedy *phlegmone* [a 1 cit]
217. emphysema [1661, Lovell] 201 The Greekes call it *Emphysema*: Auicene termeth it a windie *apostema* [a 1 cit]
218. emptying [1, 1605, Shakespeare] 162 vomiting ... purgation ... or also other accustomed emptyings [a 1 cit]
219. empyema [1615, Sylvester] 70 Empiema in Greeke signifieth a mattery spitting
220. enema [1, 1681, Willis *Rem. Med.*] 279 A Clyster or *Enema*, is a kinde of medicine the which is cast and put into the bowels by the fundament liquid and thinne [a 1 cit]
221. ephialtes [1601, Holland] 34 Ephialtes in Greeke, and in latin *Incubus* and *Incubo* [a 1 cit]
222. epinyctides [1676, Wiseman] 204 See **exanthema**, anted. [a 1 cit]
223. epithet [1, 1588, Fraunce]203 *vitiligo* ... would more aptly agree, if it were put with his epithete or addition, as to say *alba vitiligo* [a 1 cit]
224. equal [7, 1663, Gerbier] 132 matter that is whitish, light, equall and little in quantitite
225. equal [*a*, 9, 1680, Otway] 261 we apply a plate of lead equall for the tumour
226. equally [1, 1634, Herbert, Sir T.] 2 aboundance of all foure humours equaly
227. eradicate [2, 1647, Cotterell] 283 matter cholericke and filthie (as one would say) vitelline, the which causeth feuers hard to be eradicate and taken away
228. erect [*v*, 4, 1626, Bacon] 31 those medicines that haue power to erect the yard
229. erigeron [1601, Holland] 224 grownswell, called in Greeke *erigeron* [a 1 cit]
230. erosion [1b, 1710, Fuller, T.] 149 you must take good heede, that some erosion and gnawing be not engendered in the wombe
231. errhine [1, 1626, Bacon] 50 you must drawe fleume out of the head by Masticatories, sternutaments, and *Errhinis* [a 1 cit]
232. eruption [*sb*, 6a, 1596, Shakespeare] 69 if ther be much eruption of bloud
233. erysipelatous [*a*, 1646, Browne] 227 They ... fall into a feauer ... sooner, then they, which are vexed with *Phlegmone Erysipelatosa* [a 1 cit]
234. essera [1706, Phillips] 204 Plinie termeth them bluish pushes, disquieting specially in the night time. The Arabians call them *essere*, *sere*, or *saire* [a 1 cit]

235. ethmoida [B, 1842, Col. H. Smith] 53 the passages which be in the bones called, *Ethmoida* [a 1 cit]
236. evaporate [8, 1610, Barrough] 147 Moreouer the wombe must be euaporated and fomented with odiferous thinges
237. evaporating [*vbl sb*, 1, 1630, Taylor, J.] 254 The fifte ... consisteth in the euaporating and drying vp of that waterish humiditie [a 1 cit]
238. evaporation [3c, 1626, Bacon] 131 The best evaporation and sweating is in a tonne
239. evaporative [1668, Wilkins] 237 applying outwardly digestiue or evaporatiue medicines [a 1 cit]
240. evict [*v*, 5a, 1591, Horsey] 39 the tunicles by sundrie Anathomistes haue bene euicted
241. exacerbation [2, 1625, Hart] 135 continuall exacerbations and fittes are caused
242. exact [I, 1, 1633, Herbert] 188 neither is there any exact and perfect rest from being feuerous
243. exact [*v*, 3, 1592, West] 209 Nowe the course of our treatise doth exact, that we should adde the signes and tokens
244. exanthema [1657, *Phys. Dict.*] 204 those, which we have rehearsed and touched alreadie, are reckened by the Greekes *ionthi*, *epinyctides*, *hidroa*, *psydraces*, *exanthemata*, *celsi papule*, and *Pliny mentagra* [a 1 cit]
245. exasperate [*v*, 2, 1611, Cotgrave] 63 whatsoeuer doth exasperat the *trachea arteria*
246. excedent [*sb*, 1811, Black, J.] 235 And of choler which besides nature is caused of adustion, by reason of the thinnes or thickenes of the substaunce thereof there are engendred either *herpetes estiomeni* (that is) *excedentes* [a 1 cit]
247. exclusion [4, 1646, Browne] 120 he must vse meates of easie digestion and extenuating [a 1 cit]
248. excretion [2a, 1640, *Erotomania*] 141 *Gonorrhea* in Greeke, *seminis profluuium* in Latine, it is excretion and shedding of seede or sperme against the patientes will
249. exedent [1883, *Syd. Soc. Lex.*] 201 See **miliary**, anted. [a 1 cit]
250. exhalate [1a, 1598, Sylvester] 74 They which through thinne vices which doe [*sic*] swiftly exhalate and flye vp [a 1 cit]
251. experiment [*sb*, 1b, 1586] *vii^r^ a few experimentes which passed from hand to hand
252. expirate [1615, Crooke] 145 little foode, that little doeth expirate and breath out streight [a 1 cit]
253. exquisite [2c, 1610, Barrough] 170 A pure and exquisite Tertian
254. extension [1b, 1612, Woodall] 150 For in women the wombe, when it is retched and stretched out, it runneth not to an other place like a wandering beast, but is drawen backe through the extention
255. extensive [3a, 1706, Phillips ed. Kersey] 250 windinesse throughout

the whole bodie, sometime running this way, sometime that way, which causeth extensiue paine [a 1 cit]

256. extenuating [*ppl a*, 1607, Topsell] 28 Ther diet must be altogether extenuating and naturall [a 1 cit]

257. extenuative [A, 1610, Barrough] 67 They haue more need of extenuatiue meates [a 1 cit]

258. extinguishing [1677, Hale] 230 the extinguishing and destroying of life in them [a 1 cit]

259. extirpation [2b, 1706, Phillips ed. Kersey] 244 we haue mencioned as remeadies for the extirpation of *myrmecia* and *acrochordones*

260. extort [*v*, 2, 1601, Shakespeare] 199 This definition they haue extorted out of Galene his wordes

261. exustion [1610, Barrough] 233 After exustion, minister the iuyce of leeks, and other such thinges, which doe drie, bind, and stop fluxe [a 1 cit]

262. falern [1601, Holland] 230 Let them be taken in *mulsum* made of *Falernum* [a 1 cit]

263. fatty [4, 1615, Crooke] 98 The excrementes first are cholericke, diuerse, and fattie, by reason of the fatte that cleaueth within in the bowells being melted

264. fatuity [2, 1621-51, North] 21 If reason be lost together with memorie, then the affect is called *Fatuitas* or *stultitia*

265. fay [sb^2, 1747, Hooson] 257 a certain humour like vnto hony, or fae, or sodden meale, or water [a 1 cit]

266. filling [*ppl a*, 1626, Bacon] 229 it must be healed with filling medicines [a 1 cit]

267. filmy [1, 1661, Lovell] 234 that filmie and thinne skinne which inwardly compasseth the internall parts [a 1 cit]

268. fistulous [1, 1611, Cotgrave] 258 some tumours are scaly, fistulous, and cancerous

269. flax-hurd [8, 1673, *Phil. Trans.*] 42 make a plaister of flexenherdes

270. fotus [1586, Bailey] 295 *Fotus* is a medicine nourishing or keeping warme [a 1 cit]

271. frequency [4, 1641, Digby, Ld. J.] 186 the swiftnesse and frequencie coming in the fittes

272. frontal [1c, 1601, Holland] 300 Frontale or *Splenium* be plaistres made to apply to the forehead ... to cease paine

273. function [*sb*, 3a, 1590, Shakespeare] *vi^r to preserue the body of ma[n] ... in respect of the varietie of his seuerall functions

274. fur [v^1, 3, 1593, Nashe] 10 noisome humours doe cleaue ... to the filmes and tunicles of the stomake, and dothe so furre them

275. furuncle [1676, Wiseman] 201 ... a kinde of *phlegmone* ... which Celsus doth call *furunculi*, felons [a 1 cit]

276. galange [1599, Hakluyt] 30 Rx ... galange [a 1 cit]

277. ganglion [1, 1671, Salmon] 202 the euils called of Greekes *ganglia*, of Auicen *glandulæ* [a 1 cit]
278. ganglion [2, 1732, Arbuthnot] 255 *Ganglium* ... is a gathering together of the sinowes [a 1 cit]
279. glandule [3, 1656, Whitley, R.] 200 those inflammations which we terme *glandulæ* and *bubones*
280. glans [2, 1704, Harris] 255 *Glandula* ... took his title of the likenesse of *Glans*, an acorne [a 1 cit]
281. gluten [2, 1597, Lowe] 215 these also do stuffe & stop the passages *farina* called *volatiles*, the white of an egge, *amylum*, *gluten*, & the kindes of gummes [a 1 cit]
282. gravity [6, 1610, Healey, *St. Aug.*] 12 The paine that inuadeth the sicke with grauity and heauines, declareth plenitude and aboundance of humours
283. gurgulio [1630, Randolph and ns] 58 first of this *Columella* appeareth a certaine fleshie peece, hanging in the vpper parte of the mouth ... By old time it was called *Gurgulio* [a 1 cit]
284. gutta serena [1657, *Phys. Dict.*] 41 The first kynd of Cataracts vncurable the Phisitians call *Gutta Serena*
285. heap [5e, 1653, More, H.] 122 them, which through vntimely drincking of colde water, haue their liuer cooled on heapes [fpl]
286. heartburn [2, 1597, Gerarde] 15 a gnawing in the stomacke, as it were the hart burne
287. heating [*a*, 1591, Percivall *Sp. Dict.*] 66 he must knowe ... whither the paine doth mitigate and dissolue with heating medicines [a 1 cit]
288. helcoid [1854, Mayne] 206 spottes in the face ... called of the Greekes *helcodes* [a 1 cit]
289. hemicrania [1657, *Phys. Dict.* and ns] 1 *Hemicrania*, which occupieth but the one half of the head [a 1 cit]
290. herb [4, 1662, Davies] 117 the roote and herbe of *Tamariscus*
291. herbary [3, 1634, Jackson] 225 wild cucumber (which is commonly called in herbaries and shoppes *cucumer asininus*)
292. homotonous [1775, Ash, and ns] 169 some of them [fevers] doe endure of an equall vehemencie, and force from the beginning vntill the ending: those the Greekes call *homotonos* and *acmasticos* [a 1 cit] [fpl]
293. husked [2, 1607, Topsell] 4 barley husked
294. ilium [1590, Barrough] 103 the said dong of the wolfe, easeth the collicke being bound to the Ilions
295. ill-disposed [4, 1771, Goldsmith] 90 if anie be ... ill disposed to drinke coulde thinges
296. imminution [1590, Barrough] 211 the tokens of a stonie hardnesse of the tumour are, imminution of the tumour [a 1 cit]
297. impertinent [3, 1590, Barrough] 42 Many ignorant practicioners ... haue endeauoured to cure this infirmitie with many impertinent medicines

298. impossible [3, 1858, Carlyle] *iii[r] to excuse my selfe, in that I haue not laboured to fit your affection in the presentme[n]t of this my labour, which is so impossible, in respect of your singular knowledg

299. inconvenient [A, 4, 1651, Hobbes] *iii[r] the earnest affaires of the Common wealth ... togeather with the inconuenient vneasines of the studie hath kepte your Honor from being acquainted with

300. incorrigible [3, 1596, Spenser] 106 Brode wormes do bring continuall gnawing of the stomach, and an impotent, and incorrigible appetite to meate

301. incursion [1, 1615, Crooke] 50 If daefnes [*sic*] come of cholericke humours specially after feuers, then it is wont with suddain incursions to runne to the brain

302. indagation [1589, Nashe] *iiii[r] The painfull indagation of the secretes of nature [a 1 cit]

303. indic [*a*, 1877, Rawlinson and ns] 6 barkes of mirabolanes citrinorum, indorum, chebulorum [a 1 cit]

304. indicatory [1, 1590, Barrough] 94 If the fluxe ... be indicatorie, the signes are rehersed in another place [a 1 cit]

305. inequality [3a, 1607, Topsell] 106 they that are thus diseased there followeth slendernesse and weaknesse of the body with inequality

306. infamously [b, 1695, Dryden] *vi[r] many ... are of this minde, that the time of their youth is infamously ouerslipped [a 1 cit]

307. inflamed [3, 1599, Buttes] 84 whether it be an oyle that the inflamed member be nourished withall

308. influxion [1, 1605, Bacon] 210 the influxio[n] of humours [a 1 cit]

309. infrigidation [1590, Barrough] 290 if ... we thinke that there be greater neede of infrigidation and cooling [a 1 cit]

310. inglorious [1, 1591, Spenser] *iiii[v] Did not he make Coos ... of an inglorious Iland, a famous coutrie [*sic*] [a 1 cit]

311. insensible [1b, 1584, Cogan] 208 [Naturall humours] sometime by an insensible ayer inwardely infused ... doe excite sweatinges

312. insession [1, 1652, French] 85 Also insessions to be applied to the loins & share

313. insist [2, 1586, *Let. Earle Leyc.*] 220 Wherfore in curing tumours ... we may chiefly insist, and be occupied about that most, which ... is most vrgent [a 1 cit]

314. intend [4a, 1603, Heydon] 252 For according to the difference of these things, the power or facultie of those medicines, which are ministred, ought to be intended and remitted

315. interception [1c, 1597, Wotton] *vi[v] the interception and præscision of diseases is very availeable [a 1 cit]

316. interjection [3a, 1598, Florio] *v[v] the interiection of these few lines hath not made me to forget

317. intermit [2b, 1665, Boyle] 180 the fittes in a burning feuer do not intermit or slake

318. intermitting [*ppl a*, 1626, *Art ag. Duk. Buck*] 136 remedies for intermitting feuers [a 1 cit]
319. internal [A, 1a, 1590, Spenser] 17 The internal senses, which be … imagination, cogitation & memory
320. intestines [*sb*, 1a, 1597, A. M. *Guill.*] 8 clisters … empty out such things as are contained in the intestines [a 1 cit]
321. involucrum [2, 1753, *Chambers's Cycl.* and ns] 27 *epithymum*, (which the Romaines call *inuolucrum*) [a 1 cit]
322. irrigate [2b, 1876, *Clin. Soc. Trans.*] 162 irrigate and sprinckle the aggrieued place with oyle of rewe
323. irrigation [2b, 1612, Woodall] 12 You must applye to the head irrigations and oyntmentes [a 1 cit]
324. irritation [3, 1685, Boyle] 61 After the irritations and chafinges made by medicines, you must appease it with decoction of lycorice [a 1 cit]
325. ischiadic [1727, *Chambers's Cycl.*] 162 The Latines call this disease *Ischias*, and they that are afflicted with this disease, are called *Ischiadici* [a 1 cit]
326. ischium [1646, Browne] 162 the ioint, which the Greekes do call *ischion* [a 1 cit]
327. ischuria [1675, Baxter] 289 *Ischuria* … retention and with-holding of vrine [a 1 cit]
328. issue [4b, 1607, Topsell] 226 If … there is no hope of resolution, you must make an issue for that which yeeldeth not vnto digestion in that place especially, where it is highest
329. lacedæmonian [B, 1780, Cowper] *ii^{v} Polis the Lacedemonian marchaunt [a 1 cit]
330. languishing [*ppl a*, 1b, 1611, Shakespeare] 234 somewhat raising the member into a tumour with a languishing inflammation
331. lapidous [1610, Barrough] 273 commit the cure of a scirrhous splene and a lapidous liuer, to the wisdome of the Physition [a 1 cit]
332. lapis [1641, French] 31 The perfume or smoke of *Bitumen*, or *Lapis gagatis* [a 1 cit]
333. lapis hæmatites [1741, *Compl. Farm Piece*] 52 Rx … *lapis hæmatites* [a 1 cit]
334. lapis indiacus [1646, Browne] 129 those thinges that breake and teare the stone in the reines … *lapis indiacus*, *xanthium* [a 1 cit]
335. lappet [2b, 1609, Holland] 64 The Asthma is caused when as grosse and clammy humoures be gotten in aboundantlie into the gristells or lappetes of the loungs [*sic*]
336. latus [1702, Ralphson and ns] 105 There be three kindes of wormes … The second … called *Lati*, be brode and longe [a 1 cit]
337. leek [6, 1688, Holme, R.] 243 Those little tumours … the common sort call … porra, leekes, because sometime they have certaine threads lying betweene them not much vnlike vnto the rootes of leekes

338. leet [*sb*^{4}, 1744, Ellis, W.] 286 make a syrupe boyled vpon a leate fire [a 1 cit]
339. lenticule [1884, Ogilvie] 215 the thinges following doe represse by refrigeration ... *lenticula palustris* [a 1 cit]
340. leucophlegmacy [1657, *Phys. Dict.*] 253 a waterish humour running betweene the skinne and the fleshe, called *Leucophlegmatia* [a 1 cit]
341. lichen [3, 1657, *Phys. Dict.*] 203 that light infection of the skinne, called of the Greekes *licene*, of the Latines *impetigo*, in English the ringworme [a 1 cit]
342. lienary [1684, *Bosset's*] 186 You must cut the innermost veine of the left arme, which is called *lienaris vena*, the spleene veine, or *mediana* [a 1 cit]
343. ligament [1, 1599, A. M. *Gabel.*] 144 you must keepe them vp with conuenient trusses, and ligamentes
344. loosener [2, 1630, Braithwait] 297 applie only dissoluers, and looseners [a 1 cit]
345. loosening [*vbl sb*, 1665, Hooke] 84 Therefore those which do attempt the cure with loosening remedies onlie ... cause perill of death [a 1 cit]
346. loosing [*ppl a*, 1665, Lauder, Sir J.] 75 you must vse oyle solutiue and loosing [a 1 cit]
347. lupulin [1826, Henry] 270 some purging medicine ... as ... *lupulus* [a 1 cit]
348. lymphate [1610, Barrough] 40 but if his body be weake, let him drinck wyne well lymphate [a 1 cit]
349. magistral [2a, 1605, Bacon] 281 Practitioners doe put a double vnderstanding in syrupes ... *simplex*, which is called vsuall, and *compositum*, which is called magistrall
350. manchet [1b, 1590, Barrough] 87 Giue them manchet made of fat brothes without honie
351. maniple [1, 1632, Johnson] *iii^v Manipulus. is a great handfull
352. manual [1d, 1591, Gerard] 229 to roote out a malicious carbuncle by actuall or manuell instrumentes
353. marasmoid [1895, *Funk's Stand. Dict.*] 189 Euen such is the feuer which is altogether *marasmodes* (that is) consuming [a 1 cit]
354. marasmus [*a*, 1656, Trapp] 170 if this feauer doeth so increase ... then it is called *Hectica marasmodes*, and *marasmus* [a 1 cit]
355. masticatory [*sb*, B, 1611, Cotgrave] 33 minister sternutaments, *masticatories* and such things as do purge [a 1 cit]
356. mattered [*ppl a*, 3, 1590, Barrough] 217 such kind of mattered tumours [a 1 cit]
357. medulla [1, 1651, *Raleigh's Ghost* and ns] 288 the playnest and simplest waie of making it [Bolus], is of *medulla, cassia fistulæ* [a 1 cit]
358. melancholiousness [1610, Barrough] 35 these be thre diuersities of melancholiousnes, according to the thre kinds of causes [a 1 cit]
359. melanthy [1595, Chapman] 280 dissolue ... *mel anthos* [a 1 cit]

360. menstruous [2a, 1599, Moufet] 153 much menstrous blood flowing into the matrice
361. mentagra [1802, Turton] 205 Mentagra a Latine word vsed ... to haue altogeather meant another thing from *impetigo* [a 1 cit]
362. mentha [1846, *Penny Cycl.*] 223 Rx ... of *mentha*, which is called *Glaucium* [a 1 cit]
363. mesentery [3, 1626, Bacon] 110 carried to the liuer by the veynes *mesentery*
364. metrenchyte [1601, Holland] 156 cast them in with an instrument called *metrenchita* [a 1 cit]
365. miliary [2, 1737, Hamilton] 201 But vnto *erysipelas* are referred *herpetes*, whiche in kinde be two manner of wayes ... *miliares* and *exedentes*, byting and gnawing
366. millipede [2, 1651, French] 13 vse oyle, wherin sowes, called in Latin *Millipede* be boyled [a 1 cit]
367. misty [1c, 1859, Tennyson] 42 som which by the occasion of the Ophthalmy are greatly troubled in their eyes, and haue them fumous & mistie
368. mithridatum [1603, Dekker] 10 to minister inwardly to the sick ... triacle, or *Mithridatum* proffiteth [a 1 cit]
369. mitigating [*ppl a*, 1612, Webster] 252 you shall rather vse a more mitigating remedie [a 1 cit]
370. moderating [*ppl a*, 1673, Leigh R.] 238 refrigerating and moderating helpes [a 1 cit]
371. mola [1, 1601, Holland] 153 Mola ... is ... a swellinge that is hardened, sometime in the mouth and entrie of the matrice [a 1 cit]
372. mole [1611, Cotgrave] 153 Of the mole in the matrice [a 1 cit]
373. mollifier [1592, *Misc. Hist. and Philol.*] 51 commix drawing thinges with mollifiers
374. mollifying [*ppl a*, 1590, Barrough] 59 you must minister mollefying medicines [a 1 cit]
375. morbilli [1693, *Blancard's*] 205 thicke humours stuffed in the skin, which are commonly called *morbili* and *variolæ* [a 1 cit]
376. mordacity [2a, 1601, Holland] 63 medicines which do ... stop sharpnesse and mordacitie [a 1 cit]
377. motion [2e, 1602, Shakespeare] 18 the body being much weakened by veheme[n]t motion
378. moulting [*vbl sb*, 2, 1610, Barrough] 179 A bath ... bringeth foorth excrementes or moltinges, if anie sticke within the Skinne
379. nasal [*sb*, 2, 1601, Holland] 301 Of making Nasale or Erthinum
380. necrosis [1, 1665, Needham] 231 *Gangrena* and *Syderatio*, which the Grecians call *necrosis* and *sphacelus* [a 1 cit]
381. nefresie [1590, Barrough] 295 a particular bathe, which is applied for paines of the nefresie

382. neoteric [B, *sb*, 1, 1598, Meres] 198 according to the opinion of the Neoterickes [a 1 cit]
383. Nestor [1588, Shakespeare] *ii[v] rather as a Nestor vnto his Agamemnon, as a Zenophon vnto his Cyrus, & as a Plutarch vnto his Traian which thought it not so glorious to tie their enemies to them by forced feare [a 1 cit]
384. nitrous [1, 1601, Holland] 246 it is made both salt, nitrous, and corrosiue [a 1 cit]
385. nodulus [1651, Culpeper] 278 Of making Nodulus [a 1 cit]
386. obdurate [*v*, 2, 1597, A. M. *Guill.*] 202 the skinne being obdurated & hardened through much labour
387. obscure [4b, 1597, A. M. *Guill.*] 74 See **rare**, anted.
388. obstinate [2, 1638, Rawley] 269 a harde and stonie tumour, verie obstinate, and resisting touching
389. obstruction [4, 1597, Shakespeare] 48 medicines which doe deuide and take away obstructions and stoppings
390. obstructive [2, 1620, Venner] 179 obstruction and abundance of obstructiue humours [a 1 cit]
391. obturation [1610, Barrough] 128 About the beginning of obturation and stopping [a 1 cit]
392. obvert [1, 1623, Cockeram] *iii[v] I will obuert and turne against all the venemous bitinges [a 1 cit]
393. occasion [*v*, 4, 1634, Herbert, Sir T.] 41 other maladies of the eyes caused and occasioned of the four humours
394. occlude [1, 1597, A. M. *Guill.*] 215 shutting & occluding the poores [a 1 cit]
395. ocyme [1621, Burton] 244 the leaues of ocymum
396. œdematous [1641, Browne] 247 These œdomatous tumours are rather excited in the winter time [a 1 cit]
397. ophioglossum [1881, *Sat. Rev.*] 99 See **ophrys**, unrec. [a 1 cit]
398. ophrys [1785, Martin] 99 Restrictive thinges be ... *ophrys*, *ophioglossum* [a 1 cit]
399. opiate [*sb*, B, a, 1603, Jonson] 293 Hote conserues respecting the vertue animall be ... almost all *Opiatæ* (that is) liquid thinges, as *Mithridatium* Treacle
400. orange-tawny [1602, *Narcissus*] 234 yellow or red, declining vnto a certaine colour like orengetaunie
401. orthopnic [1610, Barrough] 64 Those which be properly astamatickes, or orthopnickes, they haue no feauer at all [a 1 cit]
402. outward [2b, 1612, Woodall] 14 you may come to local & outward medicines
403. oxycratum [1597, A. M. *Guill.*] 83 such are best healed with *oxycratu[m]* that is) a drink made with vineger & water sodden together [a 1 cit]

404. oxyrrhodin [1639, J. W. *G's Char.*] 20 apply to the head oxyrhodium, (that is), vineger of roses [a 1 cit]
405. ozæna [1, 1656, Blount] 51 Ozænæ in greek be vlcers in the nose, that be deepe and rotten [a 1 cit]
406. panax [1617, Middleton] 233 the roote of *panax* [a 1 cit]
407. papule [1706, Mayne] 204 Those which are called of the Greekes *hidroa*, the Latines terme *sudamina*, and of Plynie *papule sudorum* [a 1 cit]
408. paracmastic [1892, *Syd. Soc. Lex.*] 169 Some [fevers] doe decrease and deminish by little and little those the Greekes call *paracmasticos* [a 1 cit]
409. paraplegia [1657, *Phys. Dict.*] 26 the word *Paralysis* is a more generall name then *Paraplegia* [a 1 cit]
410. paregoric [B, a, 1704, Harris] 225 those thinges, which because they mitigate and lenifie paine ... are properly called *Anodyna* & *paregorica* [a 1 cit]
411. parotis [2, 1693, *Blancard's*] 50 Parotides in greeke be inflammation which are wont to issue out in the kernelles, which be by the eares [a 1 cit]
412. perfusion [c, 1848, *Ecclesiologist*] 161 apply about the priuities, foments, perfusions, and ointementes
413. persic [B, 2, 1599, Gerarde] 106 Rx ... leaues of persica [a 1 cit]
414. perspirable [3a, 1646, Browne] 87 Let the sicke remaine in an ayer, that is cold and perspirable [a 1 cit]
415. perspiration [1, 1611, Cotgrave] 179 perspiration and breathing out [a 1 cit]
416. pestilent [2, 1613, Cawdrey] 197 the pestilent aire doth readily creepe into the body
417. petasite [1771, *Gent. Mag.*] 198 Rx. ... *petasitio* [a 1 cit]
418. petroseline [*a*, 1727, Switzer and ns] 251 take *apium hortense* (which is commonlie called *petroselynum*, parsley) [a 1 cit]
419. phagedæna [1657, *Phys. Dict.*] 235 there are engendered *phagedæne*, which doe somewhat deepely gnaw the flesh [a 1 cit]
420. phenomenon [b, 1605, Bacon] 193 The second [sign of the Pestilence] is often *phænomena* in the ayre, specially in Autumne [a 1 cit]
421. phlegmagogue [1657, *Phys. Dict.*] 248 some medicine that can purge fleume called *phlegmagogon* [a 1 cit]
422. phlegmonoid [1755, *Gent. Mag.*] 201 because of melancholie gouerning, *Erysipelas* is saide to be *phlegmonodes* [*sic*] [a 1 cit]
423. phlegmonous [1666, Harvey, G] 215 in the beginning of these phlegmonous humours [a 1 cit]
424. phlogosis [1693, *Blancard's*] 214 euerie hote and flaming disposition, which the Greekes call *phlogosis* [a 1 cit]
425. phlyctena [1693, *Blancard's*] 201 There commeth also of choler almost those diseases called of the Greekes *phlyctænæ* [a 1 cit]
426. phrenitis [1621, Burton] 17 Phrenitis in Greeke and in Latin is a disease, wherin the mind is hurte [a 1 cit]

427. phyma [1693, *Blancard's*] 200 the inflammation of the eye, the squince, the inflammation of the throte, *phyma, phygethlum*, and those inflammations which we terme *glandulæ* and *bubones* [a 1 cit]
428. pinching [1, 1693, Evelyn] 30 If any pinching or binding of the synowes cause resolution
429. plausibly [2, 1612, Hall, Bp.] *ii[r] Poetes wer wo[n]t to pen such Enterludes, as they thought would be plausibly heard of their auditory
430. plethoric [1a, 1620, Venner] 215 in a plethoricke or full bodie [a 1 cit]
431. pleuritic [*a*, 2, 1652, Benlowes] 170 that feauer, which is engendred through inflammation of the filme or caull, that girdeth in the ribbes, it is called *pleuretica febris*
432. polygonum [a, 1706, Phillips] 35 iuice of *Poligonum* [a 1 cit]
433. pompholyx [1, 1678, Phillips ed. 4] 276 *pompoligos,* [*sic*] which is commonly called *tuthia* [a 1 cit]
434. pomum [1760, Lee, J. and ns] 196 Rx. *Lapdanum* ... *storax* ... cinnamon, mace ... mirrhe, masticke, frankensence ... commix them & make a *pomum odoratum* [a 1 cit]
435. pregression [1623, Cockeram] 207 Primitiue causes, which we cal both *prægressæ* & *euidentes* [a 1 cit]
436. prescission [1589, Nashe] *vi[v] See **interception**, anted. [a 1 cit]
437. prescript [2, 1603, Harsnet] 46 the tunicle must be saued by this forenamed prescript
438. presentment [1607, Shakespeare] *iii[r] the presentme[n]t of this my labour
439. pretergress [1, 1596, Barrough] 267 it keepeth within the precinctes of his libertie, which if it shall once pretergresse ... it is no longer to be called melancholie
440. priapism [11, 1590, Barrough] 140 *Priapismus* ... is whe[n] the yeard is stretched out in length and breadth, nothing provoking the patient to lust and desire [a 1 cit]
441. profluence [1, 1633, Fletcher] 47 The watery profluence of teares
442. profusion [1, 1604, Cawdrey] 259 the incision ... oftentimes ... causeth great profusion of bloud [a 1 cit]
443. propagation [4, 1586, *Reg. Priv. Counc. Scot.*] *iii[v] the furtheraunce and propagation of good learning
444. psora [1681, *Willis's Rem. Med.*] 202 *scabies*, which is called ... *psora* [a 1 cit]
445. psydracium [1693, *Blancard's*] 205 *Psizacion* is not truly read in Celsus for *psydracion* [a 1 cit]
446. putrefact [*a*, 1597, A. M. *Guill.* and ns] 110 putrifact blood which is curded [a 1 cit]
447. quality [II, 7d, 1704, Swift] 5 By drynes is ment in this place a drie distempure of the qualitie alone, and by moisture, a moist distempure of the bare qualitie

448. quilt [3, 1601, Holland] 5 a quilt made in this sorte profiteth much R. leaues of laurell, serpillum

449. radicle [1, 1671, *Phil. Trans.* and ns] 129 those things that bring downe vrine vnto the Reines: as is ... *apium* and *radicula* [a 1 cit]

450. ramex [1608, Middleton] 143 *ramex intestinorum*: that is, the ruptire of the bowelles [a 1 cit]

451. rare [3d, 1707, Floyer] 74 the pulse is rare and obscure

452. rarefying [*vbl sb*, 1648, Hammond] 251 wee make perfect ... the raryfying of the thicke bodie [a 1 cit]

453. rectified [*ppl a*, 2, 1605, Timme] 197 it is better and more holesome to vse frictions at home in a rectified aire

454. refrication [1590, Barrough] 97 The eating of sharpe thinges ... causeth a certaine refrication and rubbing open againe of the scarre [a 1 cit]

455. refrigerating [1634, Herbert, Sir T.] 238 refrigerating and moderating helpes [a 1 cit]

456. refrigerative [B, *sb*, 1706, Phillips ed. Kersey] 242 those refrigeratiues, which can also greatlie drie vp [a 1 cit]

457. reinforce [3b, 1659, *Gent. Calling*] *iii^{v} offring to reenforce my ouer presumptuous determinatio[n] [a 1 cit]

458. remission [6b, 1685, *Willis's Lond. Prac.*] 169 the feauer doeth not leaue the patient, but it hath a certaine remission and slaking in euerie fitte

459. remit [*v*, 6c, 1615, Burton] 250 you shall both mitigate the paine ... & remit the tumour also

460. remit [*v*, IV, 15b, 1685, Sandys] 232 the furie of the euill [is] somewhat remitted and slaked

461. remitting [*ppl a*, 1693, *Phil. Trans.*] 216 resoluing and remitting medicines [a 1 cit]

462. remollition [1590, Barrough] 297 for the cure of *Oedema*.... it is necessary to haue remollition with discussion [a 1 cit]

463. repel [2c, 1719, Quincy] 13 To the head it selfe you must first apply thinges, that doe repell and dryve back

464. repellent [*sb*, B, 1, 1661, Lovell] 222 those [medicines] which are called *repellentia* and *regerentia* repulsives, and restrictives [a 1 cit]

465. repelling [1597, A. M. *Guill.*] 215 the whole order of applying of repelling medicines [a 1 cit]

466. repulsion [2, B, 1725, Bradley] 215 the matter is thicke, and not pliable to repulsion

467. repulsive [*a*, A, 1, 1611, Chapman] 51 medicines that be repulsiue and discussiue [a 1 cit]

468. repulsive [*sb*, B, 1, 1656, Ridgeley] 215 there be two kinds of repulsiues both amongst the late Physitions & also the Arabians (that is to say) common & proper [a 1 cit]

469. resistance [3b, 1656, Hobbes] 220 There is furthermore resistance of the member if it be touched

470. resolution [3c, 1783, Cullen W.] 210 These kinde of tumours … should be comprehe[n]ded vnder one of these foure either vnder insensible exhalation or resolution, or vnder suppuration, or putrefaction, or induration & hardning
471. restriction [3b, 1758, J. S. Le Dran] 3 The payne of the head caused of heat, is cured with such thinges as doe coole, without manifest restriction, especiallie yf they be of thinne and percing substance
472. rheum [1753, *Chamb. Cyc. Supp.*] 99 Restrictiue thinges be these … *rheum ponticium* [a 1 cit]
473. rhodium [2, 1678, Phillips] 223 oile of roses is marueilously effectuall, (the Greekes call it rhodinon.) [a 1 cit]
474. rhus [1611, Florio] 223 *rhus*, that is, *sumach* [a 1 cit]
475. ripening [*ppl a*, 1, 1592, Shakespeare] 248 it shall be cured by ripening medicines [a 1 cit]
476. rostrum [1753, *Chambers's Cycl.*] 279 Rx … of lettuce, scarioll, *rostrum porcinum*
477. rove [*sb*[1], 1b, 1590, Barrough] 61 pull away the scabbe or roue
478. rubefacient [B, *sb*, 1805, *Edin Rev*] 65 vse those medicines which can exulcerat the skinne … as those be which are named *rubefacientia*. For this purpose the breast must be rubbed with nettles, brayed or beaten [a 1 cit]
479. rubeola [1, 1676, Cooke, Jas.] 205 But the French men preposterouslie abusing the names haue called the lowe and broade kinde *rubeole*, but the higher sort *variole* [a 1 cit]
480. ruff [*a*, 1651, Barker] 110 Moreouer thirst doth trouble the[m], their vrine is ruffe, and the pulse is swift [a 1 cit]
481. sacculus [1, 1621, Burton] 297 *Sacculus*, *videlicet*, a little bagge [a 1 cit]
482. salvatrice [1590, Barrough] 39 two coates the one whereof they terme *Salvatrix* because it saueth and keepeth the humours
483. sapa [1624, Middleton] 49 *Sapa* is newe wine sodden till it come to the third parte [a 1 cit]
484. satyriasis [1, 1657, Coles, W.] 140 Priapisimus … is whe[n] the yeard is stretched out in length and in breadth … and if there chaunce to the yeard panting or beating, then the euill is called *Satyriasis* [a 1 cit]
485. scene [II, 8b, 1662, More, H.] *iii[r] can the whole Scene of mans life so gorgeouslie & stately set forth by the historia[n]s of seueral ages, shew vs at one time, on one stage, two such notable actors
486. scirrhus [1a, 1615, Crooke] 27 a *Scirrhus* (which is a hard swelling without sense) [a 1 cit]
487. scissible [1626, Bacon] 242 alume scissible [a 1 cit]
488. scope [4, 1590, Barrough] 222 We now dispatch the third scope or intention, in the beginnings of *phlegmone*
489. scourer [*sb*[2], 6, 1719, Quincy] 176 Stronger scourers then these, be the froth of salt Peter, the salt Peter it selfe

490. scouring [*ppl a*, 2, 1597, Gerarde] 114 decoction of cicers, & other like things, which haue an abstersiue & scouring vertue [a 1 cit]
491. scraped [*ppl a*, 1, 1597, A. M. *Guill.*] 130 Rx. … lycorice scraped [a 1 cit]
492. scrofulose [1753, Russell, R.] 246 other vlsers which they call *scrufulosa* [a 1 cit]
493. scrupulous [5, 1638, Junius] 201 let it be lawfull for euerie man to impose what titles or names they will, so that (as Galene saith) they doe not swarue or straie from the naturall meaning of the thinges them selves: but leauing all the scrupulous and scholerlike contentio[n]s, which some doe vse in the intreatie of this subject
494. scutum [3, 1771, *Enc. Brit.* II and ns] 81 For this purpose also Cerotes are commended, which the Phisitions commonly do call *scutum stomachale* [a 1 cit]
495. semicupium [1634, Johnson T.] 295 *Semicupium* … is a particular bathe, which is applied for paines of the nefresie, for the cholicke, and for the iliacke [a 1 cit]
496. semitertian [1661, Florio] 191 It is called in Greeke *hemitritæus*, and in Latine semitertiana, in English halfe a tertian [a 1 cit]
497. sense [12, 1586, Sidney] 127 if the feuers and paine wax lesse, and sense of heauinesse remaine about the reyne that is affected
498. septic [B, 1608, Topsell] 266 wast the humour by applying of gnawing medicines which the Grecians call *Septica* [a 1 cit]
499. sequestration [5, 1898, *NSSL*] 209 true apostemes … which maladie the Grecians call *cacoethia* and also in the greater or lesser sequestratio[n], *determinata*
500. serous [1, 1594, T. B. *La Prim.*] 253 And these kindes of tumours which doe proceede of waterish fleame, or of the aforesaid serous encreasing, they doe also call vnlawfull and vntrue *ædemata* [a 1 cit]
501. sideration [2, 1612, Cotta] 201 Likewise *gangrena* of some member … mortification but not absolute, and also sphacelus which is called of the Latines *syderatio*
502. simplex [A, 1594, Blundevil] 281 See**compositum**, anted.
503. sinapsism [1601, Holland] 29 you maie vse sinapsismes or cauterizatio[n] [a 1 cit]
504. skink [*sb*, 1, 1590, Barrough] 143 Also the partes of scinces which embrace the reynes, are drunk to raise a stiffenes of the yarde [a 1 cit]
505. sluggish [4c, 1899, *Allbutts*] 185 cast into the bellie not verie easie clisters, that they may bring fourth the sluggish and hurtfull matter
506. solution [11, 1681, Willis's *Rem. Med.*] 147 See **dejection**, anted.
507. somnoriferous [1590, Barrough] 19 some somnoriferous compounde [a 1 cit]
508. sopor [1, 1675, Burthogge] 24 deade sleep … is called simply *Coma* or *sopor* [a 1 cit]

509. soporiferous [1, 1590, Barrough] 24 The soporiferous and sleepy *Coma* [a 1 cit]
510. sorbus [1706, Phillips ed. Kersey] 58 soure apples, and *sorbus* [a 1 cit]
511. spather [1597, Gerarde] 301 stirre it a long time with a spater [a 1 cit]
512. species [9b, 1620, Granger] The first species, which is aloft and superficiall ... is called of the Greekes *alphos*
513. spleen vein [9a, 1611, Cotgrave] 66 the inner vaine of the arme, which they call the liuere vaine, or the splene vaine [fpl]
514. spontaneous [3a, 1664, Power] 240 which vlcers they call *spontanea*, because the humour which causeth them, is stayed and tarieth still in their going out or issue [a 1 cit]
515. stable [*a*, 1c, 1666, Boyle] 87 You must giue vnto them meates that be stable, durable, and hard to corrupt
516. steatoma [1599, A. M. *Gabel.*] 202 there be three such kindes of *abscessus ... atheromata, steatomata, melicerides* [a 1 cit]
517. sternutament [1677, Gale] 32 minister sternutaments [a 1 cit]
518. stillicidium [2, 1791, Wallis, G.] 137 Strangurion in greeke, *stillicidium vrinæ* in Latine is a disease wheras the vrine distilleth downe by drops [a 1 cit]
519. stomachic [1a, 1656, Blount] 74 Also sometime it chaunceth to the stomach (that is) when humours abounding or heaped together or crude, either els sharpe and gnawing be in it: that kind of *sincope* is called *stomachica* [a 1 cit]
520. stomachic [B, *sb*, 1753, Bracken] 16 pilles that be good for the stomake, called *stomachica* for that cause [a 1 cit]
521. strain [sb^2, 7, 1616, Chapman] 47 the streyns of egges
522. strigment [1646, Browne] 271 *strygmenta gymnasiorum* (which they call the filthines of bathes) [a 1 cit]
523. strike [*v*, 42, 1590, Barrough] 19 Ther [*sic*] pulse is greet, and stryketh sceldome
524. strumous [1, 1590, Barrough] 260 *King Edward* also ... was wonte marueilously to cure Strumous persons onely by touching them [a 1 cit]
525. strumous [2, 1590, Barrough] 258 See **diuretical**, anted. [a 1 cit]
526. struthion [1587, Newton, T.] 151 thinges that cause sneezing, as be pepper, *castoreum, struthium* [a 1 cit]
527. stupefact [*v*, 1598, Florio] 102 those thinges that doe stupefact and astony strongly [a 1 cit]
528. suckling box [1679, Nesse] 20 droppe it into his mouth with a suckling boxe
529. sudamina [1671, Salmon] 204 these *sudamina* ... come (as their name doth declare) by many bilious swettes [a 1 cit]
530. suffiment [1650, Brooke, H.] 271 remeadies only, which can fitly both mollifie, and also digest: as ... *suffimen* [a 1 cit]

531. suffite [1, 1621, Burton] 301 Suffitus (in English a perfuming) is made of dry thinges to stoppe distillations [a 1 cit]
532. sulphur vivum [1651, French] 124 you must vse emplaisters of ... *sulphur vivum* [a 1 cit]
533. sulphur water [7, 1665, *Verney Mem.*] 122 washed with alomme water, or sulphure water [a 1 cit]
534. sulphurous [1b, 1815, Smith, J.] 121 The bodie being purged, let him vse chieflie waters that spring by them selues of alome and salte peter, and afterwarde sulphurous waters
535. superficial [1d, 1804, Abernethy] 202 Besides these tumours ... there chaunce other also, affecting oftentimes the superficiall partes of the bodie
536. suppression [5, 1601, Holland] 123 if the euill be engendred of suppression of hemorhoides or menstruis
537. suppurated [1612, Woodall] 218 the incision of a suppurated abscession [a 1 cit]
538. suppuration [2, 1603, Holland] 127 these sometime do breake the suppuration, and purge out the matter with the vryne
539. symptomate [1590, Barrough] *v[v] the varietie of diseases, the causes, signes, and symptomates of the same [a 1 cit]
540. synulotic [1657, *Phys. Dict.*] 229 it must be healed with filling medicines (which the Greekes call *Synulotica*) [a 1 cit]
541. tabes [1651, Biggs] 253 But in those daungerous dispositions or diseases they call it *Tabes*, which name *Hydrope* and *Cachexia* doe require [a 1 cit]
542. tabulate [*a*, 2, 1826, Kirby] 288 Rx. ... suger roset tabulate as much as sufficeth [a 1 cit]
543. talpa [2, 1693, *Blancard's*] 257 if it groweth in the head, it is called *Talparia* or *talpa*
544. tardiness [*a*, 1605, Shakespeare and ns] 49 Noyse and tincklinge in the eare ... is caused through an exquisite tardinesse of the sense of hearing [a 1 cit]
545. taxis [2, 1727, *Chamb. Cycl.*] 262 the diseases called *Strume*, *Taxi*, and *Parotides*
546. tenebricose [1730–6, Bailey] 15 *Tenebricosa vertigo*, and that is when the patient doth thinck that al that he seeth turneth about, and sodenlie with it, his sight faileth him [a 1 cit]
547. terra lemnia [1613, Harcourt] 52 Trochiskes of *terra lemmia* [a 1 cit]
548. terrestrial [5, 1638, Rawley] 269 let him flie and auoide ... the flesh of all terrestriall creatures
549. tetrapharmacon [1727–41, *Chambers's Cycl.*] 216 *Tetrapharmacum* consisteth of foure thinges ... of waxe, of rosen, of the gumme of the herbe *colophonia* ... and of bulles tallow [a 1 cit]
550. thymus [2, 1693, Blancard] 202 See **almismar**, unrec. [a 1 cit]
551. tonsil [1, 1601, Holland] 59 Of inflammacion of the tonsilles [a 1 cit]

552. tormina [1656, Robinson, R.] 98 The Latynes call this disease *tormina*, because through it, the bowells are tormented and fretted verie much with payne [a 1 cit]
553. tracheal artery [1a, 1710, Fuller] 63 whatsoeuer doth exasperat the *trachea arteria* [a 1 cit]
554. tremor [2a, 1611, Shakespeare] 37 Tremor in latin, in English trembling or shaking
555. tubercle [2, 1661, Lovell] 64 If ther be a crude and rawe tubercle and botch ingendred
556. tuberculome [1903, *Nature*] 201 a kinde of *phlegmone, phygethon*, which is called *panus* (Celsus being the author) but of our men *phyma* and *tuberculum* [a 1 cit]
557. tunic [4a, 1661, Blount] 39 the eye hath seuen coates, which they call *Tunicæ*
558. twitch [*sb*, 3, 1596, Barrough] 45 Take therfore a twiche of silver and therwith lift vp subtellie the vngle from the tunicle
559. typhoid [1, 1800, *Med. Jnl.*] 170 That which chaunceth through inflammation of the stomach, the liuer, or the longes, is called in Greeke typhodes (that is) inflaming or burning [a 1 cit]
560. typic [*a*, 2, 1601, Holland] 170 Of the aforesaide feauers, some be *Typicæ*, (that is) certaine and ordinate: and some be, *erraticæ*, (that is) vncertaine and vnordinate [a 1 cit]
561. umbilicus [1615, Crooke and ns] 215 These thinges following do represse flux by refrigeration & cold, sengreene, lettuce, *psillium, cotyledon* (that is to say) *umbilicus Veneris* [a 1 cit]
562. uneasiness [2a, 1594, Ashley, R.] *iii[r] a subiect ... which ... the inconuenient vneasines of the studie hath kepte your Honor from being acquainted with
563. unfrequented [1588, Shakespeare] *v[v] let him ... not leaue the poorest house vnfrequented [a 1 cit]
564. ungle [3, 1590, Barrough] 45 sometime it also happeneth that another vngle ariseth in the other corner [of the eye]
565. unpure [3, 1590, Barrough] 192 but if one feuer do exceed the other, the[n] it is called an vnpure hemitrice
566. unulcerate [1590, Barrough] 274 It shall therfore be sufficient to hinder the encreasing of vnulcerate cancres [a 1 cit]
567. usnea [1597, Gerarde] 249 of *Vsnea* (that is) of the mosse of trees [a 1 cit]
568. ustion [2, 1588, Read, J.] 274 the cure of these cancres either by section or vstion
569. vacuation [2, 1590, Barrough] 6 exercyses, bathes, sweetings, and other naturall and other artificiall vacuations
570. variola [1771, *Enc. Brit.* and ns] 205 See **morbilli**, anted. [a 1 cit]
571. varus [1822–7, Good] 204 little swellings and those harde which arise

in the outwarde skin and *superficies* of the face ... The Latines call them *vari* [a 1 cit]

572. vastness [2b, 1622, Fletcher] *v[r] the laborious difficultie and confused vastenes of this arte [a 1 cit]

573. vena cava [1598, Florio] 113 the veyne which is called *Vena cava* [a 1 cit]

574. ventricle [4, 1641, Milton] 128 The stones be in the reynes, nigh their ventricles either little or great

575. viall glass [1647, Hexham] 41 keepe it in a viall glasse

576. vicious [7a, 1597, Gerarde] 106 But when the wormes were killed by the aforesaid medicines you must driue them out without delay, for there proceedeth a vicious exhalation from them

577. viscus [*sb*, 1, 1643, Steer, J.] 263 Rx. ... *viscus quercinum* [a 1 cit]

578. visual [2, 1603, Holland] 15 The visuall spirites beholding a wheel that turneth about, or any such like thing, doth also turne about in like sorte

579. vitelline [*sb*, 1891, *Cent. Dict.* and ns] 234 whenas vnnaturall choler called *vitellina*, is throughly concocted

580. vitiligo [1657, *Phys. Dict.*] 203 *Vitiligo* ... is a filthie colour of the skinne ... which doth infect the skinne onely with certaine markes, which doe cleaue fast vnto it like vnto little scales [a 1 cit]

581. volatic [2, 1684, *Bonet's* and ns] 203 called ... of the Latines *impetigo*, in English the ringworme and commonly of some ... *volatica* [a 1 cit]

582. volatile [*a*, B, 1597, A. M. *Guill.*] 215 And these also do stuffe & stop the passages *farina* called *volatiles*

583. volvulus [*a*, 1679, J. Smith] 103 See **convulvulus**, ns. [a 1 cit]

584. vulpine [1, 1789, Phillip *Voy. Botany Bay*] 29 stronger medicines as be oiles *costiuum vulpinum* [a 1 cit]

585. white dittany [1605, Timme] 194 the roote of white diptayne [a 1 cit]

586. yellowish [*v*, 1590, Barrough] 115 his tongue is yellowished [a 1 cit]

2. New senses

1. addition 203 *vitiligo* ... would more aptly agree, if it were put with his epithete or addition, as to say *alba vitiligo*

2. alteration 7 digestio[n] that we speak of now is no thing els but an alteration of the humour that causeth the disease

3. anointing 233 butter or some other anointing thing

4. cenchrine 241 the other kinde of *herpetes* ... we haue saide to be called in Greeke *miliaris* and *cenchria*

5. complication 171 Complicatio[n] is when the feauers invade the patient at diuerse houres

6. compositum 281 Practitioners doe put a double vnderstanding in syrupes ... *simplex*, which is called vsuall, and *compositum*, which is called magistrall

7. compost 278 a Suppotary [*sic*] made of hony, which if you thincke so weake that it will not moue the compost or ordure
8. conceivable iii[r] he [God] had infused into man a conceauable minde
9. constitution 135 continuall exacerbations and fittes are caused, and long constitution of the euill
10. convulvulus 103 The *Iliaca passio* ... The Latines do call ... *vuluulus*, & *conuoluulus*
11. dacryd 237 iuice of *scammonium*, called of new Greece, *dacrydion*
12. declining 154 Conuulsion and cramp of the armes, the fingers, and the necke, and declining of them contrarie
13. deduction 62 Take heed also that ther be litle diduction of the veine
14. deprehension 23 Catoche or *Catalepsis* in Greeke, in Latin may be called *Occupatio*, *Detentio*, *&* *Deprehensio*
15. discolorate 39 the second they terme *discolorata* (that is, hauing no colour)
16. distillation 149 Uteri *fluor*, in Latine, fluxe of the matrice in English, is a continuall distillation, and flowing out for a long time, of the whole bodie, purging it selfe
17. dracontion 202 Vnto choler there seemeth to partaine this euill, which the grecians call *dracontion*, the Latines *dracunculus*, according to the liuely similitud [*sic*] ... of that name, Auicene calleth it *vena medeni*, Haly Abbas, *vena saniosa*
18. dracunculus 202 See **dracontion**, unrec.
19. empirica 260 There are also very many remedies called *Empirica*, consisting in practice described and celebrated of the auncient Physitions
20. fasting 205 if it be dayly rubbed with fasting spittle, it waxeth whole
21. fistolo 47 I speak of watery eyes & of corrupt humours like teares, which the Phisitians call *fistoles*, to discerne betweene the *fistula* and the watery profluence of teares
22. glandulous 256 *Scrofa* ... haue thicke and glandulous neckes and commonly they be strumous and full of kernells
23. gurgulio 58 See **gurgulio**, anted.
24. hemicrania 14 medicines which of the old Phisitions were called *Hemicrania*, for that they were vsed for the migrime
25. hepatic 110 they which haue weake facultie and strength of the liuer they are called *hepatici*, as Galen sayeth
26. homotonous 169 some of them [fevers] doe endure of an equall vehemencie, and force from the beginning vntill the ending: those the Greekes call *homotonos* and *acmasticos*
27. inclination 174 in the inclination of the fitte, you must bringe them straight vnto a bath
28. indic 6 See **indic**, anted.
29. inflation 250 Tumours aboue nature, which the Latines call inflationes ... commonly called windie Apostemes

30. intemperance 165 wine if the intemperaunce of the sicke may suffer it
31. involucrum 275 *epithymum*, (which the Romaines call *inuolucrum*)
32. ischiadic 126 The Latines call this disease *Ischias*, and they that are afflicted with this disease, are called *Ischiadici*
33. judgement 54 Hote distempure is knowen by the tempure of the whole body ... the face is redd ... cold is knowen by contrary iudgmentes
34. latus 105 There be three kindes of wormes ... The second ... called *Lati*, be brode and longe
35. medulla 288 the playnest and simplest waie of making it [Bolus], is of *medulla*, *cassia fistula*
36. myrtine [also postd] 69 sprinckle the breast ... with ... oiles of roses, quinces, and myrtines
37. nude 46 put a litle of it into the eye, and it wil knit together, and make so nude againe the tunicle if it be broken or hurt
38. pannicle 41 There be other diseases alsoe of the eye engendred of bloud, as the ophthalmy and pannicles
39. pending [cf. v^2, a] 160 If sore trauaile in childbirth be caused of ... adarctation and pending in of the child
40. petroseline 251 take *apium hortense* (which is commonlie called *petroselynum*, parsley)
41. pomum 196 See **pomum**, anted.
42. prassina 234 vnnaturall choler ... the colour of leeks which they also call *prassina*
43. precinct *vi[r] there is no arte or science, be it neuer so difficult, but might be perfectlie knowen within that shorte precinct
44. putrefact 110 like putrifact bloud which is curded
45. radicle 129 See **radicle**, anted.
46. releasing [*ppl a*] See **dissolving**, anted.
47. repressive [*sb*] 216 onelie pure repressiues are to be vsed
48. sciatici [*sb*] 162 The barbarous sort call this disease *Sciatica*, & they cal the[m] that be diseased with it *Sciatici*
49. sclerotica 220 a stony and almost indissoluble hardnesse, commonly called *Sclirotica*
50. scutum 81 See **scutum**, anted.
51. second table 122 Let them eschue much fruites and second tables
52. spina 234 This affect is properly called of Galene, a true and exquisite *Erysipelas* ... Auicene calleth it *spina*
53. tardiness 49 See **tardiness**, anted.
54. taxis 262 the diseases called *Strume*, *Taxi*, and *Parotides*
55. trochiscate Rx of Agaricke trochiscate
56. tuberculome 201 a kinde of *phlegmone*, *phygethon*, which is called *panus* (Celsus being the author) but of our men *phyma* and *tuberculum*
57. twilt 32 make a twilt with .iij. sheetes of graie paper
58. umbilicus 215 See **umbilicus**, anted.
59. usual [*sb*] 281 See **compositum**, anted.

60. variole 215 See **rubeola**, anted.
61. visible 38 the influence of the visible Spirits
62. vitelline 234 whenas vnnaturall choler called *vitellina*, is throughly concocted
63. vngula 45 There is another infirmitie also which proceedeth by the aboundance of melancholy, and that they call *Vngula*: for it is much like the Naile of a finger
64. volatic 203 See **volatic**, anted.

3. Unrecorded

1. abscessus 200 the abscessions are those tumours which the Latines call *Abscessus*
2. acatia 58 (Acacia?) Rx ... *sumach*, *hipociscidis*, *acatia*. ana
3. acmastica 169 those the Greekes call *homotonous* and *acmastic[os]*, (that is) remaining still in the same force and vigoure
4. adarctation 160 If sore trauaile in childbirth be caused of ... adarctation and pending in of the child
5. aedema erysipelatoides 246 See **aedema phlegmonoides**, unrec.
6. aedema phlegmonoides 246 three other humours may be commixed therewith and these be they: *ædema phlegmonoides*, *ædema erysipelatoides*, and *ædema schirrhoides*
7. aedema schirrhoides 246 See **ædema phlegmonoides**, unrec.
8. aesipum 157 made of æsipum, that is, oyle tried out of woll in sheepes flanks or necks
9. Agamemnon Aii^v rather as a Nestor vnto his Agamemnon, as a Zenophon vnto his Cyrus, & as a Plutarch vnto his Traian which thought it not so glorious to tie their enemies to them by forced feare
10. agrippa 163 you must apply more effectuous medicines ... as ... *agrippa*
11. alba vitiligo 203 *vitiligo* ... would more aptly agree, if it were put with his epithete or addition, as to say *alba vitiligo*
12. albae 242 See **verruncula**, unrec.
13. albara 203 that which is saide of [Auicene] and almost of all the Physitions of Africke to be *albara*, is named of the Greekes & of Celsus also *leuce*
14. alcola 51 See **aphtha**, anted.
15. aldaron 232 Trochiskes ... which are called ... *Aldaron*
16. alephangina 7 Also you may vse *Pilula aurea*, and *Alephanginæ*
17. alhasaphum 204 See **almansorus**, unrec.
18. alica 68 hulled wheat, called *Alica*
19. alipta 151 Trochiskes of *gallia* and *alipta moschana*
20. almansorus 204 Auicene *planta noctis*, & *almansorus* & *alhasaphum*
21. almatium 206 certaine whelkes, which he calleth in the same place, *bothores iuncturarum*, & in lib. 4. he calleth them *almatium*
22. almismar 202 in forme ... like to a harde rounde pillar ... of Auicene ... called *almismar*, *Thymion* or *thymon*

23. amphymerinon 188 *Qvotidiana febris intermittens* (that is) an intermitting quotidian feuer ... called of the Greekes *amphimerina*
24. amylum 215 See **gluten**, anted.
25. anadendromalache 270 the barke of the roote of *Althea*, (which the common sort ... call *Anadendromalache*
26. anagallis 112 iuice of **Anagallis** the female
27. andron 229 Trochiskes of *Andron*, *Polyida* & *Musa*
28. andron musa 228 See **pasio**, unrec.
29. anini 112 Among simple medicines these that follow do take away obstructio[n]s ... lupines, capares, *anini*, with wind parsley
30. antecedens materia 236 The second [scope] concerneth the auersion of the humour that floweth to the affected member, which they [Chirurgians] call *antecedens materia*
31. antispasis 214 Nowe *Antispasis* (that is) a reuulsion the contrarie way, is a common remedie against all these kind of tumours
32. apium 122 Let those thinges that be ministered ... that haue vertue to attenuate and heate: as is *Apium*, percelie
33. apostema 201 The Greekes call it *Emphysema*: Auicene termeth it a windie *apostema*
34. apostema ventosum 246 *apostema ventosum*, a windie aposteme
35. apthe 55 The vlcers which are bredde, in the ouermost parte of the mouth ... ar called *Apthe*
36. aqua mellis 67 Minister those thinges that do clense and purifie matter and filthe (as is) *aqua mellis*
37. aqua mulsa 17 *aqua mulsa* (that is) water & hony sodden together
38. aranea 39 all those overcurious diuisions, (namelie, *Iris*, *Cornea*, *Aranea*, and *Vuea*, and the residue)
39. archoticon 28 See **plicis**, unrec.
40. argenti spume 141 Rx. ... *argenti spume*
41. arnoglossa 281 Rx. the iuyces of plantayne, *Arnoglossa*
42. aromaticum rosarum 72 Rx ... aromaticum rosarium. ana
43. arthretica 289 of the which vertue also be *Arthretica maiores* and *minores*
44. asarum 37 these thinges that provoke vrine, as anyse, *daucus*, *asarum*, *smirinon*
45. ascachilos 201 *gangræna* of some member, necrosis ... and also *sphacelus*, which is called of the Latines *syderatio*, & of Auicene *ascachilos*
46. aspanar 269 For pothearbes, let him vse that which the Arabians call *Aspanar*, but we ... do call it spinach
47. athanasia 260 Galen willeth vs to minister ... *Athanasia*
48. athera 256 *Atheromata*, which consist of a certaine kind of matter like vnto a pulse, which the Greekes call *Athera*
49. attery 135 vrine that is bloudie, atterie, and stinking
50. aurea alexandrina 22 After purging it is good to minister vnto them ... *aurea Alexandrina*
51. bausci 44 R. spynache, bansci [*sic*]

52. benedictæ laxitiua 8 dissolue therin *benedictæ laxitiua*
53. bismallow 280 Rx. mallowes, bismallowes
54. bismalva 280 Rx. mallowes, *bismalua*
55. bizantijs 123 For which purpose minister also syrups ... of Agrimony and bizantijs
56. blitum 9 iuyce of maiorame, blitum, coleworts
57. bothor 200 those little tumours (which they call *bothor*)
58. bruscus 112 both the endives, sperage and bruscus
59. bulimos 87 Bvlimos in Greeke is nothing else, but great and vehement famine
60. buphthalamum 120 Also chammomill is most profitable, which is called *leucanthemus*, and also *buphthalamum*
61. bursa pastoris 9 walwort, bursa pastoris
62. bursa pastria 56 knottgrasse, *bursa pastria*, bryer leaues
63. caliacus morbus 121 a continuall *Dysenteria*, and the disease called *Caliacus morbus*
64. calidicon 232 Trochiskes ... being thoroughly brayed and beaten togither, and then washed in vinagre and wine: as that either of ... *calidicon*, *Aldaron*
65. caphura 215 See **cotyledon**, anted.
66. capnos 270 *fumus terra*, (which of the Grecians is called *Capnos* or *Capnios*
67. capparis 291 trochiskes of Reubarbe, or of *Capparis*
68. carbo 227 Whenas in very deed *ανθϱαξ* among the Greekes is the very same, that *Carbo*, or *Carbunculus* is among the Latines
69. carbunculus 227 See **carbo**, unrec.
70. carnici 202 *cancri*, which of the Greekes be called *carnici*
71. catalepsis 23 See **deprehension**, ns.
72. cataputia 41 Turbith, *cataputia minor*
73. cataputia minor 41 See **cataputia**, unrec.
74. cauda equina 281 *cauda equina*, horsetayle and such like
75. causa coniuncta 208 that, which they terme *causa coniuncta*
76. causos 178 a continuall Tertian, which the Greekes call *causos*
77. celsi papule 204 those, which we have rehearsed and touched alreadie, are reckened by the Greekes *ionthi*, *epinyctides*, *hidroa*, *psydraces*, *exanthemata*, *celsi papule*, and *Pliny mentagra*
78. cephalaea 12 Cephalaea both in Greeke and Latine is the name of headache which is exceeding painfull
79. cephalica 6 The vttermost vaine, which in the arme is called *humeralis*, or *Cephalica*
80. ceratum liquidum 141 The making of this cerote which is called *ceratum liquidum*
81. cerefolium 158 herbes that be odoriferous and sharpe, as is, *Cerefolium*, fennell
82. chalbana 266 Rx. ... *Terebintha*, *chalbana*, *opoponax*

83. chamaepityos 162 Rx ... chamæpityos
84. chancalthum 244 shoemakers bleache, (which the Greekes call *chancalthum*
85. cherva 78 the leaues of *cherua* annointed with the iuce of greene parcely
86. chœrades 202 These be called of the Greekes chœrades, of the Latines, strumæ
87. chordapson 104 some swelling of the thinne and smalle gutts sticketh out, that it seemeth wounden together, like a string called *Chorda*, whereupon manie do call this disease *Chordapson*
88. citron apple 195 barks of the citron apple
89. clavelata 262 lye made of ashes commonly called *clauelata*
90. coarctatio 156 See **obturatio**, unrec.
91. coma somnolentum 24 called simply *Coma*, or *sopor*, or els *Coma somnolentum*
92. continens causa 208 this cause called *coniuncta* or *continens causa*
93. conuulsio 30 See **spasmus cynicus**, unrec.
94. conuulsio canina 30 See **spasmus cynicus**, unrec.
95. corarium 242 the shrub *corariu[m]* (which of the late Physitions is called *Sumach*)
96. cordial bagges 195 it is better to vse cordiall bagges
97. cornus 58 a fruite called *Cornus*
98. costum 251 let the stomach be annointed with oyle of speke, of *Costum*
99. costus 92 Rx. Costus
100. cretica calaminthe 260 that medicine also, which is made of *cretica calaminthe*
101. cucufa 300 Cucufa is made for the cure of the euill called Cœphalalgia
102. cuscuta 120 Also iuice of *cuscuta* profiteth maruelouslie
103. cyaneus 260 See **cerule**, anted.
104. cyclaminus 16 Poure into the nose iuyce of chickweed, betes or cyclaminus
105. cynosbatos 269 the wilde eglantine brier which the Greekes call cynosbatos
106. Cyrus *ii^{v} see Nestor, anted.
107. damosonium 129 roote of damosonium
108. darke vertigo 15 The *Scotoma* or darke vertigo becometh most vehement in winter
109. daucus 129 seede of *daucus*
110. deficiens febris 169 most aptly called in Lataine *febris interpolata* because the fittes come and renewe at their times: some call it *deficiens febris*
111. determinata 209 But they are not counted to be true apostemes in deed, which we haue termed *pustule* & *abscessus*, besides that tumour, which maladie the Grecians call *cacoethia* and also in the greater or lesser sequestration, *determinata*

112. deustion 268 of unnaturall melancholie thorough deustion, are all the kindes of Cankers ingendred
113. diabrion 52 pouders of *Diabrion santalon*
114. diacarion 57 comixe *mel rosarum, diacarion*
115. diacotoneon 17 some restrictiue thing as is *Diacotoneon sine speciebus*
116. diactrilon 51 medicinnes altogither discussiue, as is *Diactrilon*
117. diacurcuma 123 See **diarrhodon**, anted.
118. diairis 290 with one Lozenge of ... *Diairis Salomonis*
119. diairis salomonis 290 See **diairis**, unrec.
120. dialactia 138 the antidotes of *diacalaminthes, dialactia*
121. dianthon 37 *Galens dianthon,* and such like
122. diaria 168 there be two kinds of diaries: Or, which is named *Diaria* simplie and without adiection or putting to of anie word, which feauer doth not extend aboue the space of a naturall day
123. diaria febris 168 Diaria febris, (that is) the one day feauer
124. diasaccha 112 *diasaccha, diacurcunia* [*sic*] are good
125. diayreos 64 *Diayreos salomonis*
126. diospoliticum 90 for the same, *Diacotoneum* is good, *and diospoliticum*
127. dipsacos 215 The medicines repressing which of nature are cold are these ... *dipsacos, virga pastoris*
128. dispneas 294 See **apnœa**, anted.
129. dispuras 287 Also the decoction of a cocke may conueniently be given for diseases in the breast & of *dispuras*
130. distempure 1 a simple distempur without any humours
131. distempure 145 which thing chaunceth to the wombe sometime through hote or colde distempure of the same
132. dolis 284 Dolis otherwise called *Potus*, or *Potio*, is a medicine laxatiue dissolued in some kinde of licour and given in drinke
133. dothienes 201 they be called *dothienes*, which Celsus doth call *furunculi*, felons
134. dracontion 202 this euill, which the grecians call *dracontion*, the Latines *dracunculus* ... Auicene calleth it *vena medeni*, Haly Abbas *vena sanosa*
135. drageta 251 this confection following, which they call *Drageta*
136. dubelata phlegmatica 202 certaine tumours, comprehended of the Greekes vnder the name of *apostema* which be called of Auicene *nodi*, of Haly abbas, *selaa*, and *dubelata phlegmatica* of the Latines *abscessus*
137. duplex tertiana 182 if the feuer doth inuade the patient daily with vehement rigour and cold ... then it is called *duplex tertiana*, a double tertian
138. durities 201 See **sephirus**, unrec.
139. earwarde 45 in the corner of the eye to the earwarde
140. effectious 93 an effectious remeady
141. electuarium 97 See **electuarium de gemmis**, unrec.
142. electuarium de gemmis 9 Rx. pouder of *Electuarium de gemmis*

143. electuarium de nuncibus 198 that medicine, that is commonly called *electuarium de nuncibus*
144. electuarium nidum 123 the Antidotes *diaphœnicon*, and *Electuarium nidum* be good
145. elephantia 202 See **ulcus nigrum**, unrec.
146. elephantus 202 See **ulcus nigrum**, unrec.
147. elychnion 249 If there be no plentie of new sponges, it is better … to vse that which the common sort call, *elychnion*
148. epacmaticos 168 Some [feuers] alwaies encrease and augument by little & litle, those the Greekes do call, *anabaticos*, & *epacmaticos*, (that is) encreasing and augumenting more and more
149. ephelide 206 the disease ephelide (that is to saie) for the roughnes and swartnes of the face
150. ephemera simpliciter 171 Ephemera simpliciter, or Diaria one day feauer
151. epialos febris 188 a feuer called *Epialos febris*: in which the patient is feuerous, and vehementlie cold together
152. epidermida 234 that little outward skinne, (which the Greekes call *Epidermida*)
153. epino 64 Rx. *Loch*, *epino*
154. epithema 52 apply to the forehead an *Epithema*
155. epolotica 233 But in tender and yong bodies for the separation of the crust, and detersion of the filthie corruption, the meale of tares mingled with honie … procure a scarre: the Grecians call them *synulotica* and *epolotica*
156. erisymo 158 *erisymo*, & other such like
157. ernum 147 z .j. of the meale of *ernum*
158. erthinum 301 Nasale and Erthinum be medicines which be cast into the Nose for many causes
159. erubinosa bilis 234 See **porracea**, unrec.
160. esula 41 R. of the best aloes, red Sanders, *Esula*
161. excitore 32 oile of excitore
162. exsiccatory 151 and let all their diet be exciccatorie and drying up
163. febris interpolata 170 See **deficiens febris**, unrec.
164. fera 205 the skinne is made more sharpe, and is exulcerate, and groweth verie vehemently, and looketh red … this is termed … in Latine *fera*
165. ferinos 269 Such tumoures … are truelie *scirrhi* … but … do leaue that member, which they did first infest, and afterwarde doe passe ouer to … another … then Auicene calleth the euill *ferinos*
166. flos æris 244 See **viride æris**, unrec.
167. formicule 202 To this kinde also may be referred myrmecia, as if one should call them formiculæ
168. fugillinus bubo 258 *Guido* … doth register *Fugillinus bubo* amongst the number of flematike abscessions

169. fumaria 270 some purging medicine, which can expell melancholie as are ... *Mesua Epithymum* ... *fumus terra* ... called ... of the Latines *fumaria, lupulus*
170. gallia 5 Rx ... gallia moschata
171. gallicum malum 206 that disease which ... some do call *Gallicum malum*, some *Neapolitanum*, other some ... *venereum*
172. glandosæ 206 certaine pushes ... rehersed euen now out of Auicene, lib. 4. called *glandosæ*
173. glaucium 223 Rx. ... *menntha* [*sic*], which is called *glaucium*
174. granedo 53 Granedo is when the humour falleth into the nose, and causeth the pose
175. gutturosi 257 our countrey men call it *Hernia gutturosi*, whereup[o]n they also call them *Gutturosi*, which doe labour of that disease
176. hailefolk 64 For distillation doth also chaunce in hailefolke
177. handy cure 161 but if it do not come foorth, because the infant is dead, or hath a very great head ... you must come ... to cutting ... [but] it is not our purpose to teach handy cure heare
178. hectica febris 170 both in Greeke and Lataine *Hectica febris*, and in English, the feauer ethicke
179. hectica marasmodes 170 if this feauer doeth so increase ... then it is called *Hectica marasmodes* and *marasmus*
180. hemitrice [*a*] 191 Of an hemitrice feuer
181. hemitrice [*sb*] 192 when a feuer is ingendred of an intermitting tertian, and a continuall quotidian being equall of like force ... it is called an exquisite hemitriteus ague, but if one feuer do exceed the other, the[n] it is called an unpure hemitrice
182. hemitritaeus 171 Another is, when an intermitting Tertian is ioyned with a continuall Quotidian. This is called by a peculiar name of the greekes *Hemitritæus*
183. herd 44 lay on a plaister of herdes & the white of an egge
184. hernia gutturis 255 See **bronchocele**, anted.
185. herpetes estiomeni 235 See **excedent**, anted.
186. hidraleum 33 nourish with hote oyle or *hidraleu[m]*
187. hidroa 204 See **exanthema**, anted.
188. hiera ruphi 270 *Cæruleus, Diasene, diacatholicon, hiera Ruphi*, all which things do purge foorth melancholike humours
189. hiera simplex 7 Pilles of Rewbarbe, or of *Hiera simplex* and such like
190. hircina 249 branke vrsine, or *hircina*, which is called *Achantus* or *achanta*
191. humeralis 6 See **cephalica**, unrec.
192. hypochymum 217 those humours called hypochymum, (that is to say) the webbe in the eye
193. hypocischidos 107 pomegranate rindes, *hypocischidos*
194. iberis 163 the roote of the hearbe called iberis

195. ignes sacri 234 swellings ... called of the Greekes ... *Erysipelata*, but of the auncient Latines *Ignes sacri*
196. ignis sancti antonii 230 This kinde of corruption being perfect in the affected part, and altogether depriued of sence, is called commonlie in Fraunce *Ignis Sancti Antonij*. In another place *Ignis Sancti Martialis*
197. ignis sancti martialis See **ignis sancti antonii**, unrec.
198. indorum 6 barkes of mirabolanes, citrinorum, indorum
199. ininacotoueorum 70 those thinges which can alter and make thicke the thinne and sharpe humours ... as ... *ininacotoueorum*
200. iniubarum 285 Rx. ... prunes damascene, *iniubarum*
201. insolencicity *iv[v] the insolencicity and pride of auncient Physitions
202. ionthi 204 See **celsi papule**, unrec.
203. ionthosus affectus 204 Galen maketh mention ... of an affect which he calleth *ionthosus affectus*, which he sayth is the beginning and foundation of *elephantiasis*
204. ischias 162See **ischiadic**, anted.
205. lapatium 249 sorrell, (which our countriemen do call *lapatium acutum*)
206. lapis gagatis 31 See **lapis**, anted.
207. lapis molaris 272 the stone called *lapis molaris*, which the Greekes call *mylites*
208. laserpitium[8] 32 put into ther mouth *Castoreum*, or *laserpitium* with *oxymell*
209. laxus tumour 201 the Greekes call it *œdema*, but our Phisitions terme it *laxus tumor*
210. lenticula palustris 215 See **cotyledon**, anted.
211. lepus 235 that part of the nose, which is commonly called *lepus*
212. leucanthemus 120 Also chammomill is most profitable, which is called *leucanthemus*
213. leuce 203 that [disease] which is saide of him [Auicene] ... to be *albara*, is named of the Greekes & of Celsus also *leuce*
214. leuisticum 249 of *leuisticu[m]*, or *ligusticum*
215. licium 55 drying medicines, as is *licium*
216. lienaris vena 186 You must cut the innermost veine of the left arme, which is called *lienaris vena*, the spleene veine, or *mediana*
217. ligusticum 249 See **leuisticum**, unrec.
218. long pepper 9 Rx ... long pepper and nuttmegs
219. lupia 256 they do greatly erre which do make this euill called *Lupia*, to be all one with that disease called *Lupus*
220. lypiria 170 a feauer, in Greeke called *Lypiria* ... there is heate fealt within, and in the bowelles and entrailes
221. macedonicum 233 that medicine ... also called *macedonicum*
222. mala 205 This perhappes is that scabbe, which certayne of the Frenchmen call *mala dartra*

223. mamia 22 dissolue therin of fine mamia Z.ij
224. materia coniuncta 236 The third [scope] consisteth in the emptying out of the humour ... which they [Chirurgians] also call materia coniuncta
225. mel 280 See **mel violatum**, unrec.
226. mel anacardinum 163 Rx. *Mel anacardinum*
227. mel violatum 280 dissolue therein *Cassia fistula*, *mel violatum*
228. memoria deperdita 20 Memoria deperdita, the losse of memorie
229. memytha 242 those medicines ... which haue the nature and force of *glaucium* (that is) of *memytha*
230. menstruis 121 retention of hemorhoides or menstruis
231. mesue 262 the same effect likewise that hath diachyton called magrum mesues
232. mirmeciæ 201 those *verrucæ*, which the Greekes call *mirmeciæ*, the Latines *formicæ*
233. miua 302 Rx ... *Miua*
234. molybdos 276 leade, which he himselfe calleth in Greeke *molybdos*
235. morbus comitialis 31 Epilepsia ... the Latines call this disease *Morbus comitialis*
236. mulsum 122 But they must eschue sweete wines, and *mulsum*
237. muscilaginis 298 Rx. *Muscilaginis* of the seede of *Althea*
238. myamis 276 *myamis*, a certaine ointment inuented of *Apollonius* for vlcers
239. mylites 272 the stone called *lapis molaris*, which the Greekes call *mylites*
240. mysos 242 more sharpe medicines, and those which haue euen the power of fire, as is, *mysos*
241. myxaria 106 you must adioyne ... *myxaria*
242. napta 202 But vnto *stratomata* doth belong a certaine swelling without paine, which they do call *nata*, or *napta*
243. nardinum 4 rewe, cammomill, and nardinum
244. nata 202 See **napta**, unrec.
245. neapolitanum malum 206 See **gallicum malum**, unrec.
246. nex 295 medicines ... to prouoke menstruis, as ... nex
247. nitisalba 48 the roote of *nitisalba*
248. nitrum 16 Also nitrum beaten with nigella
249. numularia 99 walworte, *pedelion*, *numularia*
250. nux cupressi 215 *nux cupressi*, and such like thinges
251. nux indiæ 42 R ... *nux Indiæ*
252. obturatio 156 Phinosis in greeke, *obturatio*, or *coarctatio vteri* in Latin, is a stopping or streightening in the mouth or necke of the matrice
253. ocinium 233 Bread also beate[n] & brayed with *apiu[m]* or *ocinium*
254. ointment of alabaster 46 annoynting ... the temples of the patient with the ointement of Alabaster

255. oleum de Lateribus 21 oyle made of tyle stones, called *Oleum de Lateribus*
256. oleum melinum 116 take oyle of roses, or *oleum melinum*
257. oleum nardinum 22 annoint the head, whith [*sic*] *Oleum nardinum*
258. oleum omphacinum 215 oyle of roses, *oleum omphacinum*
259. one day fever 168 in Latine *Diaria febris*, and in English it may be called one day feauer
260. orcaselinum 129 These that follow drawe much vrine ... *orcaselinum*
261. orminum 158 *orminu[m]* it is an herb like vnto horehound
262. oxalme 269 seasoned either with brine, or with *oxalme*
263. oxis 99 See **sanicula**, unrec.
264. oxymel scylliticum 8 Rx ... of *oximel scylliticum*
265. oxymel simplex 8 oxymell simplex and compositum and scilliticum
266. pannicum vitreum 43 the eyes appeare troubled and full of veynes, so closed with a pannicle that the patie[n]t cannot well see, nor discern any thing, & this siknes is called pannicu[m] vitreu[m]
267. panus 201 See **tuberculome**, anted.
268. papule sudorum 204 See **papule**, anted.
269. pasio 228 some strong medicine which ... can greatly drye ... *Andron Musa*, *Pasio*, or *Polyida*
270. pasta regia 294 Of making Pasta Regia or Marzapane
271. pelidnon 268 This *Scirrhus* when it happeneth in the partes of the bodie, manie of the Phisitions ... do call it *pelidnon*
272. pencedanum 32 Also pencedanum, or dogge fennell
273. pensiles verrucæ 202 See **acrochordon**, anted.
274. phantasticall cell 38 sent from the phantasticall Cell by a senowe
275. philonium 49 the Antidote *Philonium*
276. phinosis 156 See **obturatio**, unrec.
277. phrisarcotion 34 those thinges which strengthen the head, as ... Phrisarcotion
278. phthoe 245 the euilles called *phthoe*, & *cachexia*
279. phygethlum 200 See **phyma**, anted.
280. pill of Jerusalem 47 purge the patient his stomak with Pilles of Ierusalem
281. pilula alephangina 7 See **alephangina**, unrec.
282. pilula aurea 53a medycyne purging choler as is, *Pilulæ aurea*, *alephangina*, *azairet*
283. pilula azairet See **pilulæ aurea**, unrec.
284. pilula bechicæ 63 Rx. ... *pilulæ bechicæ*
285. pilula rufi 196 the pilles that are called *pilulæ rufi*
286. pistax 143 sweete almondes, *pistax*
287. pistolochia 55 R. ... *pistolochiæ*
288. pixis plunubra 266 lay on *pixis plunubra*, with the distilled lye
289. planta noctis 204 Auicene *planta noctis*, & *almansorus*, & *alhsaphum*

290. pleuretica febris 170 that feauer, which is engendred through inflammation of the filme or caull, that girdeth in the ribbes, it is called *pleuretica febris*
291. plicis 28 Rx. of *diambra, plicis, archoticon*
292. plirisarcoticon 143 Rx. *Dianthos, pliricarsoticon*
293. Plutarch *ii^r See **Nestor**, anted.
294. politricum 283 Rx. … *politricum*
295. polyida 229 See **andron**, unrec.
296. pomum odoratum 196 See **pomum**, anted.
297. porra 202 *verrucæ*, which be swellinges like vnto little hillocks appearing in the skinne, whereof they haue this name, being called of the common sort, *porra*
298. porracea 234 *porracea* & *erubinosa bilis* are engendred oftentimes in the stomach, of naughtie and corrupted humours
299. posca aquosa 242 neither in sweete wine, nor in *posca aquosa*
300. potio 284 See **dolis**, unrec.
301. potus 284 See **dolis**, unrec.
302. prassium 294 Horehound called *prassium*
303. preparating 130 the preparating of the goats bloud
304. pritching [*vbl sb*] 203 itching & pritching in the bodie
305. procured 265 swelling of the procured crust
306. psillium 3 night shade, or sorrell, or psillium
307. psizacion 205 *Psizacion* is not truly read in Celsus for *psydracion*
308. pugillus *viii^v Pugillus is a small handfull
309. pulvis 42 this powder, which many, in respect of the notable vertue thereof, do call *Puluis benedictus*
310. pulvis benedictus 42 See **pulvis**, unrec.
311. pulvis nabetus 43 the pouder called *Puluis Nabetus*
312. pustulæ corrosiuæ 235 maliganant vlcers, which are called of the late chirurgians *pustulæ corrosiuæ*
313. ramex aquosus 143 *ramex aquosus*: that is, waterie rupture
314. ramex carnosus 143 ramex carnosus, that is a fleshie rupture
315. ramex inguinis 143 *ramex inguinis*, that is, the rupture aboue the priuie members
316. ramex intestinorum 143 See **ramex**, anted.
317. ramex ormenti 143 *ramex ormenti*: that is, the rupture of the filme
318. ramex varicosus 143 *ramex varicosus*: that is, the rupture of the swollen veines
319. raucedo 53 *Raucedo* is when the humour chaunceth to distill to the sharpe arterye
320. regerentia 222 See **repellent**, anted.
321. regines 19 some somnoriferous compounde as is regines *Nicolai*
322. repressing [*ppl a*] 215 We may rather vse repressing medicines
323. roberibes 69 Rx. … of *Roberibes*

324. rubia 261 *rubia maior*, ana

325. ruptorium medicamentum 212 that medicine which they call *ruptorium medicamentum*

326. rupura 143 See **cele**, anted.

327. sacer ignis 201 They terme this euill *Erysipelas*, but these name it *sacer ignis*

328. saire 204 See **essera**, anted.

329. sanguinea pustulæ 226 Of a Carbuncle, and a Cancre, and of the maladie named Sphacelus, all which they call sanguinea pustulæ, 1. bloud pushes

330. sanicula 99 Restrictive thinges be ... *oxis, sanicula*

331. sarcites 121 There be three kindes of the dropsie ... the thirde *Anasarca, Yposarca, Sarcites*

332. sarcocolcastoreum 30 Rx. ... sarcocolcastoreum

333. scabiosa 229 Some also do declare wonderfull things of *Scabiosa*

334. scincus 143 Rx. ... *scincus*

335. scirrhon 201 See **sephirius**, unrec.

336. scirrhosis 201 they be grieued with the disease *Scirrhosis*

337. scolopomacherion 245 that instrument made to the forme of a mirtle leafe ... which the Greekes call *scolopomacherion*

338. scrofa 256 *Scrofa* that is to say, *Sues* haue thicke and glandulous neckes

339. selaa 202 tumours caused of phlegm ... called of Haly abbas, *selaa*

340. semicucufa 300 it is called *Semicucufa*, when we prouide but for one parte of the head

341. semiss *viii^{v} Semiss. is the halfe of euerie weight

342. sephirus 201 They call this *Scirrhon*, the Latines, *Durities*, the Arabians *sephirus*

343. sere 204 See **essera**, anted.

344. serica 264 those threedes which are called *serica*, or small lute stringes

345. serpens 239 For *ιϱτα* (?) in Greeke is all one with *serpo* in Latine, whereupon /S/*ιϱπυσ*/S/(?) is called *serpens*

346. serpentia vlcera 239 so called *serpentia vlcera*, creeping vlcers

347. serpo 239 See **serpens**, unrec.

348. seryphium 106 these simples are good ... *seryphium*, which is a kind of wormewood growing in the sea

349. sidiorum 101 .iij. *sidiorum*

350. siligna 58 decoctions of ... *siligna*

351. silplinum 32 iuice of *silplinum*

352. sinapsismus 20 It profiteth to apply a sinapsismus

353. sium 133 seede of *althea, sium*

354. smaras 244 the heade of the fish *smaras*

355. smirinon 37 See **asarum**, unrec.

356. solatrum 282 the lesse morell, called *Solatrum*

357. soldana 124 Colewortes of the sea called *soldana*

358. spasmus cynicus 30 There is an affect of the face called in Greeke *Spasmus Cynicus*, & in Latin *Conuulsio canina*, or of some *Torturaoris*
359. spasmus torturaoris 30 See **spasmus cynicus**, unrec.
360. specillum oricularium 156 Therefore if the vlcer may be seene, it may be knowen by an instrument called *specillum oriculariu[m]*
361. sphecle 266 Rx. ... of *sphecle*, (that is) of the burnt dregges of wine
362. splenium 300 See **frontal**, anted.
363. spuma maris 254 Rx. ... *spuma maris*
364. stechas 4 flowers of stechas
365. straight gut 100 inflammation engendred in the streight gut
366. stratomata 202 But vnto *stratomata* doth belong a certaine swelling without paine, which they call *nata*
367. strygmenta gymnasiorum 271 vse ... *strygmenta gymnasiorum*
368. stubium 18 *Mathiolus* doth greatly commend *stubium*
369. stultitia 21 See **fatuity**, anted.
370. subpale 66 if his spittle be ... yellow and subpale
371. subrufe 172 An vrine, that accordeth with nature, is subrufe in colour
372. succida 252 vnwashed wool (which they call *succida*)
373. sues 256 See **scrofa**, unrec.
374. sustument 54 For the same purpose it is good to minister sustuments
375. symphyton 229 comferie (which the Greekes call *symphyton*)
376. synechis 169 in a feauer *Synochus*, there is no remission or slaking of the heate, but in the feauer *Synechis*, there is sensible remission and slaking in euerie fitte
377. syrupus 7 Iulep of Roses and Violettes, or *Syrupus acetosus*
378. taberzet 282 In one ounce of the strayning dissolue sugar taberzet
379. talparia 257 if it groweth in the head, it is called *Talparia* or *talpa*
380. tarsecum 243 See **tusium**, unrec.
381. tecolithus 132 the stone of *tecolithus*
382. teretes [*sb*] 104 There be three kinds of worms. The first be round and long, named *teretes*
383. termina 98 Dysenteria ... The Latynes call this disease *termina*
384. terminthis 108 They which haue the hemmorhoides, neither be vexed with ... *terminthis*, nor with the leprie
385. terra cimolia 223 Rx. ... *terra cimolia*
386. testa sepia 266 Rx. of a burnt hedghog, of *testa sepia*
387. testiculus canis 143 *orchis*, called also *testiculus canis*
388. theriaca 195 apply *theriaca* to the botches
389. theriaca andromachi 195 fill it with *Theriaca Andromachi*
390. thuris purgamenium 218 that medicine, which the Greekes call *Mamia*, which is *thuris purgamenium*
391. thymion 202 See **almismar**, unrec.
392. tonsila 59 Tonsillæ be infla[m]macions of those things which lye betweene the mouth and the throte

393. Trajan *ii[r] See **Nestor**, anted.
394. tria 291 the powder of *Tria sandalorum*
395. triphera 147 commixe them with honie or *triphera*
396. triphera magna 147 Rx. of *Triphera magna*
397. tritura 194 beate them all to a verie fine powder, and make a *Tritura*
398. tunica 194 roote of *betonica altilis*, commonly called *tunica*
399. tusium 243 Auicene seemeth to haue named this kinde of *verruca*, *tusium*, or … *tarseum*
400. ulcus nigrum 202 The same Celsus deuideth *cancer* into many parts or kindes (that is to say) into *erysipelas*, *gangrena* & *vlcus nigrum* of this kind also is *elephantus* or, *elephantia*, or *elephantiasis*
401. unguenti populeon 3 Rx. *vnguenti populeon*
402. unguentum 29 you may adde these ointmentes, *vnguentum aregon*, *vnguentum agrippa*, and *vng. martiaton*
403. unguentum aegypticum 218 *vnguentum aegypticum*
404. unguentum agrippa 29 See **vnguentum**, unrec.
405. unguentum alabastrum 46 annoynt the temples of the patient … with *vnguentum Alabastrum*
406. unguentum apostolorum 218 you must come to the applying of … *vnguentum Apostolorum*
407. unguentum aregon 29 See **vnguentum**, unrec.
408. unguentum martiaton 29 See **vnguentum**, unrec.
409. unguentum subtile 46 vse the oyntment before rehearsed, which they call *vnguentum subtile*
410. unthicked 261 alume *zuccharinum* vnthicked
411. vena medeni 202 See **dracontion**, unrec.
412. vena sanosa 202 See **dracontion**, unrec.
413. venereum malum 206 See **gallicum malum**, unrec.
414. verbasculi 162 minister … *verbasculi odorati*
415. verruncula 243 They be called of Auicene *claui*, but the Latines doe terme them *claui*, *verruncula*, *albæ*
416. veternus 19 some call this disease, in Latin *Veternus*
417. vigilans sopor 24 The other euill called *Vigilans sopor*
418. virga pastoris 215 See **dipsacos**, unrec.
419. viride æris 244 the ruste of brasse (which of the late Physitions is called *viride æris & flos æris*)
420. vmbilicus veneris 215 These thinges following do represse flux by refrigeration & cold, sengreene … *Veneris*
421. vndimia 201 the Greekes call it *edema* … the interpreter of Auicene *vndimia*
422. vngula caballina 287 horsehofe called *vngula caballina*, which is an herbe called of some little clote
423. vulgalpus It is grauelly, and avoideth out always filth. This sore is called *vulgalpus*

424. well of the head 38 set in the well of the head
425. wind parsley 112 See **anini**, unrec.
426. xanthium 129 See **lapis indiacus**, anted.
427. yealking 81 Of yealking and vomiting
428. yrisilarica 48 bitter thinges which purge and clense without Erosion, as is *yrisilarica*
429. Zenophon See **Nestor**, anted.

4. Postdatings

1. acetose [1547, Borde]minister vnto the patient syrupe of vyolettes, and *acetosus simplex*
2. affect [1538, Starkey] 121 The liuer is affecte by the spleene being colde
3. bocion [1547, Borde] 255 See **bronchocele**, anted.
4. cardiaca [1561, Hollybush] 73 a corrupt motion of the heart, or a stretching out of it against nature. The new sort of Phisitions do wrongfullie call it *Cardiaca*
5. carene[1] [*c.*1420, *Pallad. on Husb.*] 280 Rx. ... anise, fennell, and *careum*
6. clammishness [1578, Lyte] 256 clammishnesse and thicknesse of the humour
7. cochee [1547, Borde] 256 afterward purge with purgations (that is) with *pilulæ cochiæ*
8. consolid [1480, Caxton] 69 the roote of *consolida maior*
9. defrut [*c.*1420, *Pallad. on Husb.*] 223 wine boiled either to the halfe or thirde parte, (one we call *sapa*, the other *defrutum*)
10. descend [10b, 1471, Ripley] 89 do not eate before some moderate exercise, or before yesterdays meate be well discended
11. epilency [1540, Borde] 32 the cure of a new & sharpe epilence
12. esthiomene [1541, *Guydon's Quest Chirurg.*] 230 But Auicene calleth it Estihomenon, when as the corruption therof doeth passe to the continuall partes
13. febris [1535, Stewart] 170 It may most aptly be called in Lataine *febris interpolata*
14. incourage [1550, Nicoll] 160 you must comfort and incourage a fearfull woman
15. mespile [1545, Raynold] 56 mespilers, vidz. medlars or open arses
16. myrtine [*sb*, 1545, Raynold] 69 sprinckle the breast ... with ... oiles of roses, quinces, and myrtines
17. pestilential [2b, 1460, *Bk Quintessence*] 197 the pilles that are called *pilulae rufi* or *pestilentiales*, or els *communes*
18. piste [*sb*[1], 1420, *Pallad. on Husb.*] 72 it is good to eate ... pistay
19. preparate [*ppl a*, 1575, Turberville] 3 a litle Cynamon in it, or Coriander sead preparate
20. preparate [*v*, 1569, Androse] 146 minister medicines which can cut & divide the aforesaide humours and preparate them

21. serpille [1558, Warde] 5 See **quilt**, anted.
22. slay [14a, *c.*1425, *Stockh. Med. MS*] 282 syrupes that be acetose and sharpe are not to be ministered, because they excoriate, rase, and slea
23. tenasm [*c.*1425, Arderne's *Treat. Fistula*] 98 this beginneth after *Tenasmus* sometime
24. unwise [3, 1480, *Morte Arthur*] 31 Ther goeth before this euill an vnwyse state of the body and mind
25. virtue [6a, 1325, *Prose Psalter*] when the feuer waxeth more moderate, and vertue is stronger

5. Other

1. cypress nut [ncit] 215 the hote repulsiues are, allome, Cipresse nuttes
2. diamargariton [ncit] pouder of *diamargariton*
3. digestive [nd, ncit] 10 oyle of roses, which is both repulsiue, digestiue, and discussiue
4. erysipelatoid [ncit] 201 we will call *phlegmone* the principall, to be *erysipelatodem*
5. incourage [ncit] 160 You must comfort & incourage a fearefull woman
6. inflammate [new last date, 1590, Barrough] 67 the breast within be inflammate

B[OSTOCKE], R[OBERT], *The difference betweene the auncient Phisicke … and the latter Phisicke*, 1585

1. Antedatings

1. abstergent [A, 1612, Woodall] Eii^r the Chymicall Physitions consider the nature of things … whether they be *Attractiua, Anodymæ, Abstergentia, Aperitiua Constringentia contrahentes.* [a 1 cit]
2. accident [7, 1621, Burton] Cvi^v Humors and qualities … are but onely dead accidents
3. action [3, 1600, Cornwallis] Bii^r all our actions, artes and Sciences
4. actor [3, 1603, Shakespeare] Aii^v there must be an Actor before there be action
5. adulterate [2, 1592, Daniel] Fiii^v other bastard, adulterat, sophisticat stuffe [a 1 cit]
6. aerial [I, 1, 1664, Power] Aiii^v æryall, waterie, and earthly thinges [a 1 cit]
7. afflicted [2, 1680, Temple, Sir W.] Cvi^r things, which nature in the place afflicted doeth require for the cure
8. agend [1, 1753, Chambers] Iviii^r *quies*, bringeth forth nothing but *motus*, & *agendi operatio* doth frame to it self, that thing which is [a 1 cit]
9. agent [*a*, A, 1600, Melton] *6^v neither doth his Philosophie teach any agent cause of those thinges which it affirmeth to be eternall
10. alimentary [A, 2, 1620, Venner] Ev^v he ministreth not the substance

and grosse quantitie or bodyes as the other doe, vnlesse it bee in some *Alimentary* diseases [a 1 cit]
11. ancient [3, 1605, Bacon] Ciiii[v] as the auncient Philosophers haue taught
12. apply [10, 1790, Paley] Fviii[r] meditations applied to *Astrologie*
13. arcanum [1, 1599, Sandys] Dvi[v] their *arcana*, inward and secret thinges remayning for the phisition to iudge vpon [a 1 cit]
14. arcanum [2, 1646, Browne] Dv[r] the three substanties of each thing and his *Arcanum* [a 1 cit]
15. argonaut [1, 1596, Spenser] Hii[r] the golden Fleece brought from *Colchos* by *Argonautae* [a 1 cit]
16. asclepiad [*sb*, 1, 1656, Blount and ns.] Gv[v] his sonnes which were called *Asclepiades* after their father *Æsculepias* [a 1 cit]
17. assation [1605, Timme] Fi[v] Which of them doth knowe the seuerall maners of *Calcination, Reuerberation, Cementation, Inceration, Imbybytion, Pastation, Liquefaction, Ablution, Sublymation, Exaltation, Contrition, Resolution, Putrifaction, Circulatio[n], Inhumation, Distillation, Ascention, Fixation, Lauatio[n], Coagulation, Assation, Co[n]gelation, Fermentation, &c* [a 1 cit]
18. assyrian [B, 1591, Spenser] Fv[r] the *Chaldea[n]s*, *Mesapotamians*, and *Assyrians* [a 1 cit]
19. astrological [1a, 1591, Percivall] Giiii[r] He left diuers rules of *Astrologicall* prognostication [a 1 cit]
20. atheism [1587, Golding] Hi[v] naturall thinges being remoued from diuine, mans mynde is turned from them, which is the right way to *Atheisme* [a 1 cit]
21. attribute [7, 1599, Thynne] Fviii[v] *Apollo* ... to whome *Ouid* and some others attribute the first inuention of Phisicke
22. aurum potabile [1644, Quarles] Lii[v] the common *Aurum potabile* and such like ... be mediciens warranted by this Arte [fpl]
23. authority [8, 1665, Glanvill] Dvi[r] *Paracelsus* ... [i]n comparison of which al other Aucthorities in those matters are small or none
24. balsamum [3, 1631, Donne] Eii[v] as when in a Mynerall desease the toe or foote is growing towardes mortification, because *Balsamu[m] humanum* that shoulde keepe vnitie betweene the three *principia* ... is oppressed
25. barbarian [2, 1604, Shakespeare] Gii[r] other Nations, which the *Grecians* doe call *Barbarians*
26. bather [1636, Healey, and ns] Hv[r] our later Phisitions ... in steade of ... healers ... are become warmers, or coolers and bathers [a 1 cit]
27. binary [A, a, 1766, Croker] *2[r] Of the Medicin *Binarij* or *Vulgaris*
28. body [22b, 1594, Plat] Eiiii[v] sometimes the very bodies of some Mettals
29. breach [5a, 1605, Bacon] Ciiii[r] breach of unitie and seperation
30. bring [18f, 1602, Shakespeare] Fvii[v] Also in his first Booke of 15. intituled *libri Hermeicorum*, he bringeth in a priest saying thus
31. bringing [2, 1603, Shakespeare] *4[v] a peculiar power ... of generation, and propagation, and bringing foorth

32. bristle [3, 1731, Miller, P.] Kvi^{r} in a little corne or grayne, all thynges be inuizible at one tyme, whiche in processe of tyme doe appere in the stalke and eare, as the roote, stalke, knottes or ioyntes, blade eare, blossom, chaffe, brissels, and corn

33. cabbalistic [1624, Middleton and ns] Hi^{r} They excelled in secrete Scyences, which they called *Cabalisticæ* [a 1 cit]

34. caution [3a, 1605, Shakespeare] *3^{v} Certaine notes and cautions giuen, for the better vnderstanding of this Chimicall Phisicke

35. cementation [2, 1595, Plat] See **assation**, anted. [a 1 cit]

36. centre [*sb*, 1b, 1600, Shakespeare] Aii^{r} thou art sayd (as it were) to sit in the center of all thinges that bee

37. centre [*sb*, 6b, 1606, Shakespeare] Cv^{v} the true *Center* of vnion

38. centre [*sb*, 11b, 1628, Spencer, T.] Hiiii^{v} *Rationales*, whose foundation doth depend vpon a false Center of dualitie and contrarietie

39. chemical [*a*, 2, 1621, Burton] *3^{r} Of certaine Phisitions that vsed Chimicall medicines

40. christianlike [*adv*, B, 1593, Shakespeare] Fiii^{v} sincerely, charitably and Christianlike

41. circulate [5, 1656, *Hobbes's Elem.*] Liiii^{r} and in suche deseases if they be not long circulated nor in the remote parts

42. circulated [*ppl a*, 1641, French] Evi^{r} they proceede without respect of the right difference betwixt diseases, vehement, long, circulated [a 1 cit]

43. coagulation [1, 1605, Timme] Fi^{v} See **assation**, anted.

44. coagulation [1b, 1683, Robinson] Avii^{r} the lothsomnesse of heates, tastes, smelles, coagulations, &c

45. cohobate [*v*, 1641, French] Ciii^{r} distill it, then cohobate the same three time [a 1 cit]

46. coloured [*ppl a*, 1c, 1855, Macaulay] Hiii^{v} such other Poeticall Fables, darke speeches and coloured tales, doe secretly hide and couer this whole Arte

47. comment [*v*, 4a, 1591, Shakespeare] Hiii^{v} Galen folowi[n]g *Hypocrates* 600. yeres did comment vpon him against his meaning and words

48. condition [2a, 1588, Fraunce] Dii^{r} the condition of the band being read

49. consolidant [A, 1755, Johnson] Eiii^{r} *potiones vulnerariae* and *consolida[n]tia* ought to be vsed

50. constringent [1603, Heydon, Sir C.] Eii^{r} See **abstergent**, anted. [a 1 cit]

51. consultation [2c, 1800, Duncan] Eii^{v} the followers of the Heathen … after their consultations, either knowe not what to doe, or els determine often the worst rather the[n] good for their patient

52. contrition [1, 1594, Plat] Lii^{r} he that would learne what this worde *Alcool* meaneth, he must knowe what *Contritio Philosophica* is, so shall he find that it doth not signifie a powder stamped and most finely serched, though he did wash it in water, and take the powder after the water be dried awaie

53. contrition [9, 1594, Plat, *Jewell-ho*] Fi^v See **assation**, anted.
54. conversant [3b, 1595, Shakespeare] Giiii^r he was conuersant with the Priestes of the Jewes
55. corroding [*ppl a*, 1605, Timme] Eiii^r any corroding Salt [a 1 cit]
56. corrosiveness [1611, Cotgrave] Eiii^r Likewise in Caukrose and corrosiue Vlcers they purge and euacuate moysture out of the body which should mitigate the corrosiuenesse of the Salt [a 1 cit]
57. count [2, 1596, Shakespeare] Ii^v the mightie Prince *Otto*, Cou[n]ti-palatine of *Rhene*
58. deep-rooted [1669, Woodhead] Eviii^r the deepe rooted spiritual tynctures [a 1 cit]
59. diffuse [*v*, 2, 1590, Spenser] Ivi^r the incorporall soule is diffused and dispersed into all the members & partes of the bodie
60. direction [8, 1658, Phillips] *7^v the Orbes and celestiall bodies of contrary motions from the East to the West, and from the West to the East, and in retrogradation and direction, and stationarij
61. distinguished [3, 1736, Butler] Fv^v so goodly and beautifull distinguished varietie [a 1 cit]
62. distribution [2, 1589, Puttenham] Bv^v if ... the Stomacke or any part of the body be faultie in attraction, separation, resolution, digestion, distributio[n], or expultio[n]
63. doctorship [2, 1598, Florio] Iii^v thei are ashamed after their doctershipp [a 1 cit]
64. duncical [2, 1588, Harvey, J.] Fi^r opinion or dunsicall wrangling and arguing
65. dynamic [2, 1862, Tyndall] Hv^r such things [tha]t haue power to worke, which he calleth /S/δψναμειζ/S/ [a 1 cit]
66. effect [8, 1588, Parke, R.] Gviii^r He also did write one excellent worke ... in effect like vnto that of *Hermes Trismegistus*
67. effected [*ppl a*, 1, 1604, Hieron] *8^v it placeth the effected cause in the steede of efficient [a 1 cit]
68. element [1b, 1724, Watts] Bvii^r it is *Aethereall*, separated from the inferiour Elements
69. energumen [2, 1702, Mather, C.] Cii^v in the Primatiue Church, those that were *Catechymeni* and *Energumeni* [a 1 cit]
70. equal [8, 1626, Bacon] Gi^v the Egle ... is gently and quietly brought a sleepe with *Apollo* his golden Harpe, that is by equal sweete and temperate motion in the sayd fire
71. equally [1, 1634, Herbert, Sir T.] Diiii^v *unarii* ruling equally in three
72. esse [2, 1640, Dering, Sir E.] Ivi^r the fountaine and originall of liuing things, the which from him that is, *Esse*, doeth giue *Esse* [a 1 cit]
73. ethereal [A, 1, 1598, Barkley *Felic. Man*] Bvii^r It is not moyst, could, drie nor hotte, but it is *Æthereall*, separated from the inferiour Elements
74. exactly [2, 1612, Brinsley] Giii^v the first that is remembred to haue written of Hearbes (as some say) exactly

75. exalted [*ppl a*, 5, 1594, Plat] Eiii[r] any corroding Salt in the bloud exalted hath frett through some vayne within the body [a 1 cit]
76. exist [1, 1605, Shakespeare] Aiiii[v] Thou ... sustayneth all things that they may exist and liue [a 1 cit]
77. experiment [1b, 1586, Cogan] Gvi[v] the experiments of olde wives, men and women of the Countrey and Citie
78. explicate [*v*, 6, 1622, Heylin] Iiii[v] I will breefly explicate some obiections that be made against him
79. extract [4, 1594, Plat] Ei[r] cure the desease by extracting out of things in the greate worlde that which is wholesome
80. false-imagined [D, 2b, 1625, Milton] Avi[v] their false imagined naturall causes [a 1 cit] [fpl]
81. feeling [5, 1588, Shakespeare] Biii[v] See **sense**, anted.
82. fiat [2, Donne, 1631] Kii[r] he confesseth accordyng to Gods holy worde that *Prima materia mundi* was *Fiat* [a 1 cit]
83. fixed [*ppl a*, 4b, 1651, French] Bviii[v] a Stone or fixed matter that could conuert and turne al other base metals into materiall Gold
84. founded [1, 1605, Shakespeare] Dvii[r] It is otherwise in Ginger, because his heate is stable, liuely and fou[n]ded in his naturall seede [a 1 cit]
85. framing [*ppl. a*, 1876, Eliot, George] Lvi[r] not fit for framyng timber [fpl] [a 1 cit]
86. fugitive [*a*, 4b, 1678, Russell, R.] Dvi[v] See **radically**, anted.
87. galenist [1594, Nashe *Terrors*] *3[r] And that the Chimical Phisitions, ought rather to bee called *Rationales*, then the *Galenists* [a 1 cit]
88. great [II, 6d, 1594, Blundevil] *2[r] in the greate worlde, and in the little worlde, which is man
89. green dragon [A, 12c, 1840, Paxton] Cii[v] Take the greene dragon and bath hym in warme liquor [a 1 cit] [fpl]
90. helm [5, 1594, Plat] Hii[v] *Mercury* ... which by often sublimation, doth so rise out of the matter co[n]tained in the Alembeck, into the helme or head
91. impassable [2, 1780, Madan] Aiii[v] Thou art the vniuersal Word remayning impassible and not turning
92. impure [2b, 1613, Purchas] *5[r] by the fal ... or our first parent Adam, the earth was accursed, and impure seedes added and ioyned to the pure
93. impure [II, 3a, 1626, Bacon] Avi[r] See **tincture**, anted.
94. impurity [3, 1605, Timme] Dvi[v] The Chymicall Phisition ... first spoyleth them of all their outward formes, qualities, impurities, and accidents
95. inceration [1610, Jonson *Alch.*] Fi[v] See **assation**, anted. [a 1 cit]
96. indigested [*a*, 3, 1642, Wotton] Evii[v] The followers of the Ethnickes ... doe minister rawe and indigested medicines [a 1 cit]
97. inflict [1a, 1593, Shakespeare] Avi[r] See **originally**, anted.
98. influency [1641, French] Ci[r] These Mines are as it were Starres or

Seedes, therefore they make influencies & blomings, which are the fruites of Starres and Seedes [a 1 cit]

99. inhumation [3, 1612, Woodall] Fi[v]. See **assation**, anted. [a 1 cit]

100. intelligent [B, 1, 1601, Gill] *6[r] *Aristotle* ... assigneth to certaine myndes, Intelligentis, or vnder straunge natures and essenties

101. invention [II, 6b, 1613, Purchas] Fiiii[v] two Pillers, in which they did ingraue their learning, knowledge, and inue[n]tions

102. lavation [1627, Hakewill *Apol.*] Fii[r] See **assation**, anted. [a 1 cit]

103. lesion [3, 1747, *Astruc's Fevers*] Ei[v] some greefes doe come to man which be not properly deseases but *lesiones* or hurtes

104. lively [4c, 1604, Grimstone] Lvi[v] liuely artificiall proofe by fire

105. liver [4, 1694, Salmon] Ciii[r] take this liquor and distill it with the Liuer of Mars

106. loose [B, 1, 1849, Hannay, J.] Hiiii[v] all maner cure doth consist in binding the loose, & in loosing that is bounde

107. magisterium [1, 1593, Harvey, G.] Fii[r] these seuerall works and operations, whereby *Regeneration, Tyncturs, Arcana, Magisteria, Quintumesse*, and *Elixirs* be had and gotten [a 1 cit]

108. magnalia [1645, Howell] Iv[v] suche like *Magnalia dei* ... procede onely from God [a 1 cit]

109. mangling [1652, Smith, J.] Eiii[r] See **regenerant**, anted. [a 1 cit]

110. manifesting [1603, Knolles] Aiii[r] the manifesting of the power is action [a 1 cit]

111. mastery [7, 1668, Hale] Fi[r] palpable sensible and visible experience, which is the maysteries of Artes and Sciences

112. mechanical [*a*, 7, 1664, Power *Exp. Philos.*] Avi[v] And because the heathnish Philosophie doth attribute the cause of thinges to dead qualities, of heate, cold, &c. and not to the liuely vertues and powers in thinges, therefore that heathnish Phisicke seeketh by like dead qualities, to cure liuely and mechanicall spirites

113. medium [5, 1605, Bacon] Bvii[r] it is agreeable with our *Anima* (the *Medium* aforesayd)

114. mesopotamian [1880, Poole, R. S. and ns] See **assyrian**, anted. [a 1 cit]

115. method [2b, 1662, Evelyn] Fii[v] he had first learned all their decrees and determinations perfectly, and had gotten a briefe method to iudge them

116. meum [1594, Greene and Lodge] Biii[v] Unquietnesse beginneth in things, where *Meum* & *tuum*, is become to be knowen in them [a 1 cit]

117. mind [17e, 1612, Bacon] *6[v] he alloweth that mynde or essence which is the elder: that is, God to bee onely so much the more excellent then the rest

118. mineral [*a*, 4, 1599, Jonson] Bv[r] The beastes ... because ... they be nourished with the vegetables and minerall resolutions, haue like impurities as they haue

119. mineral [*sb*, 4, 1602, Warner] Biiii^{v} all liuing creatures, Hearbes, Plants, Mynerals
120. misplace [1, 1594, Shakespeare] Lv^{v} wordes may esely escape and be misplaced
121. mitigating [*ppl a*, 1612, Webster] Giii^{r} mitigating Balmes or Oyntments [a 1 cit]
122. mixture [1c, 1597, Hooker] Ciiii^{r} the badd is seperated from the obedience and mixture of the good
123. monarchy [5, 1609, Butler, C.] Diiii^{r} the Monarchie of mans body must be preserued by harmony
124. mundifying [1610, Healey] Eviii^{r} by mundifying and clensing of *Balsamum* [a 1 cit] [fpl]
125. non esse [1654, Whitlock] Iviii^{v} and of *esse* cometh *non esse* [a 1 cit]
126. obedience [1b, 1671, Addison, L.] Cv^{r} the bad doe no longer abide in obedience of the good
127. occult [4b, 1633, Austin] Dvii^{r} eche thing hath two natures, that is *occultum* and *manifestum*
128. onus [1, 1640, Smith, J.] Kiiii^{r} neither is God in part any where but in *singulis totus* and in *onibus omnis* [a 1 cit]
129. operation [4, 1594, Hooker] Aiii^{r} not cut from the first power in the operation
130. order [*v*, 2d, 1642, Rogers] Iviii^{r} so saieth the Psalmist ... thou gouernest, conteinest, makest, orderest, and bearest me
131. originally [3, 1654, Bramhall] A6^{r} those diseases that bee either originally or inflicted into the inuisible parte of man *Anima* or *Limbus*
132. paracelsical [1602, Hering] Di^{v} this *Paracelsicall* Phisicke [a 1 cit] [fpl]
133. particular [B, 5, 1600, Shakespeare] Bi^{v} See **universal**, anted.
134. persist [4, 1760, Lee, J.] Biiii^{r} The worlde did persist in this vnion, and did obserue the nature of vnitie
135. potentia [1601, Copley] Kvii^{v} God made heauen and earth not because it was so presently, but because it was so *potentia* [a 1 cit]
136. potential [B, 1, 1656, Blount] Ivii^{r} God the Father whiche is principal *Vivere*, and *Potentia vivendi*
137. potentially [2, 1625, Jackson] Aii^{v} All thinges dwell in thee, potencially [a 1 cit]
138. pre-exist [*v*, 1, 1599, Moufet *Silkwo.*] *iv^{r} God, which of nothing, that is hauing no matter, preexisting, or goying before, hast created al the world [a 1 cit]
139. prepare [6, 1722, De Foe] Bviii^{r} this vniuersall medicine, wherewith they digest and expell the corruptions out of their naturall bodyes, wherby the body was so prepared, that therein was made a perfect vnion betweene *Corpus*, *Anima*, & *Spiritus*
140. preserver [2, 1615, Latham] Gvi^{r} tradition of doctrine without writing ... is no faithfull preseruer of the trueth therof

141. principium [1a, 1600, Watson, W.] Ci^{v} three *Principia*, of mans body
142. progression [4, 1586, Day, A.] *2^{v} See **succession**, anted.
143. propagator [*sb*, 1, 1686, Good *Cel. Bodies*] Av^{v} it assigneth no Author nor propagator vnto the essences or natures [a 1 cit]
144. radically [1, 1624, Donne] Dvi^{v} impurities ... doe come to bodies accidentally and not borne in them, in their first nature, nor bee in them radically, therefore they are fugitiue ... it is possible to spoyle them of their accidents [a 1 cit]
145. rational [C, 1b, 1756, D'Israeli] *3^{r} the Chimical Phisitions, ought rather to bee called *Rationales*, then the *Galenists*
146. reducible [1b, 1646, Browne] Eiiii^{v} they are not reducible into mettall againe, but bee volatill spirits
147. regenerant [1855, Bailey] Eiii^{r} Then *regenerantia* and *renouantia*, & not that paynefull cutting and mangling of that parte of the body [a 1 cit]
148. renovant [1610, Folkingham, W.] Eiii^{r} See **regenerant**, anted. [a 1 cit]
149. resting [2, 1601, Shakespeare] Aii^{r} thou ... O God ... art the resting and quiet fountaine of al thinges
150. rise [IV, 26, 1601, Holland] Hii^{v} The golden Bow which *Virgil* doth speake of, which being cut of, an other like to it did immediately rise in his place
151. rooted [2c, 1744, Berkeley] Evi^{r} euen in such rooted diseases
152. sacrum [1753, Chambers] Bi^{r} See **ars sacra**, unrec. [a 1 cit]
153. scope [4, 1590, Barrough] Bi^{v} Medicines [whose] ... scope and end is to bring the sicke person to vnitie in himselfe
154. sense [*sb*, 16a, 1604, Shakespeare] Biii^{v} griefe, which is a sense or feeling
155. separate [5a, 1617, Moryson] Bv^{v} they be tempered, seperated, resolued and expelled out of mans body
156. sickly [5, 1604, Grimstone] Evi^{r} medicins grosse, grosse, grosse, and sickly
157. simplex [A, 1594, Blundevil] Gi^{r} he hath his name of /S/*Aπλουν*/S/, that is *simplex* simple [a 1 cit]
158. spagyrical [2, 1652, anon. *Herm. Ban.*] Ei^{r} such an one is to bee accompted a Chymicall or Spagyricall Phylosopher and Physition [a 1 cit]
159. speculation [5c, 1796, Horsley] Eiii^{v} So that experience and practise ought not to proceede of speculation, but speculation ought to be deriued out of practise
160. speech [9c, 1596, Spenser] *2^{r} the darke speaches of the writers therof
161. spirit [21a, 1610, Jonson] Ciiii^{v} you may perceiue by wine ... as long as his spirite doth abide in him mingled with the tarte vineger in unitie and peace, the wine is sounde pleasant and perfect
162. starry [2, 1594, Barnfield] Hviii^{r} the starry motions
163. substitute [2a, 1588, Shakespeare] Biiii^{r} [God] substituted him [man]

in the place of his other creatures which were cast out of heauen

164. succession [10b, 1653, More] *2[v] The first Authors of the auncient Phisicke, and of the succession and progression therof to *Hermes Trismegestus*

165. sugar [3a, 1652, French] Dvii[r] a pleasaunt sweete Sugar wilbe drawen out of it [lead]

166. swing [*sb*, 6b, 1856, Dixon, H. H.] *7[v] there was and is one that hath coupled, vnited, and ioyned together, such and so diuers contrary thinges: otherwise, such diuers and contrary thinges and motions, by their owne swing, course and mouing, would bee dissolued one from an other

167. synteresis [1, 1594, Plat] *v[v] the better part of the Soule or *Spiritus*, which some call sinteresis doeth perswade to that is good [a 1 cit]

168. tartareal [1602, Hering *Ob. Anat.*] Ev[r] the Agewes ought to be called the disease of Sulphur, of salt peter kendled, for this cause diuers diseases are called tartareall diseases [a 1 cit]

169. tincture [5, 1610, Holland] Avi[v] defectes doe proceede of the mechanicall spirites and tinctures of impure seedes

170. tincture [6a, 1599, Moufet, T.] Dviii[r] from thence flow Tynctures, *Arcana, Quintumesse* [*sic*]

171. tincture [7, 1610, Jonson, B.] Ci[v] the tinctures of *Gold, Mercury* & *Antimony*

172. transfer [1c, 1646, Daniel, G.] Aiii[r] not by locall motion, neither by transferring into place, but by a better and diuine motion

173. transplantation [1, 1601, Holland] Kiiii[r] These seeds saith *Paracelsus* haue receiued by the diuine worde the power of multipliyng and transplantation their essence and properties [*sic*] [a 1 cit]

174. trifle [1774, Trinket] *viii[r] Reason can not comprehende this worde, therefore it must needes childishly trifle off the causes of such things

175. universal [B, 4, 1656, Smith, J.] Bi[v] This auncient and true phisicke consisteth of Medicines of two sorts. The first is *Vniversalis* or *unarii*. The second is *ternarii* or *particularis*

176. vegetable [2, 1767, Young, A.] Dvi[r] [th]e foode which wee receiue for nourishment ... of the vegetables which receiue their nourishment of the resolued spirites of the Myneralles

177. venthole [*sb*, 2, 1612, Sturtevant] Hii[r] the purging and preparing of the matters and substaunce of the medicine, in the furnaces that breath out fire at the venteholes continually

178. vim [1850, *Odd Leaves*] Di[r] they attribute *vim vitæ*, to accidents and dead qualities

179. vitrum [1657, *Phys Dict.*] Lii[v] *Vitrum antimonii* (which purgethe and shaketh the bodie so sore) [a 1 cit]

180. volatile [*a*, 3, 1605, Timme] Eiiii[v] See **reducible**, anted.

181. vulnerary [A, 1a, 1599, A. M.] Eiii[r] *potiones vulnerariae* and *consolida[n]tia* ought to bee vsed [a 1 cit]

182. warmer [1, 1595, Southwell] Hv[r] See **bather**, anted. [a 1 cit]

183. well-being [1b, 1702, Calamy] *6^{v} the world ... needeth none other to prouide for his being or well being [a 1 cit]
184. working [1b, 1586, Marlowe] A6^{v} thy working power doth preserue and maintaine all thinges
185. wrangling [1b, 1612, Brinsley] Fi^{r} See **duncical**, anted.

2. New senses

1. asclepiad Gv^{v} his sonnes which were called *Asclepiades* after their father *Æsculepias*
2. bather Hv^{r} See **bather**, anted.
3. beautiful Fv^{v} so goodly and beautifull distinguished varietie
4. cabbalistic Hi^{r} They excelled in secrete Scyences, which they called *Cabalisticæ*
5. drake [= dragon, 14] Bv^{r}. See **transplantation,** ns.
6. excess Hviii^{r} *Ptolomeus* ... whose Tables of motions of the starres by long excesse of time grewe to be vnperfect
7. flower Cvi^{v} onely flowers and colours of diseases and not the very matter, cause, substance, or nature of the disease
8. goldish Bviii^{v} by this meanes they make no more Gold, then that weight of Gold was, fro[m] whence they tooke their medicine, because the medicin had no more goldish nature, then serued onely for an ounce
9. increate *3^{v} how all things created were at one time in the increate
10. limbus A6^{r} See **originally**, anted.
11. mesopotamian Fv^{r} See **assyrian**, anted.
12. star Ci^{r} The excrements comming of his Gold be called Mynerall excrements, of the likenesse of the drosse which is about the Gold, before it be fyned with *Antimony*. These Mines are as it were Starres or Seedes, therefore they make influencies & blomings, which are the fruites of Starres and Seedes
13. surgery Giii^{r} *Petrus Hasardus*...in his French Epistle before the great Surgery of *Paracelsus*
14. ternary Bi^{v} See **universal**, anted.
15. terrestre [not as *sb*] Evi^{r} some diseases be *Cælestes*, other some be *Terrestres*
16. transplantation Bv^{r} some grounde will make transplantation of one seede into an other, as from Wheate to Drake or Darnell
17. visible Cv^{r} make them manifest to visible and palpable experience
18. vulgar Bi^{v} The Ethnikes or heathen haue ... deuised a third kinde of phisicke or Medicine which is *binarii* or *vulgaris*

3. Unrecorded

1. actio A4^{v} See **agens**, unrec.
2. agens A5^{r} there must be *Agens* before there be *Actio*
3. anima Bvii^{v} the nourishment of our naturall fire or *Amina*

4. **aploun** Gi^{r} he hath his name /S/*Απλουν*/S/, that is *simplex* simple
5. **apnus** Giiii^{v} a medicin that hee vsed to minister, called *Apnus*
6. **ars magna** Bi^{r} See **ars sacra**, unrec.
7. **ars sacra** Bi^{r} The true and auncient Phisycke ... is called by auncient name, *Ars sacra*, or *magna*, & *sacra scie[n]tia*, or *Chymia*, or *Chemeia*, or *Alchimia*, & *mystica*, & by some of late, *Spagirica ars*
8. **ars signata** Dv^{v} *Ars Signata* also hath his place to giue euidence of the properties of things
9. **astructum** Hiiii^{v} See **laxum**, unrec.
10. **astrum** Ci^{r} See **philosopher's gold**, unrec.
11. **athenian** *3^{v} The true meaning of *Paracelsus* in dedicating his Booke ... to the *Athenians*
12. **balsamum humanum** Eii^{v} See **balsamum**, anted.
13. **batefulness** Eiiii^{r} Æthereall fyre, which nourisheth and quickeneth mans body, whose property is to consume all corruptions, caused by the elementall fyre, and with his batefulnesse to restore the naturall moysture which was consumed by the Elementall Fyre
14. **botrion** Hiiii^{r} Aechines of Athens did vse to helpe & cure the disease called Qwinsie ... with the Ashes of a brunt man. This medicin he called *Botrion*
15. **bursy** Lvi^{r} thei be like knottie and bursie woode, not fit for framyng timber
16. **caukrose** Eiii^{r} See **corrosiveness**, anted.
17. **chemeia** Bi^{r} See **ars sacra**, unrec.
18. **chymia** Bvi^{r} manifested and made plaine to the eye, touch and taste of them that haue skill to seperate the pure from the unpure, by his auncient Phisicke or Chymia
19. **curing** A6^{v} thy curing vertue
20. **decipe** Eviii^{v} the Chymicall Phisition calleth such receiptes, *decipe*, and willeth their followers to leaue such receiptes
21. **deuberation** Av^{v} some thinges that bee done are done without cause: as deuberation, &c
22. **dulcedine** Eiii^{r} *Sanguine[m] renouantia, dulcedines* out of apt things rightly extracted
23. **ex motu** Iviii^{v} all thynges that bee ... made or begotten *ex motu*
24. **fons vitæ** Cvii^{v} *Anima* wherein *Fons vitæ* consisteth
25. **gratian** Cvi^{v} See **repugnant**, postd.
26. **humidum radicale** Evii^{v} such Purgations do withall purge *humidum radicale*
27. **laxum** Hiiii^{v} They reduce all particalar [*sic*] affects, vnto two generall, that is to say, to *Astructum* and *Laxum*
28. **lex** Fiii^{r} the lawe called *Lex Aquilia*
29. **lex aquilia** Fiii^{r} See **lex**, unrec.
30. **long-exercised** Iii^{v} their ... long exercised weening practice

31. **lumen naturæ** Dv^{r} Then may he vse *Lumen Naturæ*

32. **manifestum** Dvii^{r} See **occult**, anted.

33. **materia prima** *3^{v} How *materia prima* and *mysterium magnam*, was the beginning of all thinges

34. **materia ultima** Kvi^{v} God ... formed, out of *materia prima materias ultimas*, [tha]t is to saie all creatures

35. **medicina** Ei^{r} For *Chymia* and *Medicina* may not be seperated asunder

36. **misteria** Kv^{r} sometymes he calleth the seedes, the receptacles of the vertues, by the name of *Misteria* likewise

37. **motus** Iviii^{r} See **quies**, unrec.

38. **mysterium magnam** *3^{v} See **materia prima**, unrec.

39. **mystica** Bi^{r} See **ars sacra**, unrec.

40. **partel**[9] Cv^{v} For seeing that all thinges doe hang together in one chayne ... & man is partell of that chaine

41. **particularis** Ciii^{r} Of the Medicine Ternarij or perticularis

42. **pastation** Fi^{v} See **assation**, anted.

43. **philosopher's gold** Ci^{r} in my opinion, the Philosophers Gold is such a temperate medicine as I haue declared, which in deede is *Astrum* seperated from his impediments and grosse sustance

44. **potiones vulnerariae** Eiii^{r} *potiones vulnerariae* and *consolida[n]tia* ought to bee vsed

45. **preservant** Eiii^{r} the naturall Balme inwardly ought to be clensed, and outwardly *preservantia*

46. **putrefactio philosophica** Lii^{r} he that knoweth the worke and effect of *Putrefactio Philosophica*

47. **quies** Iviii^{r} *quies*, bringeth forth nothing but *motus*, & *agendi operatio* doth frame to itself, that thing which is

48. **rationales medici** Hv^{r} the Chimicall Physitions ... ought rather to be called *Rationales medici*

49. **sacra scientia** Bi^{r} See **ars sacra**, unrec.

50. **sal resolutum** Eii^{v} for the Dropsie those thinges are not to be taken which doe expell *Sal resolutum*

51. **sanguinea** Lii^{r} he that can skill to resolue ech thyng into his three substancies ... maie find what *Sanguinea*, *Cheri*, *Anthos*, & such like be in *Paracelsus*

52. **semina essentiæ** Kiii^{r} Of these *Semina Essentiæ* of their naturs, vertues, & properties, and their separations doth he here intreat

53. **spagirica ars** Bi^{r} See **ars sacra**, unrec.

54. **spiritus** *v^{v} See **synteresis**, anted.

55. **substancy** Aiii^{v} Christ ... by whose power all things doe come forth and proceede into generation, and consist according to their matters and substancies

56. **summa natura** Iviii^{r} the workyng of *summa natura* in his creatures

57. **tartishness** Dv^{v} By this is fou[n]d in Honey a venomous tartishnesse

58. ternarium Biiii^{r} Also by his bountifull goodnesse and prouidence he created *Microcosmum* or little worlde, vz. man, his *ternarium* and last creature
59. thracian *2^{v} *Democritus Abderites* a *Thracian* did write of this art, whose Bookes are yet extant[10]
60. trismegistus Fvi^{r} This *Hermes* or *Mercurius* was called *Trismegestus*, as some say, because he was the greatest Phylosopher, the greatest King, and the greatest Priest
61. unary Bviii^{r} This Medicine *Vnary*
62. vim vitæ Di^{r} they attribute *vim vitæ*, to accidents and dead qualities
63. vita Ivii^{r} the Sonne whiche is *Vita*
64. vitrum antimonii Lii^{v} See **vitrum**, anted.
65. vivere Ki^{r} his proper mouing … from *Vivere* and *Vita*

4. Postdatings

1. essentie [1552, Huloet] *6^{r} See **intelligent**, anted.
2. ministration [3, 1579, Fulke] Cii^{v} the ministration of the Sacraments
3. multiplier [3, 1560, Daus] Cii^{r} when they had wasted their owne substance they proceeded to exercise deceite … which mooued Princes in their countreyes to make Lawes agaynst Multiplyers as they were termed
4. repugnant [A, 2b, 1568, Skene] Cvi^{v} We ought not to seeke helpe in things contrarie and repugnant: who findeth medicine for the Liuer in *Gratian, Agarick*, or *Colocinthis*
5. unary [1576, Fleming and ns] Bi^{v} See **universal**, anted.
6. weening [1579, Fenton] Iii^{r} the folowers of the Ethnickes, who[m] hee calleth wenyng great *Docters*

5. Other

1. image-maker [ncit] Kvii^{r} the Carpenter and image maker maie forme out of one peece of timber what he list
2. partel [listed as spurious] Cv^{v} man is partell of that chaine
3. second cause [ncit] they tye and bind God to the second cause, and take away his prouidence ouer his creatures

CLEVER, WILLIAM, *The flower of physicke*, 1590

1. Antedatings

1. absolutely [1644, Quarles] 73 *Theophrastus Paracelsus*, who absolutely granteth a larger sustenance to children, then adolescencie
2. absume [*v*, 1596, Barlow *Serm.*] 93 those bodies … commonly preserued with naturall feuers all the daies of their life, doo not onely absume in the tenuity of their flesh [a 1 cit]
3. abundant [3, 1725, Pope] 36 the more aboundant those excrements be purged out

4. access [II, 7, 1642, Howell] 80 the humours haue such large accesse thereunto

5. accession [3, 1655, Vaughan] 25 the second course of sicknesse, it is called *Accessio*

6. active [4, 1640, Mervin, Capt.] 58 a man of a thin bloud, by reason he had no actiue increase in heat

7. active [5, 1597, Shakespeare] 43 heat among other qualities is actiue

8. affected [III, 1619, Donne] 96 other affected partes

9. affliction [3, 1598, Shakespeare] 28 the disease is caried by so large a compasse without stay into many afflictions

10. affluence [1, 1600, Holland] 114 the affluence of heate, and bloud in the body

11. aggravate [6a, 1597, Daniel] 29 vnnaturall choller, which most vehemently aggrauateth the cause in sicknesse

12. agitative [*a*, 1687, More, H. *App. to Antid.*] 24 Therefore by thys molifieng, humou[r]s are thereby made more agitatiue, and the poores to receiue such comfort, are redilie opened, so that both bodie and nature yeeld together more flexible [a 1 cit]

13. alienated [3, 1605, Verstegan] 18 moste dangerous feuers, so alienated, and estranged in their natures

14. alienation [5, 1615, Crooke] 22 when the disease beginneth to giue ouer ... then an vniversall alienation sheweth the same

15. alteration [3, 1621, Burton] 9 any fresh alteration to the body by infection

16. application [2, 1601, Shakespeare] 118 outward applications, very sensibly doo freate

17. approve [2b, 1674, Clarendon] 123 purgatiue medicines ... lenitiuely doe approue and molifie the body

18. approved [3, 1667, Milton] 32 many approued writers affirme

19. arteriac [B, *sb*, 1661, Lovell, *Hist. Anim.*] 85 also the arterick vaines, where the spirit of life recourseth [a 1 cit]

20. artful [II, 4, 1615, *Latham's Falconry*] 75 these distempered bodies are reformed by artfull knowledge [a 1 cit]

21. artificer [4, 1605, Bacon] 96 naturall heat is the artificer and instrument of all liuing thinges

22. ascendent [A, 1, 1591, Greene] 127 See **descendent**, anted.

23. ascending [1, 1667, Milton] 91 the ascending moysture [a 1 cit]

24. assenting [*vbl sb*, 1651, Hobbes *Lev.*] 19 Hypocrates in his first booke of Aphorismes, sayth the approching, assentings, and constitutions of diseases doe shewe both the passing away of the yeare, and a successiue increase of diseases [a 1 cit]

25. attend [4c, 1611, *Bible*] 90 Let somewhat more, in this our treatise, be attended vpon

26. attend [10b, 1606, Shakespeare] 77 There are diuers sortes of these

feauers, hauing diuers natural inconueniences attending vpon them
27. augmentation [7, 1853, Mayne] 25 an augmentation to a more supreame power
28. bark [*sb*, 3, 1601, Holland] 118 whether the rind and barke of the vaines be wrinkled
29. black [10, 1659, Hammond] 52 a fleame which is manie times incident to verie blacke and chollericke persons
30. choke [6b, 1599, Shakespeare] 11 I doo not speake herein ... to choke nature
31. claw-footed [8, 1667, Hope, R.] 88 claw-footed beasts
32. cloven-hoofed [1646, Browne] 88 clouen hofed ... beasts [a 1 cit]
33. coagulate [1, 1611, Cotgrave] 52 greedie eating of rawe fruites before the naturall heate of the sun, be perfectly coagulated therein
34. colliquation [5, 1662, Stubbe] 3 manie times colliquation or destruction inuadeth the mind [a 1 cit]
35. colour [*v*, 1c, 1637, Humfrey, R.] 59 See **dip**, anted.
36. combination [2, 1597, Hooker] 90 there must altogether fall out a perfect sympathie, or equall combination vnder the temperatures of countries
37. commixture [2, 1593, Shakespeare] 46 the intemperature of heate and moystnesse is an vnequall commixture [a 1 cit]
38. commoderate [*a*, 1647, Ward *Simp. Cobbler*] 62 such members which are insigned vnder any one of these humors are commoderated one by an other [a 1 cit]
39. commoderate [*v*, 1647, Ward *Simp. Cobbler*] 44 Then herein is to be required a commoderate difference of these bodies [a 1 cit]
40. comprehensible [2, 1598, Florio] 1 their iust and comprehensible manner of dyet
41. concrete [*v*, 2, 1677, Hale] 78 those thinges which easilie concreat are speedilie drie [a 1 cit]
42. condensate [2, 1605, Topsell] 120 odours ... which doo condensate into substance
43. condignity [b, 1a, 1605, Sylvester *Du B.*] 26 And all such medicines which disgrace the disease, are ordinarie and of high condignitie with nature
44. conflux [*v*, 1662, Chandler *Van Helmont*] 29 Therefore when these partes cannot bee scowred by naturall action in the qualitie of the breath, must in these seasons of infection be concocted & seasoned together by medicine, so that the one with the other may be confluxed out of the body
45. congealment [2, 1606, Shakespeare] 83 These men are in a most dangerous case, if there be a colde congealement in the vaines and other members
46. congest [2, 1859, Taylor, I.] 38 raw flegmatike humours congested the winter before
47. congested [2, 1856, Kane] 36 congested bloud in the sides
48. conjunctive [2, 1604, Shakespeare] 64 inward temperance is a cause coniunctiue

49. consociety [1624, Heywood *Gunaik.*] 27 But there is a consociety of very daungerous persons in this our age [a 1 cit]

50. constitute [5, 1646, Browne] 25 more aptly constituted for the perfect expelling and fluxing of the same

51. constitution [4, 1601, Holland] 43 the elements shoulde fall out in contrarie order, which otherwise haue an equall constitution in the rest of the bodies one after an other

52. construction [2, 1707, *Curios. in Husb. & Gard.*] 45 all necessarie causes to the construction of euery one body

53. contagion [3, 1603, Lodge] 77 these rotten feauers doo growe vpon adolescencie in the contagion aforesaid

54. contagiously [1615, Sandys] (To the reader) contagiously nourishing manie vncleane diseases [a 1 cit]

55. contemperate [*v*, 2, 1605, Timme *Quersit.*] 95 whereas sommer is verie hot in the one, and winter verie colde in the other, so an inward heat is comtemperated vnder the condition or estate of either temperance [a 1 cit]

56. contemplation [4, 1725, Strype] 14 it is a most excellent contemplation for euerie man

57. contentment [2b, 1651, Fuller] 11 appetite, and nature subdued with a sufficient contentment one with an other

58. contract [*v*, III, 7, 1620, Venner *Via Recta*] 101 a hot tyrannous fretting humour generated & contracted to the eyes

59. controller [4b, 1630, Johnson] 24 the controller of sicknesse

60. contumacious [1b, 1605, Timme] 2 extreame thirstinesse of the body … becommeth contumacious and without remedie [a 1 cit]

61. correct [6, 1620, Venner] 13 fluxes and blaines, which may most ragingly ouerspread mans bodie, for that the inward cause was not before perfectly corrected

62. corrugated [*ppl a*, 1, 1623, Cockeram] 7 for vpon these diseases the vaines become corrugated [a 1 cit]

63. created [1667, Milton] 68 The soule is a created substa[n]ce [a 1 cit]

64. critical [4, 1601, Holland] 17 these inflammatiue feuers must … haue a chryticall expulsion [a 1 cit]

65. crooked-backed [5, 1865, Trollope] 64 his body most deformed, as being goor-bellied, bowe-legged, crooked-backed [a 1 cit]

66. crop [*v*, 3, 1601, Jonson] 62 the Physitian … croppeth all these hearbes of the field

67. crud [2, 1811, Thomson, T.] 51 a certaine vnnaturall and mucilaginous fleame, grosse and thicke, the which fleames are crud, proceeding from distemperate seasons

68. dangerous [3, 1611, Tourneur] 27 there is a consociety of very daungerous persons in this our age

69. deduct [*v*, 3, 1621, Burton *Anat. Mel.*] 16 so there is another kind of feuer which vnnaturally is kindled at the heart, deducted from thence by the vaynes

70. defensible [3, 1600, Blount, E.] 2 a strong bodie ... is ... defensible against sicknesse

71. deflation [1891, *Strand Mag.*] 128 and for the exceeding thicknesse of his skinne, the deflation of heate was repressed [a 1 cit]

72. deflux [*v*, 1647, Needham *Levellers*] 101 *Rasis* affyrmeth, that although greate inundations and intercourses ... defluxing and galding the eies, yet the pretious eie-sight may long be preserued [a 1 cit]

73. dejection [1b, 1594, Plat, *Jewell-Ho.*] 74 And therefore when the humours of the body be deiected eyther by nature or art, both moystnesse and coldnesse ... are possest in the body. Yet these colde humid deiections vpward, manie times infeebleth the stomackes of children

74. deleterious [1643, Browne] 124 *Galen* calleth euerie distemperate action (in propertie) deleterion, that is, venomous [a 1 cit]

75. denunciate [*v*, 1593, Nashe *Christ's T.*] 77 These feauers haue diuers secreet [*sic*] perils depending vpon them, and oftentimes when their constitution is inwardly drie, doo denunciate great outward moystnesse [a 1 cit]

76. descendent [A, 1, 1644, Digby] 127 the saide hearbe in growth is alwaies ascendent and discendent, with the increase and decrease of the moone

77. detrimental [A, 1656, Blount *Gloss.*] 78 euery detrimental mischiefe [a 1 cit]

78. difference [*v*, 3, 1598, Barret] 96 nature hath differenced the chollericke man from the flegmatike

79. difflate [*v*, 1620, Venner *Via Recta*] 71 For a moyst bodie in a man is easily ingurged, difflated, puffed

80. dip [3, 1667, Milton] 59 dipt and coloured euery day in wicked practices

81. direct [1b, 1706, Phillips] 42 See **irradiate**, anted.

82. direct [5c, 1668, Pepys] 38 I cannot finde no direct agreement

83. direct [6a, 1596, Shakespeare] 33 the medicine hath no direct operation

84. direction [9, 1665, Hooke] 19 the cleare sunne ... is ... not able to indure so strong a course anie longer, vntill a fresh direction be renued from one degree to an other

85. discoverture [1818, Cruise *Digest*] 31 And yet in all sharpe sicknesses the same is no consequent discouerture [a 1 cit]

86. discrepate [*v*, 1, 1623, Cockeram] 82 So that discrepating fro[m] his first propertie, vtterly [c]orrupteth, decayeth, beco[m]meth absumpt in the degree of death [a 1 cit]

87. disequal [*a*, 1622, Mabbe *Aleman's G.*] 45 then all passiue actions were dispropriated and vnperfectly disequalled [a 1 cit]

88. disflourish [*v*, 1640, Sedgewicke *O Chr. C.*] 20 or els disflorisheth the laudable generation of bloud in grosse bodies [a 1 cit]

89. disframe [1629, Layton] 49 their courses vtterly diffcramed [*sic*] one from an other [a 1 cit]

90. disliking [1, 1596, Norden] 123 all foode ministred vnto the bodie should be medicinable, sheweth some naturall effect eyther of liking or disliking propertie [a 1 cit]
91. dismatch [*v*, 1591, Sylvester *Du B.*] 100 For mordicat rewmes are hurtfull to all naturall operations ... astonieth hearing, dissmacheth tasting [a 1 cit]
92. dispropriate [*v*, 1613, Purchas *Pilg.*] 45 See **disequal**, anted. [a 1 cit]
93. disseason [*v*, 3, 1628, Greville, F. *Poems M.*] 11 the elements thereby so offended in their naturall courses poure downe superaboundaunce of moisting showers, disseasoning the earthlie fruites of mans mortall estate
94. dissociate [*v*, 1a, 1623, Cockeram] 42 when they [the elements] were disframed and dissociated from their equall places [a 1 cit]
95. dissolution [2b, 1727, *Chambers's Cycl.*] 20 their bloud cannot with easie dissolucion ascend and descend
96. distinguish [*v*, II, 8c, 1592, Smith, H. *Works*] 4 some busie medlers, repayring vnto sicke pacientes, doe not in anie perfect skill, distinguish vpon the disease
97. disturb [1b, 1599, Buttes] 87 the body is disturbed by any fuliginous or smokie vapours
98. domify [*v*, 1603, Florio, *Montaigne*] 18 These and such like feuers in their strong operations, are chiefly domified by vomites in the superiour partes of the stomacke
99. downset [1, 1610, Holland] 19 the propertie of the sunne in vprising and downe setting [a 1 cit]
100. dragon [*sb*², 1813, Milburn] 127 the hearbe Dragon is of cold operation [a 1 cit]
101. dyspnœa [1681, Willis] 22 there followeth a disease, called *Dyspnœa* [a 1 cit]
102. egredience [1635, Person] 96 the egredience thereof, proffereth litle moysture [a 1 cit]
103. elementarily [*adv*, 1643, O. R. *Man's Mort.*] 108 all these medicineable hearbes are not elementarily ingendred [a 1 cit]
104. elucidate [*a*, 1670, Hacket] 19 not sufficiently elucydat or set forth to the knowledge of men
105. enchanted [*ppl a*, 1, 1596, Spenser] 4 rather with inchaunted meates, then wholsome medicines [a 1 cit]
106. enfeebled [*ppl a*, 1649, Daniel, G.] 11 their infeebled and stuffed affections [a 1 cit]
107. enfreeze [1596, Spenser] 121 medicines many times haue an action of heate, yet of their potentiall power they doe ouercoole and infrese the body [a 1 cit]
108. engendered [1633, Herbert, G.] 16 the ingendered humours [a 1 cit]

109. engenderment [1835, Todd *Cycl. Anat.*] 28 hauing ingenderment with black fleame & yellowe choller [a 1 cit]
110. entertain [11, 1622, Heylin] 55 many of them thorow exceeding great ryot, easily do intertaine many diseases
111. equal [3a, 1674, Clarendon] 4 flux the body, by some gentle and potatiue electuary, in equall and artificiall degree
112. equal [4, 1661, Morgan] 90 See **combination**, anted.
113. equally [1, 1634, Herbert, Sir T.] 79 the fleshe and the fatte may bee equallye inlarded: agreeable one together with an other
114. ethiopian [A, i, 1684, *Friendly Advice*] 90 the Ethiopian yoong men
115. european [1, 1603, Knolles] 50 those Europian countries bordering vpon Affrica [a 1 cit]
116. european [B, 1632, Massinger] 95 Europians, are more fiercer then the Asians [a 1 cit]
117. exactly [2, 1612, Brinsley] 23 care to regard health from sicknesse in euerie seuerall constitution more exactlie then heretofore
118. exasperate [*v*, 2, 1611, Cotgrave *Aigrun.*] 4 without searching the cause or vnderstanding the matter of the sicknesse, doe preferre their owne hazard, and exasperating the disease, eyther with fulsome medicine, or grosse nourishment [a 1 cit]
119. exclude [I, 1b, 1598, Barret] 29 thicke thinges are easily comprehended, and swiftly excluded
120. exclusion [4, 1646, Browne] 118 the exclusion of one part more then an other [a 1 cit]
121. excoriated [1661, Lovell] 36 ptisans, made of exoriated [*sic*] and vnhusked barly [a 1 cit]
122. exhaust [5, 1631, Googe] See **punish**, anted.
123. extend [2b, 1639, Wotton] 36 There is a farther counsell to be herein extended
124. extract [4b, 1596, Davies] 117 the vaines may extract a mouing comfort
125. fashionable [A, *adj*, 3, 1630, *R. Johnson's Kingd.*] 64 *Aiax* was of a fashionable, strong, and mighty body [a 1 cit]
126. fashionable [A, *adj*, 1, 1607, Hieron *Works*] 63 those bodies cannot be temperate, which are not fashionable [a 1 cit]
127. fathom [4, 1634, Brereton] 110 for searching, searing, scowring and fadoming the deepenesse thereof
128. fatigable [b, 1656, Blount] 17 preuenting variable hazardes by fatigable wrestling [a 1 cit]
129. favourably [2, 1655, Nicholas, Sir E.] 4 some gentle and potatiue electuarie … fauourably casting out the infected humours
130. flashy [*a*, 2a, 1625, Bacon *Ess. Studies*] 88 the growth of haire in a beast, is like a flashie fresh medowe ouerfloten with a shalow water in the rootes, and the grasse therewithall ouerflorisheth

131. flux [*v*, 1a, 1666, Boghurst, W.] 4 foorthwith flux the body
132. flux [*v*, II, 3, 1638, Read, A.] 31 nature ... fluxeth off [*sic*] her owne free propertie
133. fluxible [1b, 1607, Topsell] 29 bodies which be naturally fluxible
134. fluxing [*ppl a*, 1702, De Foe] 119 some hotte fluxing humour [a 1 cit]
135. fluxing [*vbl sb*, 1,1659, Heylin] 78 liquid propertie of fluxing [a 1 cit]
136. foreign [5, 1621, Burton] 32 whether nature be ouercharged with the forraine estate of the disease
137. foreshow [*v*, 2b, 1601, Chester] 49 See **glut**, anted.
138. formity [1623, Cockeram] 64 we are to vnderstand, that formitie and fashion is an instrumentall cause [a 1 cit]
139. freezing [1, 1611, Shakespeare] 94 outward thinges vpon the north partes are cold and freesing [a 1 cit]
140. frugal [1, 1598, Shakespeare] 83 a thinne body sheweth frugal fatnesse [a 1 cit]
141. fumatic [1641, *True Ch. Unt. Bp.* and ns] 20 especially in those natures whose bodies are euermore incombred with fumaticke grossenesse [a 1 cit]
142. function [1, 1597, Daniel] 25 Many writers of the same function which *Theophrastus Paracelsus* is of
143. generable [*a*, 2, 1633, Fisher *Jasp. Fuimus*] 45 water and ayre commixed, are of generable nature, producing sustenance, agreeing with all natures indumentes
144. glut [*sb*[3], 1b, 1599, Jonson *EMOH*] 49 all which foresheweth excessiue gluttes in the vnseasonable aboundance of raine the winter following
145. gluttonous [3, 1600, Vaughan] 5 vnordered and glottonous meates
146. gracile [1623, Cockeram] 39 a gracil and thin diet [a 1 cit][11]
147. gravelly [2, 1607, Topsell] 7 a grauelly congested substance
148. greenness [3, 1649, Drummond of Hawth.] 48 there is also a chaungeableness in all things: as from moystnesse and greenesse, to ripenesse and rottennes
149. grossly [3b, 1594, Hooker] 79 in their feeding doo groslie satisfy appetite
150. grossness [4a, 1681, Dryden] 14 beware of varietie and grossnesse of meates
151. guide [*sb*, II, 5, 1700, S. L.] 89 the vaynes of the necke, beeing called the guides
152. half-sphere [1611, Jonson] 49 the halfe spheare called horyzon [a 1 cit]
153. hotly [1, 1592, Shakespeare] 78 hotly and excessiuely breathing thereupon
154. humane [2, 1691, Wood] (ep. ded.) most sweet flowers, from the pleasant garden of humaine and liberall arts
155. humid [1b, 1604, Jas. 1] 74 humid deiections vpward
156. humid [1d, 1813, Thompson, J.] 118 clammie matter impendent vpon the loonges ... alwayes belonging to such humid diseases

157. hungry [3b, 1611, Coryat] 14 subtil and hungrie airs are most best for these diets

158. hurting [1681, Flavel] 108 See **salving**, anted. [a 1 cit]

159. hypothesis [3, Browne, 1646] 76 the good and euill estate of inward thinges, are knowne & beleeued, as onely by a supposed Hypothesis [a 1 cit]

160. immediate [2b, 1624, De Laune] 107 the immediate and extraordinarie reason

161. immedicable [*a*, a, 1596, L(inche), R. *Diella*] 4 nature cannot disgest such grosse imperfections ... as commonly in the end become immedicable and mortall

162. immethodical [*a*, 1605, Powel, G. *Refut. E*] 5 it were not immethodicall so to distinguish these cold and hote diseases [a 1 cit]

163. immixed [1855, Bailey] 44 certaine immixt elementes [a 1 cit] [fpl]

164. immixtion [1653, R. G.] 45 The immixion of humours in mans bodie [a 1 cit]

165. impedimental [*a*, 1654, Montague, W. *Dev. Ess.*] 77 See **adversible**, unrec. [a 1 cit]

166. impendent [1, 1611, Cotgrave] 118 See **humid** 1d, anted. [a 1 cit]

167. impendent [2, 1592, Greene, Jas. IV *Wks.*] 110 the staying and stopping of some further impendent danger [a 1 cit]

168. imperious [2, 1592, Daniel] 43 See **ruling**, anted.

169. impermixt [1629, Donne] 55 the quality thereof is impermixt [a 1 cit]

170. impostumate [2, 1607, Markham] 21 bloud impostumated in the liuer

171. impress [*v*, c, 1657, Morice] 99 buls flesh, which impresseth and setleth rawe humours [a 1 cit]

172. improvidently [1, 1607, Donne] 5 improuidently throwne vpon many dangerous extremities [a 1 cit]

173. impure [*a*, I, 1a, 1597, A. M. *Guill.*] 98 their passage from the gall to the bowels, is ouer-little, and more larger about the stomacke, comprehending excessiue excrementes, which impureth vitall bloud ouer grosly

174. inclination [7, 1593, Shakespeare] 108 single medicines haue an appropriat inclination in themselues

175. inclineable [3, 1607, Norden] 83 there are some sanguine complexions of inclineable fat

176. incomprehensible [2b, 1604, Cawdrey] 66 The excellencie hereof is incomprehensible in a perfect vertuous man

177. inconcocted [1605, Timme] 71 hot and drie bodies of some women ... growe into many inward diseases for want of naturall deuoydance of their inconcocted superfluities [a 1 cit]

178. inconveniently [2, 1656, Hall, Bp.] 28 two offensiue causes inconuenientlie conioined in one disease

179. increasing [*ppl a?* 1597, Shakespeare and ns] 7 increasing wholesome bloud [a 1 cit]

180. increment [4, 1631, Braithwait] 126 all hearbes whose properties are ... hote, are ... compounded by an increment of the north wind
181. indicate [2, 1706, Phillips] 101 hauing a camoysed nose, indicateth much chollerike drinesse [a 1 cit]
182. indication [2, 1660, More, H.] 83 if their breath be sharpe, sweete and thinne: if their bloud be warme, sharpe and sweete, all which maketh indication of a perfect substance
183. indirection [1a, 1602, Shakespeare] 5 opilations and ventosites in the guttes, worke all contrarie indirections to health [a 1 cit]
184. indivertible [1811, Lamb] 39 their accidentes are infectious and of indiuertible substance [a 1 cit]
185. inducement [1c, 1605, Bacon] 107 all inflammations shall sensibly appeare more subdued, moderated, and seasoned, for inducement of a more higher and excellenter practise in the worke thereof [a 1 cit]
186. induction [9, 1660, Stanley] 49 no certaine nor constant induction of the weather for health and wholesomenesse
187. inequality [3b, 1626, Bacon] 95 greater inequalities of seasons
188. inflame [4, 1607, Hieron] 29 vnnaturall choller ... inflameth the disease
189. inflammative [A, *a*, 1730, Bailey] 17 These inflamatiue feuers must eyther haue a chryticall expulsion, or els doe they alter from one degree to another [a 1 cit]
190. inflow [*v*, 2, 1886, Scott Holland, H.] 86 nature hath prepared a way ... for those excrementes, to inflowe by the ... cheekes [a 1 cit]
191. ingurge [1631, Heywood] 79 the stomach ingurged [a 1 cit]
192. insatiableness [1618, Rushw. *Hist. Coll.*] 17 the greatnesse and insatiablenesse of their accidentes [a 1 cit]
193. insignia [2, 1796, Hamilton, E.] 66 the insignes and renowmed tokens [a 1 cit]
194. insinuate [1b, 1598, Hakluyt] 110 strong medicines ... easily doo insinuate and winde themselues into all the partes of man
195. insulse [1, 1609, Barlow] 25 *Insulsum*, that is, vnsauory and without feeling [a 1 cit]
196. insult [1, 1603, Holland] 25 *Ieremias Thriuerus* doth cal the accidents of euery disease *Insultum*, a brag, in reproch of the whole body [a 1 cit]
197. insult [4, 1697, Dryden] 126 medicines which hasten the disease to become more swift, sharp, and insult the spirituall partes [a 1 cit]
198. insume [*v*, 1675, Evelyn *Tena.*] 72 [a moyst bodie] ouermuch insumeth and spendeth vpon nature [a 1 cit]
199. intendment [5b, 1626, Jackson] 122 their accidentall heate, hath supreame intendment in the one, and disgraceth the other
200. intercourse [5, 1626, Bacon] 101 greate inundations and intercourses
201. intercourse [*sb*, 6, 1598, Stow *Surv.* xxv.] 14 also stop vp the entercourses of blood

202. interdeal [*v*, 1601, Daniel *Civ. Wars*] 33 So there must be a like caution taken, in these sharpe diseases ... not to interdeale therewith by fluxing [a 1 cit]
203. interflow [1, 1610, Holland] 116 when a dispersed due interfloweth from sustenance [a 1 cit]
204. interflowing [*ppl a*, 1610, Holland *Cam. Brit.*] 92 continuall moyste interflowing vapour [a 1 cit] [fpl]
205. interjoin [1607, Shakespeare] 53 enterioyned with grosse fleame [a 1 cit]
206. intermingle [3, 1626, Bacon] 81 cholericke bloud is not intermingled therewith
207. interpose [1, 1599, Minsheu *Sp. Dict.*] 75 like as difference is interposed betweene a cleere and grosse ayre [a 1 cit]
208. intervent [1593, *Motives Rom. Faith*] 109 some effectuall propertie ... which ... can neither be interuented nor altered [a 1 cit]
209. inundate [*v*, 1, 1790, Beloe, W. *Herodotus*] 79 matery substance of waterie blood, inundating between the skinne and the flesh [a 1 cit]
210. invest [2b, 1632, Lithgow] 84 women, whose bodyes are inuested with corpulent and fattie flesh
211. invest [3a, 1604, Shakespeare] 121 cold water ... if it be inuested with an accidentall heate
212. inwardly [II, 4a, 1667, *Obs Burn. Lond.*] 129 the bloud and breath were inwardly repulsed
213. irradiate [*v*, 3, 1617, Bayne *Lect.*] 42 a direct light gleaming and irradiating from the starres [a 1 cit]
214. jellied [*v*, a] 19 colde and heate gelied together in one substaunce of drinesse [a 1 cit]
215. judicable [1647, Taylor, Jer.] 107 (margin) All indicable thinges haue a iudicable temperance [a 1 cit]
216. judication [1625, Hart] 36 it behoueth to yeeld the body some slender reliefe, so that continually it be limitted within iudication [a 1 cit]
217. kernel [7a, 1641, Best *Farm Bks.*] 79 the pyth and kernell of the bones
218. knit [5b, 1605, Bacon] 52 this fleame knitteth in the ioyntes
219. languishing [1b, 1611, Shakespeare] 2 long and languishing sicknesses
220. lenitively [1627, Middleton] 123 See **approve**, anted. [a 1 cit] [fpl]
221. limited [2, 1610, Willey] 32 in ministring of purgatiue medicines there must be called to remembrance whether nature haue ready strength ... to performe a limited dutie in purgation or no
222. linger [8, 1641, Best] 39 not able to bear that which is wished and lingred vpon
223. loose [*v*, 2g, 1760, Brooke, H.] their haire ... waxeth thin, and vtterly looseth in the roots
224. lunatical [*a*, 1599, *Broughton's Lett.*] 68 then the disease is lunaticall following the temperance, or distemperance of the moone and the elementes [a 1 cit]

225. malefaction [1, 1602, Shakespeare] 28 bodies ouertaken with any uniuersall malefaction [a 1 cit]
226. match [*v*, 8a, 1592, Shakespeare] 75 blood may according to proportion be matched in children and adolescencie alike, & yet their heate may exceed one aboue another
227. measled [2, 1634, Herbert, Sir T.] 80 But touching measelled or kernelled flesh … which … is a monstrous mishapen substance
228. medicable [2, 1658, Phillips, *Medicable*] 28 this vertuous and medicable indeuor [a 1 cit]
229. melancholic [*sb*, 2, 1647, Clarendon] 51 This fleame is not properly permanent in the complexion of man, as choller and melancholike are
230. melancholiousness [2, 1610, Barrough, *Meth. Phys.*] 119 The third is a foule sore, hard to be cured, and being poisoned with the melancholiousnesse of the humour is called, *Noli me tangere* [a 1 cit] [fpl]
231. mellow [3, 1593, Nashe] 100 a rawe or reare egge … melloweth and increaseth appetite
232. melting [1b, 1593, Shakespeare] 94 their heartes in the end, are soluble and melting with the snowe
233. membrane [1a, 1615, Crooke] 78 the parchment skin called the membrans
234. minoration [2, 1684, *Bonet's*] 24 mollefaction in stead of minoration [a 1 cit]
235. mistaken [2, 1601, Shakespeare] 60 (margin) Hipocrates is missensed or mistooke [a 1 cit]
236. mitigating [1683, Sidney] 22 minister medicine … for the easing & mittigating the rigour of the infection [a 1 cit]
237. moistly [1602, 2nd. part *Ret. Parn.*] 78 it is moistly nourishable in digestion [a 1 cit]
238. mollefaction [1822, *Good's Study Med.*] 24 *Auycen* calleth this mollefaction the libertie of nature [a 1 cit]
239. monarch [*a*, 1884, Bower and Scott, *De.*] (ep. ded.) those monarche Phisitions of the world, Galen, Hypocrates, Auycen, and Dyoscorides [a 1 cit]
240. mordicate [*v*, 1651, Biggs, *New Disp* and ns] 98 their stomackes are mordicated and ouercharged vnder vilde, monstrous and vaporous humours [a 1 cit]
241. moving [*ppl a*, 2a, 1659, Leake] 111 a whole and perfett substance of moouing power
242. mucilaginous [1, 1646, Browne] 51 a certaine vnnaturall and mucilaginous fleame [a 1 cit]
243. muddy [3, 1618, Latham] 102 the vrine muddie, bloody, blacke, and thicke
244. natively [2, 1609, Tourneur *Vere, Sir F.*] 69 yoong men, natiuely brought vp in temperate regions

245. natively [2b, 1629, Lightfoot] 90 hayrie men natiuely appertaine vnder regions hote and drie
246. nature [4b, 1597, Shakespeare] 100 (margin) A good cooke is in the nature of a good physitian
247. nurse [5, 1736, Swift] 2 a bodie almost deuoured ... cannot easily be ... nursed vp
248. observation [7, 1600, Shakespeare] 28 Here followeth an other diligent obseruation
249. obstruct [*v*, 1, 1611, Cotgrave *Oppile*] 89 the vaynes of the necke, beeing called the guides, are obstructed, doe not perfectly recourse [a 1 cit]
250. operation [3b, 1605, Bacon] 23 feuers happening in mans bodie vppon contrarie and disseasonable operations of times
251. operative [A, 1, 1603, Holland] 78 nature vtterly desisteth, and leaueth of her common and operatiue course [a 1 cit]
252. operative [A, *adj*, 2, 1598, Bacon *Let. to Pick.* and ns] 21 but if the disease hasten to concoction, may the better be curable, and operatiue, both in medicine and nature [a 1 cit]
253. over-moist [1626, Bacon] 46 thinges which be ouer moyst [a 1 cit]
254. over-tired [1634, Tyrwhit] 69 the conceit is also ouer tyred, blunted, or dulled [a 1 cit]
255. over-travel [1654, Hawks, F. and ns] 88 the poores in a mans body are ouer traveiled by a moyst exhalation [a 1 cit]
256. over-weaken [1747, *Astruc's fevers*] 49 Some new writers perswade the worlde that mans body is ouerweakened by those seasons [a 1 cit]
257. overburdensome [1614, Raleigh] 117 it is operatiue and ouerburthensome [a 1 cit]
258. overcool [1597, Shakespeare] 121 See **enfreeze**, anted. [a 1 cit]
259. overeat [1, 1599, Moufet] 119 See **unkindly**, anted.
260. overfloat [1619, Dyke, J.] 71 their primary faculties, are ouerfloted or intermixed with superfluous grosnes [a 1 cit]
261. override [3b, 1867, Francis, F.] 59 euill custome ouerrideth ouerrunneth and ouerreacheth both disposition and temperance
262. overtravel [1856, Kane] 125 coldnesse ... greatly offend us, except the strength of our nature ouertrauell the danger [a 1 cit]
263. pandect [2, 1591, Sylvester *Du. B.*] 120 How much could I here vtter in disgrace of the Pandect, for false exposition
264. penetration [1, 1623, Cockeram] 127 the Sun ... warmeth all thinges, in deeper penetration of one thing more then another [a 1 cit]
265. pentice [1600, Fairfax] 92 an outward worke, like a comely pentise [a 1 cit]
266. penurious [*a*, 1, 1596, Spenser *FQ*] 1 And a pennurious bodie is weakened, punished, exhausted [a 1 cit]
267. phagadæna [1657, *Phys. Dict.*] 119 See **chironia**, unrec. [a 1 cit]
268. pituitous [*a*, a, 1607, Topsell *Ff. B.*] 98 then the vniversall body is

infected, with fuliginous vapours, of disposition, yeelding to be pituitous and flegmaticke [a 1 cit]
269. place [11, 1639 *Arch. Maryland*] 89 in the first place, those thinges which be hearie onely are hote and moyst
270. poisonsome [*a*, 1595, Wyatt, Capt. R. *Dud.*] 120 they are poisonsome and deadly [a 1 cit]
271. positive [5, 1606, Shakespeare] 60 Galen putteth downe ... a second maner of temperance to righteousnesse, as a positiue lawe to be obserued of all men
272. positive [IV, 8, 1618, Elton, E.] 38 a positiue operation to conserue a strong estate in nature [a 1 cit]
273. possess [1b, 1605, Grimstone] 74 both moystnesse and coldnesse ... are possest in the body
274. potative [*a*, 1737, Ozell, *Rabelais*] 21 scowred and restored by potatiue vnguentes inwardly taken
275. powdered [6, 1591, Spenser] 107 powdred medicines, whose power is onely to purge
276. pragmatical [3, 1601, Godwin] 94 See **short-necked**, anted.
277. predominate [3, 1607, Shakespeare] the foure elementes are congested in euery seuerall body, predominating euery man [a 1 cit]
278. preeminently [1747, Mallet, D.] 53 if moyst humour preheminentlie be placed [a 1 cit]
279. preparation [6, 1646, Browne] 122 *Galen* ... practiseth to wash away his former obiection against the preparation of popie, seemeth to admit the vse thereof against ... hote vlcerations
280. presign [*v*, 1598, Dickenson *Greene in C.*] 61 And yet if we behold all liuing men in their order, there is not one so to be found, which attaineth that excellencie of wisedome and vnderstanding, as hee ought to the vttermost of natures indowmentes, except some few persons presigned thereunto [a 1 cit]
281. primary [3, 1631, Donne] 101 Examples hereof may be taken from the primary reason
282. principally [3, 1832, De La Beche] 6 melancholike heauinesse is generated, which moste principally offendeth
283. profiting [1605, Hutton, T.] 108 See **salving**, anted. [a 1 cit]
284. profitableness [2, 1886, Dunkeley] 61 some temperate propertie or purpose ... as the horse for swiftnes, the Cow for fruitfulness, the Sheepe for profitablenesse
285. prolix [3, 1650, Bulwer] 92 the flegmaticke and moyst man hathe a moste prolixe increment in the nayles
286. proper [B, 2, 1663, Gerbier] 76 This reason standeth verie proper to manie dispositions
287. puff [4b, 1725, *Bradley's Fam. Dict.*] 79 the bodie is ingrossed, the guttes puffed, the braines invapoured, and the stomach ingurged

288. punish [3, 1812, *Sporting Mag.*] 1 the bodie is weakened, punished, exhausted
289. pylon [1, 1850, Leitch and ns] 7 the guttes, called Colon and Plyon [*sic*] [a 1 cit]
290. qualified [1, 1596, Shakespeare] 108 single medicines, haue an appropriat inclination in themselues, but artificially qualified from their owne nature, haue a more clearer ... effect
291. raging [1b, 1695, *New Light Chirurg.*] 17 these raging diseases
292. reading [3, 1593, Harvey] 27 the learned Physitian, which in iudiciall reading is before made to vnderstand the same
293. recovery [3, 1606, Shakespeare] 93 yet many of them after any such recouery, are greatlie incumbred with a tisich
294. reduce [17c, 1741, *Cramer's Assaying*] 117 such medicines are easily reduced, and manifested in their owne nature
295. regard [3b, 1591, Shakespeare] 115 foode ought with care and diligence to be wayed and regarded
296. regenerate [*v*, 2, 1597, A. M. *Guill.*] 129 and heate herewith regenerated
297. regular [5, 1705, Addison] 7 pure and regular dyet
298. relaxation [3, 1626, Bacon *Sylva*] 129 ouergreat thicknesse of the skinne, conceiueth a free relaxation in the poores
299. relish [2, 1607, Shakespeare] 116 the body taketh good liking and relishe of the meate
300. remotive [*a*, 2, 1834, *Gent. Mag.*] 21 those singular feuers, are in their first beginning very remotiue, and giue easie place to medicine [a 1 cit]
301. repulse [1c, 1601, Dolman] 129 both the bloud and breath were inwardly repulsed
302. repulsion [2b, 1725, Bradley] 129 the same repulsion, which is made after the concoction of humours
303. resisting [1593, Q. Elizabeth] 111 the other is wilde and of more resisting vertue [a 1 cit]
304. restible [*a*, 1656, Blount, *Gloss.*] 1 preserued and renewed by some restible electuaries and such like [a 1 cit]
305. ripen [6, 1599, A. M. *Gabel.*] 32 some meete framed medicine, to ripen the disease
306. ripening [1, 1597, Hooker] 19 the sunne ... giueth ... ripening to all liuing thinges [a 1 cit]
307. ruddy [5b, 1746, Francis] 18 of ruddie black colour
308. ruling [2, 1731, Pope] 43 earth and water are imperious & ruling elements [a 1 cit]
309. salving [1748, Richardson] 108 of medicioneable and saluing condition ouer one, and nothing at all profiting but rather hurting vnto another [a 1 cit]
310. satisfied [1, 1816, Scott, J.] 1 A full and satisfied bodie is chiefly preserued [a 1 cit]

311. searching [*ppl a*, 1b, 1593, Shakespeare] 110 hot searching and inflammatiue medicines
312. season [4e, 1601, Holland] 1 such bodies ... may forthwith be tempered, seasoned, & salued by medicinable helpe
313. sense [6, 1597, Shakespeare] 28 a strong purgation in offence of the whole constitution ... corrupteth the sences
314. sense [11, 1684, Roscommon] 66 the most excellent sences of a vertuous man
315. sensibly [1b, 1675, Boyle] 118 See **application**, anted.
316. settled [4b, 1811, Morgan, Lady] 32 See **dured**, unrec.
317. shadowed [3, 1596, Shakespeare] 42 a certain dark, thicke, and shadowed fire, about the point & centre of the earth
318. shelly [3, 1593, Nashe] 97 of fishes ... there is foure sortes: as chrustie, shellie, scalie
319. short-necked [1663, Boyle] 94 a short necked man, is apt to conceiue, pregmaticall [a 1 cit] [fpl]
320. show [*v*, 4d, 1611, *2nd. Maid's Trag.*] 53 no temperature ... which sheweth some great reproch to nature
321. situation [3a, 1600, Shakespeare] 108 the high fruitfull scituation of the sunne
322. sleek-skinned [1661, Braithwait] 79 chrustie, shellie, scalie, soft and sleeke-skinned fish [a 1 cit] [fpl]
323. smoothness [1c, 1626, Bacon] 69 a man ... ought to be indifferent in all these properties, as well in colour, stature and smoothnesse, as courage, stoutnesse
324. solicit [7, 1731, Arbuthnot] 39 these infections ... ought to be sollicited more at large ... by curatiue medicine, or diet
325. sophistical [*a*, 3b, 1613, Godwyn, T. *Rom. Ant.*] 36 fountaine water, & sharpe vinegar, not sophisticall, but seasoned from the naturall grape
326. sparing [2b, 1611, Cotgrave] 1 with sparing abstinence
327. spew [4, 1598, Sylvester] 21 the gall speweth and stayneth all the superiour partes
328. squeeze [5b, 1611, Cotgrave] 120 a certain ioyce ... squeased out of the leaues of Laserpition [a 1 cit]
329. stable [3b, 1839, Moseley] 107 celestiall bodies are stable, firme and perfect
330. starched [*ppl a*, 1b, 1599, Jonson, *EMOH*] 89 there are some bodies, whose drinesse exceedeth on the contrary, and yet vnder some moysture produce a competent number of hayres: but when their drinesse becommeth combust, are like to starched earth, which without some moysture cannot bring forth grasse [a 1 cit]
331. state [6b, 1597, Bacon] 115 nourishment nothing disagreeth from wood ioyned vnto fire, which first standeth at a state, then presently altereth
332. stenchful [1615, Adams, T. *Black Devil*] 123 remedies against all venims and stenchfull corruptions [a 1 cit]

333. stiffen [2b, 1697, Dryden] 29 choller of whateuer nature soeuer it be, is ... not styfned, but drawne more thin and open
334. stone-colic [1603, Florio] 7 the wind and stone Collike [a 1 cit] [fpl]
335. stretched [3, 1605, Drayton] 88 exhalations are in their natures ouer drie, fuliginous, and stretched
336. strictly [6, 1632, Lithgow] 33 sicknesses ... may be more strickly [*sic*] regarded in their full and perfect estate
337. subdue [4, 1615, Sandys] 107 all inflammations shall sensibly appeare more subdued, moderated, and seasoned
338. subdued [*ppl a*, 2, 1835, Lytton] 93 their courage verie much subdued from inflammation [a 1 cit]
339. substract [*v*, 1, 1604, Cawdrey *T. A.*] 37 But if the disease in forceable assault runneth forward without stay, then all dyets are substracted
340. success [1c, 1606, Bryskett] 105 there must be hereunto also annexed not onely the sensible vnderstanding of these naturall causes, but a iust co[n]senting of their sensible power and vertue to haue one successe
341. successive [1b, 1597, Morley] 19 See **assenting**, anted.
342. sudden [7, 1591, Shakespeare] 64 most wittie ... in setting foorth of fayned fantasies and sodaine deuises
343. suggest [4a, 1709, Berkeley] 92 cold venerian vapours, the extreame malice whereof, suggesteth these colde and perfect diseases of feuers
344. sultry [1b, 1620, Quarles] 49 the sunne ... inforceth the mornings of those seasons to be hote, moyst, and soultrie [a 1 cit]
345. superiority [4, 1694, Luttrell] 27 concoction ought to haue a most high superioritie in gathering & preferring the vniversall corruption of the body on a heape
346. supreme [3, 1593, Shakespeare] 109 a supreame naturall substance, coagulateth in the power of all inferiour causes
347. swimming [*ppl a*, 5, 1607, Topsell] 99 greeuous swimming aches in the head
348. sympathy [3d, 1813, Southey] (ep. ded.) touching the true simpathie of my heart, which in double duetie, I and mine doe owe vnto you and your house
349. symptomatic [3, 1751, Smollett] 66 the insignes and renowmed tokens thereof are simptomaticke, for all cogitations ... are shut vp vnder sleeping [a 1 cit]
350. tart [*v*, 1, 1616, Scott, T. *Christ's Pol.*] 7 sweete meates, tarted with vineger [a 1 cit]
351. tasteful [1, 1647, Crashaw] 75 as heate in yoong menne may be more sharper, so in children more sweeter and tastefull [a 1 cit]
352. tasteful [2, 1611, Cotgrave] 84 the naturall fat in these men is both hote and tastfull [a 1 cit]
353. tergiversate [*v*, 1, 1654, Gayton *Plea. Notes*] 29 ther is a choller ... which not perfectlie digested ... altereth with the disease it selfe, and tergiuersateth from his owne propertie [a 1 cit]

354. tinsel[12] [*sb*[3], 3, 1593, Fletcher, G. *Licia*] 65 innocencie … was stayned afterwardes by mans fuller or larger corruption, like a paynters tinsell, from white to red, in the carnation of mans bloud
355. transpierce [1, 1594, Drayton] 78 nature being transpersed [a 1 cit]
356. traverse [*sb*, I, 2, 1599, Marston, *Sc. Vill.*] 17 these feuers … doe by a superfluous trauerse inuade nature
357. under [15e, 1884, Thompson] 29 those diseases which happen vnder some preposterous chrysis
358. underbend [1611, Florio] 78 thinges which easilie concreat … and will not afterwardes vnderbend to the qualitie of moystnesse [a 1 cit] [fpl]
359. unequal [2b, 1694, Tillotson] 34 whosoeuer, eyther by unequall vertue, or unequall measure … reacheth into anie such disease … is to be adiudged in a damnable estate
360. unequal [3d, 1703, Rowe] 51 crud, proceeding from distemperate seasons, as also by an vnequall substance
361. unforcible [1, 1597, Hooker, *Eccl. Pol.*] 75 Otherwise vnforceable to reach the constitution of adolescencie [a 1 cit]
362. unhusked [*ppl a*[2], 1597, Hall, Bp. *Sat.*] 36 ptisans, made of ex[c]oriated and vnhusked barly [a 1 cit]
363. union [1c, 1631, Crooke] 118 the diseased and grieued part presently altereth his yssue, yeeldeth to a sound vnion, and is presently comprehended vnder one safe substance of the body
364. union [7, 1660, Taylor, J.] 117 the vnion hereof [sowes flesh] is of a more thicke and growne substance
365. unite [5a, 1667, Milton] 55 heat and moisture were distemperatly vnited
366. unkindly [*a*, 2d, 1649, Drumm. of Hawth.] 119 some vnkindly worme breedeth and ouereateth
367. unnaturalness [2, 1605, Jonson] 47 the vnnaturalnesse of winter
368. unnourishable [*a*, 1607, Topsell *Ff. B.*] 97 Also there is some kinde of fish drie, vnnourishable, and returneth to slender excrementes [a 1 cit]
369. unsettle [2, 1651, Hobbes] 98 the humours be before vnsetled, by some preparatiue medicine [a 1 cit]
370. unsettled [2b, 1793, Abernethy] 105 contrary medicines … inforcing the griefe to become more outragious, inflammatiue and vnsetled [a 1 cit]
371. unsingled [*ppl a*, 1697, Dryden, *Aneis*] 108 an vnsingled and variable power [a 1 cit]
372. unsoundness [1b, 1660, Brooke, F.] 55 such intemperatures are … esiest suspected of their vnsoundnes [a 1 cit]
373. unvenomed [*ppl a*, 1597, Hall, Bp. *Sat.*] 16 the body vnuenomed with corruption [a 1 cit]
374. vaporous [3, 1593, Shakespeare] 14 low and vaporous ayres
375. vestal [4, 1592, Shakespeare] 42 The which fire is vestall & pure, not elementarie

376. wearisome [3, 1594, Hooker] 15 the tedious and wearisome waies of sicknes
377. weeping [*vbl sb*, 2, 1665, G. S.] 120 Rosen which groweth into a gum, by meanes of teares and weeping of the trees
378. wind-colic [1593, Nashe] See **stone-colic**, anted. [a 1 cit] [fpl]
379. world [15, 1603, Shakespeare] 49 See **over-weaken**, anted.
380. wrongfully [2b, 1743, Bukeley] 55 the authority of *Aristotle* or *Theophrastus* shall not any thing herein preuaile, who wrongfully place the life of man between heate and moisture
381. wry-necked [1, 1596, Shakespeare] 94 A wrie necked person [a 1 cit]
382. yellow-black [C, 2, 1841, Clough] 21 discoloured with yellow blacke humours [a 1 cit] [fpl]

2. *New senses*

1. accidence 27 if the beginning of the disease continue in one accidence sixe monethes
2. arabian 120 *Asafetidæ*, which the Arabians do rather seeme to put in place of Mumy
3. blunt 6 this humour ... blunteth memory
4. capillary 77 There are diuers sortes of these feauers ... some are called *Capillares*
5. carnation 65 innocencie ... was stayned afterwardes by mans fuller or larger corruption, like a paynters tinsell, from white to red, in the carnation of mans bloud
6. cast 14 it is a most excellent contemplation for euerie man to cast vp his sences, and perfectly find vnder what temperance hee liueth
7. comminution 118 a strong and hot body will verie much blunt and dull the power hereof. As first by extenuation and comminution
8. compunction 32 The phisitian ought to surpasse the disease both in wisedome, experience, and high counsell with naturall causes, both in releasing the languishing compunction of infection, as to gather all crud and raw causes together
9. consist 4 whether the disease consist and stand at a stay
10. deject *v*, 125 [vrine] is the more easier deiected
11. estate 39 the disease doo proceede ... either by ripenesse to cease, or els take safe degrees to estate
12. force 6 *Corizam* stuffeth and infarceth the nostrels with with most humid farces
13. fumatic 20 See **fumatic**, anted.
14. impressive 109 Hemlock ... hath not onely a hot propertie and troublesome effect, but an impressiue action of a colde benumming of the sences
15. increasing 7 See **increasing**, anted.
16. indirect 19 Autum is the moste dangerous ... season ... vnder *Europe*, and moste complayned of ... for the indirect temperature thereof

17. influence 10 what perilous influence doeth then trouble and foyzen the ayre
18. intentive 42 water is of more rounder and compact substance, then of an intentiue qualitie
19. liquid 78 liquid propertie of fluxing
20. luminary 126 neither the Pandect, not yet the Luminarie make any such rehearsall
21. misordering 120 the first misordering of *Asa fetidæ*
22. mordicate 100 See **dismatch**, anted.
23. oment 84 there is another oment in the head ... commonly called of the chyrurgians *pia mater*
24. omission 84 purginges, omission of bloud, choyse of meates, might be sufficient meanes, to chase away the intollerable hurtes
25. operative 21 See **operative**, anted.
26. pylon 7 See **pylon**, anted.
27. recline 116 the body ... sheweth a degeneration of nature, and the distemperance of the body [is] reclined to some forraine contagion
28. redolent 17 the more the bodie wasteth and vanisheth away, the more redolent the strength and power of these feuers abound
29. seasoning 28 Howe much the preparing and seasoning of the body auaileth, for the perfect altering of the disease
30. subtile 51 the most subtile medicines of operation in sickeness
31. waste 98 the guttes clung, the liuer and loonges waste

3. Unrecorded

1. absumpt 82 See **discrepate**, anted.
2. absumpt 100 flegmatike humours, whose often and dayly distillations, absumpt the good indowmentes of the braine
3. adversible 77 so these feauers may be more noysome, aduersible, and impedimental
4. african 51 Ethiopia and Numidia vnder the Affrican poynt
5. arctic point 50 when two elementall figures of the Articke poynt inuadeth their territories
6. barrainous 89 So there is a most vnhappie sort of men, who by excesse drinesse in their adolescencie, become bald, bare and barrainous in their braines
7. belswyn 120 the gum of the tree it selfe called Rosen, or Belswyn, and Bewguyn
8. black poppy 106 blacke poppy cannot in the fourth degree, vnawares be intertained into the body
9. bone marrow 80 that bone marrowe is perfected and made pure
10. branchus 6 cold diseases ... called by three names: *Catarrh, Branchus,* & *Corizan*
11. carnat 72 all men doo obtaine the first partes of moystnesse by carnat generation

12. caroot 64 in all the partes of his body most deformed ... with a crooked necke, the carootes thereof were both, short and slender
13. catabalsamum 120 Balsamum, Catabalsamum, frankensence
14. cataplasma 106 the power of a cataplasma
15. cheerable 85 Their sleep is sweete, chearable and restfull
16. chironia 119 some olde writers deuide these sortes of sores into foure names: *Herpes, Phagedina, Chironia,* and *Telephia*
17. cominicial 127 the cominiciall disease, called the falling sicknesse
18. compage 62 all bodies or naturall qualities appertinent thereunto, are contayned or compaged vnder one burthen
19. concoct 4 whether there be any crud and rawe matter, or concockt setled in some part of the body
20. conflexion 126 all single hearbes ... except hearbes of cold propertie, which of themselues haue no elemental attraction, the Fusun notwithstanding hath a singular conflexion vpon them
21. conjunct 49 heate and moysture are coniuncted in the variable partes of the elementes
22. consumpt 38 oftentimes such bodyes are in those seasons apt to be consumpted and vtterly wasted
23. corizan 6 See **branchus**, unrec.
24. daphnoides 112 poisoned hearbes ... as the Daphnoydes
25. defume 99 some meates ... doe euaporat and defume the braines
26. delative 66 So also by delatiue circumstance, haue we distinguished
27. destruction 2 the vitall bloud corrupted and benummed, as the spirituall partes of man distructioned
28. devoidance 71 hot and drie bodies of some women ... growe into many inward diseases for want of naturall deuoydance of their inconcocted superfluities
29. diaphragma 82 the dyaphragma is thereby safest preserued from contagion
30. diospoliticon 59 *Dyoscorides* maketh a very commendable report of a certaine excellent potion, called *Diospoliticon*
31. disapetite 77 giddinesse distempereth the head, and disapetiteth the stomach
32. disfashion 65 what fashion or disfashion soeuer the body is
33. disfashionment 102 best outwardly regarded by the outward alteration, and disfashionment of hayres
34. disframed 43 disframed conditions and qualities
35. disoner 72 a dry body ... furnisheth the bodie with good blood, disonereth the body from raw excrementes
36. disornate 86 (margin) nature wolde not disornate the beautie of the face with haire
37. disseasonable 22 by reason of a disseasonable winter or vnnaturall spring before
38. disseparate 54 they are so deseperate one from another

39. disure 44 their actiue qualitie must be disured and fall away therewith
40. dured 32 not onely crud and rawe matter, but also dured and setled matter is then principallie expelled
41. egredience 96 They are much deceiued herein: for the egredience thereof, proffereth litle moysture
42. energiacal 126 it hath an energiecall worke to moderate ... the body
43. eucraton 53 *Galen* calleth the estate of man in the spring time of the Greeke word *Eucraton*
44. everstirring 14 euerstirring nature
45. exsanguit 116 (margin) Exanguit, that is without Bloud
46. first age 51 Asia obtaineth longer life, vnder which countries the fathers of the first age liued
47. flammative 36 appease the furie of flammatiue feuers
48. foize 28 The skilfull phisitian dooth farre otherwise, that as the sweete fountaine water, or the pure celestiall showers of raine, by litle and litle purge and purifie the fulsome sauours and contagions of the earth, doo not onely keepe them vnder, whereby their fulsome smelles breake not out, but also by litle and litle taketh away both their intollerable foyzing the ayre, as the corrupt stopping vp, and poysoning, the comfortable and essentiall estate of mans health
49. foyzen 4 the poores ... doe stain, foyzen and infect others
50. fusun 127 See **conflexion**, unrec.
51. gibseum 52 See **rallium**, unrec.
52. half-settled 129 humours which were before halfe setled
53. inclinative 100 And yet manie times also, the body is inclinatiue to these rewmes
54. inclinement 6 many such complections are fluxible, and ouermuch spend nature of their owne inclinement
55. indicable 111 they are so indicible and euident
56. infectuously 13 the most fulsome and filthy diseases of the world, thorow which mans body is infectuously stained by the slimy & ryotous course of his life
57. infoison 77 those kindes of feauers are of diuers natures, which eyther by an extreame deuoydance, or defect of blood, doo aswell offend the arteries, as other principall members, the heart, the lyuer, the lunges, the stomach, and the raines, which in their vegetatiue nature are wasted and consumed: so by that the highest degree of daunger, the spirites vitall, naturall, and animall, are excessiuely infoizned
58. infrigerate 125 the force of colde poysons beeing loste vnder the action of heate, manifestly doe infrigerate the body
59. inseize 127 For as the heate of the Sun is sincere and pure in nature and propertie, so dooth it conioine with the course of starres discending by a certaine mellifluous dewe, inseaseth it selfe vpon the hearbs of the earth
60. lame-eyed 102 squint-eyed, and lame-eyed men
61. laserpitium 120 the leaues of Laserpitium

62. liver-blood 102 the liuer-bloud thereupon is made most pure
63. melancholiously 53Choller vnnaturall is ... melancholiously mingled
64. missensed 60 See **mistaken**, anted.
65. murthersome 119 that dangerous and murthersome hearbe Cicuta
66. occulus lunæ 127 a starre, which followeth the newe moone, called *Occulus lunæ*
67. oment marrow 80 the oment marrowe is liquid in the celles of the head, and void of all during substance
68. over-grossly 98 See **impure**, anted.
69. overexquisitely 32 nature sometimes ouerexquisitely purgeth of her owne propertie
70. overfatigated 11 these creatures ... ouerfatigated and in their seruice to mans corruption
71. overmelt 99 See **transmeate**, unrec.
72. overpowerful 55 that contagion is ouerpowerful
73. overprassive 99 if it [this choler] proceede from the liuer, it is yellow and pale: if it ingender vppon the stomack, it is greene, like to the colour of a Leeke: if it breede thorow a malicious corruption, it is ouerprassiue
74. overraging 49 ouerraging pestilences are inkindled in such like seasons
75. overrebellious 39 the materiall substance of the disease [is] ouer-rebellious
76. peperites 127 the hearbe Peperites hath a wonderfull and excelent operation
77. physic cup 27 the number of physicke cuppes standing vpon tables
78. polios 111 a hearbe called *Polios*
79. prassion 53 the hearb, Prassion
80. prassive 20 whose fortitude and vertue assimilatiue thereby diminished becommeth prassiue in it selfe
81. rallium 52 a most dangerous fleame called by *Cornelius Celsus*, Rallium, of others, Gibseum
82. remedious 100 redolent wines ... are both conuerted to fragrant bloud, and establishe the complexion, to become delightsome and remedious herein
83. remissiveness 96 Then fleam doth not argue no ful quantitie of heat in winter, but rather sheweth some remissiuenesse therein
84. ruddy-black 18 of ruddie black colour
85. scopa regia 127 an other hearbe called *Scopa Regia*
86. seroot 86 the excrementes in the bleather are of two sortes: the one cleare, and the other thick: the one is called Hypostasis, which by a perfect digestion is aduanced in the substance of the vrine, and either is in the blather or seroot, or strained and extenuated from the bodie
87. telephia 119 See **chironia**, unrec.
88. timpana 7 these venemous [?]pions *As[?]des, Iposarca*, and *Timpana*
89. transmeate 99 sowes flesh, or buls flesh ... setleth rawe humours moste deepely, to ouermelt & transsmead the whole body of man

90. transumpt 19 the strong heate of sommer is weakened, and transumpted vntill another yeare
91. uberious 35 a satiable, uberious, and complet dyet
92. understay 39 but if the disease exceed beyond that lymittation, is then to be vnderstaid with a plenary & stronger food
93. undisfashioned 45 Therefore if it be possible that foure humours are confounded within themselues, and yet their formes kept together vndiffaconed [*sic*], or that one forme or fashion appeareth for them all
94. unslaken 109 unslaken lime
95. unvalurable 18 if the disease be vnvalurable in estat or fashion, how can the accidents of the disease be valurable or sharpe
96. valurable 18 See **unvalurable**, unrec.
97. viduate 5 the liuer viduated and forsaken of the wholsome bloud
98. vigent 4 Forthwith after these painefull defatigations, let naturall sweate and quiet sleepe, consolidat and refresh the body, to become more vigent, and the stomacke more sharpe
99. youngmanship 69 yoongmanship, called adolescencie

4. Postdatings

1. bend [16b, 1577, Holinshed] 39 *Hypocrates* somewhat bendeth to the second controuersie
2. cling [2a, 1414, Barlow] 98 the guttes clung
3. continently [2, 1529, More] 124 all those [vaporations] which continently doe not passe ouer in agreement with nature
4. deferve [1420, *Pallad. on Husb.*] 82 the liuer bloud is deferued and strengthened
5. defoul [3, 1548, Hall] whosoeuer infarceth and inforceth nature in the first entrance of euerie such sicknes ... cherisheth the disease, weakeneth and defoyleth nature
6. deputate [1560, Rolland] 67 but there are some outwardly deputated, for continual vse to minister inward reliefe
7. devoid [*v*, 1, 1509, Hawes] 78 devoided away by the vrine
8. disseparate [1551, Nicolls] 3 These strong diseases moste commonlie happen vnder a swift chrysis, whose mightie predomination ouerruleth, disframeth, and disseperateth those bodies from due temperance
9. invapour [1566, Alday] 79 the bodie is ingrossed, the guttes puffed, the braines inuapoured
10. loathsome [2, 1579, Twyne] 4 appetite forthwith waxeth wearie and lothsome in them
11. measurable [4, 1563, *Homilies*] 83 muche good appertaineth to those men, which are perfected vnder a measurable comprehension
12. melancholious [2, 1562, Bullen] 70 replenished with melancholious coldnesse
13. misgovernance [4, 1470, *Hors, shepe & g.*] 37 if the bodye fall into present misgouernance

14. molesting [1577, Hanmer] 27 there ought to be no troubling or molesting the body
15. over-little [1568, Ascham] 98 See **impure**, anted.
16. overtravail [1563, Golding] 125 except the strength of our nature ouertrauell the danger thereof
17. profluous [1585, Stubbes] 99 if a cold liuer be warmed vnder anie accidentall heate, it increaseth and ingendreth a profluous choler
18. repugnant [2b, 1568, Skene] 14 the medicine being repugnant
19. spiritual [II, 10, 1576, Baker] 16 the disease ... entereth vpon the spirituall partes
20. stayed [*ppl a*, 1586, Pembroke, C'tess] 32 when it [euery disease] consisteth, it is more certaine and better stayed
21. strike [II, 3, 1579, Rice] 91 colouring, crisping, platting, or striking forth of their haires
22. understanding [4a, 1585, Washington, T.] 40 It is an high onderstanding: wherefore we oguht [*sic*] to deuide the least portion of euerye tempered bodie as followeth
23. unperfect [*v*, 1568, Sidney] 50 perfect man in danger to be vnperfected
24. yearthly [1581, Lodge] 79 tallow ... the which is both drie and yearthly

5. Other

1. infester [ncit] 10 infestring the inward partes with innumerable corruption
2. purple-nosed [ncit] 93 they are also purple-nosed and hayrie about the breast
3. over-soft [ncit] 74 the one being ouersoft

COTTA, JOHN, *Ignorant practisers ... of physicke*, 1612

1. Antedatings

1. abdication [6, 1618, Bp. Hall] 124 the narrow inclosures of retired silence, and abdication vnto priuate contemplation
2. abrasion [3, 1751, *Chambers's Cycl.*] 18 the dysenterie or abrasion of her guts [a 1 cit]
3. accession [III, 1655, Vaughan] 66 my selfe ... gaue ... prediction of the conuulsion which after followed, and also of the termination of her Apoplecticke accessions in the lamenesse and palsie of some parts
4. accommodation [1a, 1644, Bulwer] 132 more distinct, iudicious and truly vnderstanding accommodation from more prudent right deliberation
5. accommodation [5, 1737, Johnson] 43 neither do I commend a trembling and timorous iudgement in prescription and accomodation therof [remedies]
6. accurate [1, Hobbes, 1651] better memorie which after may better thence guide it selfe to more large and accurate consideration

7. accurate [3, 1621, Burton] 120 Nature cannot decoct, infuse, compound ... but Art is vnto her benefite and seruice therein accurate
8. acquiescence [1, 1631, Donne] 134 repaying the vnknowne inexplicable nectar of the infinite acquiescence of mind, and ample content of rich ioy of heart vnto it selfe [a 1 cit]
9. acute [2, 1667, *Phil. Trans.*] 31 whom I found by a sharpe and acute conuulsion violently distorted
10. adaptation [2, 1790, Paley] 46 euen the greatest clerkes ... haue not blushed to borrow or learne a good medicine at a simple and vulgar hand ... in their owne more excellent adaptation ... conferring the full and true perfection
11. adherent [A, 1, 1615, Sandys] 108 by some il dispositio[n] adherent to the part
12. admission [1, 1622, Bacon] 74 the benefite of a physitions seruice or admission vnto the view of practise
13. affect [4, 1632, Sanderson] 96 though man by his starres be borne to infinite miseries, diuersly mouing and affecting him continually
14. affection [12, 1625, Sir H. Finch] 58 these with their diuellish affection, and intention are certaine proofs of diabolicall power and witchcraft
15. affinity [6, 1678, R. Russell] 123 The patterne of perfection doth shew the more and lesse perfect ... fro[m] which the farthest distance is the greatest defect and, and the nearest affinitie the best excellence
16. after-life [1833, Marryat] 8 men of better sort ... desirously oft times entertaine the messengers and ministers of vnrecoveable miserie vnto their after life [a 1 cit] [fpl]
17. alleviation [1625, Hart, *Anat. Ur.*] 84 immediately ... the same side that was let bloud, found present and sensible deliuery from those accidents with great lightsomnesse and alleuiation
18. analyse [2, 1758, Johnson] 59 euery eye is not able in so various a chaos to analyse and reduce them vnto their seuerall heads
19. ancient [B, 1b, 1615, Sandys] 82 the common & vulgar readings of the Ancients (the famous and learned Grecians)
20. annihilation [1a, 1638, Mede] 67 annihilation and frustration of wholesome and proper remedies [a 1 cit]
21. anxious [2, 1667, Milton] 2 Some are manifest, some anxious and ambiguous [a 1 cit]
22. arabic [1, 1650, Worthington] 82 innumerable dissentions amongst the learned concerning the Arabicke and Chymicke remedies
23. arbitrary [3, 1646, Browne] 94 the voluntarie motions and arbitrary actions of men
24. argute [1644, Bulwer] 35 the vanities and inanities of argute and subtill cousinages
25. artificer [5, 1635, N. Carpenter] 126 the end and perfection of art, which is the honour of the Artificer, the euer-reasonable satisfaction of needfull vse and necessitie

26. artificial [3, 1650, Cowley] 3 Some of them [accidents] bring certaine knowledge, some artificiall coniecture
27. artist [2, 1667, Milton] 118 beyond all other Artists the Physition immediatly hath need & vse of exquisite knowledge of nature
28. assimilate [*v*, 5, 1613, R. C., *Times Wh.*] 59 The forme of this disease, Hippocrates hath very fitly assimilated to the shape and fashion of drunkennesse
29. attend [II, 10, 1615, Markham] 125 For studie and contemplation must necessarily attend precept and industry both
30. audibly [1635, Jackson] 16 her child was audibly heard to cry [a 1 cit]
31. aurum potabile [1644, Quarles] 34 Aurum potabile ... dissolued pearle, and the like inestimable glories and pride of Art and nature [a 1 cit] [fpl]
32. balancing [2, 1666, Tillotson] 10 See **perpension**, anted.
33. besotted [3, 1831, Scott] 6 foolish and besotted braines
34. bewitchingly [1673, Halywell] 38 how powerfully and bewitchingly it deceiueth the distressed mind [a 1 cit]
35. bigamy [1b, 1635, J. Taylor] 134 the hated name and inured note of knowne ignorance & adulterate bigamie of two callings
36. blast [8a, 1639, Fuller] 56 to be blasted by the stupiditie of euery idle feare
37. co-operate [1a, 1616, Bullokar] 58 the act of any man consenting or cooperating
38. cohesion [3, 1690, Locke] 117 The order of nature in all her works is constant, full of wonder, and vnchanged truth in the continuall cohesion, sequence and fatall necessitie of all things [a 1 cit]
39. coincidence [2, 1650, Fuller] 86 the necessarie coincidence oft times of both callings requiring them at the same moment
40. collection [3c, 1697, Bp. Patrick] 15 See **exhaust**, anted.
41. commission [*sb*, 12b, 1659, Hammond] 25 Among those that are wise, a good conscience doth stay all rash commission
42. competent [5, 1647, Clarendon] 71 Euery one in these cases is not fit or competent arbiter
43. compiled [1886, *Athenæum*] 127 the rich compiled treasure of the excellent knowledges of many ages [fpl]
44. complaint [6, 1705, Arbuthnot] 65 her former fits and complaints vanished
45. compose [5b, 1709, Steele and Addison] 68 she lay or composed her selfe to rest
46. compose [13c, 1709, Steele and Addison] 68 the mouing power or facultie composed it selfe to a true and generall cessation and rest
47. concoction [2b, 1685, Cooke, J.] 107 See **maturation**, anted.
48. concourse [4, 1628, Preston] 58 a wild and confused concourse of accidents

49. conductive [a, 2, 1666, Smith, J. *Old Age*] 124 men haue with one generall decree and consent determined a necessitie of seuen euer presupposed conductiue helpes thereto
50. congruity [1b, 1626, Bacon] 101 Where there is an vnproportioned congruitie or susceptibilitie in the bodie or humors
51. consecution [1c, 1615, Crooke] 49 betweene a cause by accident and his effect, there is a mediate consequution
52. consecution [2, 1651, Biggs] 101 not only the imminence, but the present consecutio[n] of the dropsy
53. consent [*v*, 5, 1732, Berkeley] 58 the parties consent thereto
54. consistence [1b, 1613, Overbury, *Observ.*] 129 Lastly time well dispent doth point his proofe vnto examination of his seuerall degrees of groweth, both how in childhood and youth, vnto the years of discretion, disposed, and how also after that time in manhood and confirmed age vnto consistence, disposing himselfe
55. consisting [1, 1623, Hart] 128 The seeds of vertue ... in consisting age bringeth forth ripe fruite in practise and proofe [a 1 cit]
56. conspicuous [*a*, 2, R. C. 1613, *Table A.*] 113 benefits thereby haue euer bene conspicuous
57. constitution [4b, 1655, *Vulg. Errors confuted*] 100 corrupt and hote constitutions of the aire
58. consult [5b, 1639, Fuller] 50 they can scarce containe themselues from beleeuing and consulting with such ridiculous folly
59. contiguity [1, Wilkins, 1641, *Math. Magic.*] 108 It may be obiected, that by the contiguity of the wombe & bladder, and the meare termination of their extremities [a 1 cit]
60. contingent [*a*, 5, 1660, R. Coke] 2 the necessarie from the casuall and contingent
61. contraction [5b, 1871, Holmes] 62 some obscure contractions of some parts alreadie begunne
62. converse [*v*, 5, 1615, J. Stephens] 65 most continually conuersing with her
63. convulsion [2b, 1650, Bulwer] 37 He was sodainely surprised with acute and epilepticall fits and a generall conuulsion
64. convulsive [1a, 1615, Crooke] 64 if she suruiued her conuulsiue fits [a 1 cit]
65. course [III, 16b, 1665, Sir T. Herbert] 65 the course of naturall diseases
66. credited [1790, Ham. More] 133 in his profession carrying credited assurance [fpl]
67. crucify [2b, 1621, Burton] 9 many ... act like diuels crucifying the liues of poore men
68. deceivable [2, 1646, Browne] 105 neither is the iudgement by the vrine euer infallible, or not deceiuable, euen there where it is properly and foly allowed chiefe esteeme

69. declining [4b, 1615, Latham] 6 See **marasm**, anted.
70. defendant [*sb*, B, Ib, 1655, Hooke, *Micro.*] 101 The first is continually acted by common simple deluded people, the other patronaged by obstinate defendants of vaine paradoxes
71. derivation [3, 1660, Willsford] 104 It is a common practise in these dayes, by a colourable deriuation of supposed cunning from the vrine, to foretell casualities, and the ordinarie euents of life
72. desperateness [2b, 1667, *Decay Chr. Piety*] 55 nimble cunning, by continuall practise and custome working desperatenesse into facilitie
73. dignified [2, 1667, Marvell] 79 he spent some time in trauell beyond the sea, and returned againe thence dignified [a 1 cit]
74. diruption [1656, Blount *Glossogr.*] 26 her bloud grew so furious, that breaking the wonted bounds and limits of her veines, with violence it gushed out not onely at her mouth and nose ... but also made a diruption in the veines of one of her legs [a 1 cit]
75. dismiss [9, 1698, Fryer] 71 I will ... dismisse them both with a short historie
76. dispensation [3, 1646, Browne] 2 the manner, quantity, qualitie, and times of remedies: euery one requiring a separate and distinct respect and dispensation
77. dispensation [5b, 1665, Hooke] 117 nature in her dispensation of the whole world
78. dispense [4c, 1646, Browne] 27 necessity vrging, and therefore her age dispensing, I commanded her to be sparingly let bloud
79. dispenser [3, 1858, Simmonds] 1 wholesome medicines by the hands of the iudicious dispenser, are as Angels of God sent for the good of men
80. dissolved [*ppl a*, 2, 1707, *Curios. in Husb.*] 34 See **aurum potabile**, anted.
81. distinct [3d, 1654, Z. Coke] 78 There is to euery facultie belonging, first an habit of right iudging therein, and distinct knowing
82. distort [1, 1631, Donne] 31 I was sometime solicited by a carefull mother for her child, whom I found by a sharpe and acute conuulsion violently distorted
83. distracted [3, 1633, Austin] 77 such as haue spent most part of their life otherwise distracted, and haue not had entire emploiment in their callings
84. eclipsed [1, 1633, G. Herbert] 98 either the pride or splendor of the Sunne, mounting in his glorious altitude, or his eclipsed force and lightsomnesse opposed and abased?
85. education [3, 1616, Brinsley] 19 all that by institution, educatio[n], tradition, instruction, or stolne obseruatio[n] deriue their rule, example & custome from him
86. effect [5, 1668, *Phil. Trans.*] 49 Betweene a true cause and his proper effect, there is an immediate necessity

87. emerited [1664, Evelyn] 36 an emerited priuiledge in physicke practise [a 1 cit]
88. eminence [II, 4b, 1647, Clarendon] 124 an Artist … Vnto whom … either excellence doth giue true splendor and eminence
89. employment [2c, 1648, Gage] 73 by their owne emploiment … in applications and administrations vnto the sick
90. engage [13b, 1657, S. W.] 43 another so far ingaged in the Neapolitan disease
91. epileptical [*a*, 1, 1621, Burton] 37 See **convulsion**, anted.
92. equal [8, 1626, Bacon] 26 I found (oft obseruing her pulse) a manifest, equall and constant magnitude
93. event [3b, 1644, H. Parker] 8 these barbarous medicine-mongers, (good oft in their euent)
94. everyday [B, 1, 1647, Saltmarsh] 18 the continuall vse of euery-day-glysters
95. eviction [5, 1621, Sclater, W. *Tythes*] 69 I grant the voluntary and vncompelled, or duly and truly euicted confession of a witch, to be sufficient condemnation of her selfe and therefore iustly hath the law laid their bloud vpon their owne heads, but their confession I cannot conceiue sufficient euiction of the witchcraft it selfe
96. evidence [I, 1, 1655, Boyle] 102 who comparing the one with the other, cannot see, in which truth hath more euidence, and trust securitie?
97. evidently [2, 1690, Locke] 70 It is knowne euidently vnto learned men
98. excretion [3, 1630, Braithwait] 104 many other particular parts haue their peculiar excretions
99. execration [1b, 1688, Ellis] 82 Some with execration accuse and curse them as damned and hellish poysons
100. exhaust [*ppl a*, B, 1621, Burton *Anat. Mel.*] 15 the purulent collection after the 40 day exhaust
101. exiguity [1623, Cockeram] 99 as the greater abundance thereof doth necessarily more aduance and promote his efficacie, so the exiguitie thereof must needs abridge and obscure it
102. explode [1a, 1621, Burton] 109 the prediction of conception by the inspection of vrine, which also the most ingenuous and iudicious of writers … haue euer generally exploded as impious imposture
103. exposal [1, 1651, Moore, H. *Enthus. Tri.*] 135 not falling vnder the heauie burthen of thy owne guilt in rash exposall, or carelesse neglect
104. extravagant [5, 1650, Fuller] 133 immoderate, extrauagant and impertinent curiositie too prodigally dispent in things of least moment
105. extrication [1, 1650, Discoll, B.] 35 If men would consult with reason & iudiciously consider; though their wonders were truly to be wondered, and worthy to exercise the wise and learned in their extrication … yet must it neuer be forgotten, that wonders yea and miracles themselues are solie neuer arguments of truth or sufficiencie

106. fatal [7, 1681, Dryden] 106 they may more amply after exercise & satisfie themselues, whom their owne fatall stupiditie doth not detaine
107. fatuity [2, 1621, Burton] 63 great fatuitie and defect of reason
108. fit [3c, 1621, Burton] 37 See **convulsion**, anted.
109. fix [3b, 1663, Gerbier] 50 Fancie, according vnto the nature thereof, can seldome be long fixed vpon any thing
110. fluctuate [1, 1656, Blount] 38 small fractions of Quicksiluer fluctuating and floting like white pinnes heads [a 1 cit]
111. foreconsidered [I, 2a, 1677, Otway *Cheats*] 134 so many miserable calamities as daily fall out in want of more reasonable foreconsidered care thereof [a 1 cit] [fpl]
112. forestalling [3, 1642, R. Carpenter] 134 more likely forestalling of otherwise more casuall good
113. frequent [2b, 1632, tr. *Bruel Praxis Med.*] 62 With these fits (oft in the meane season first frequenting) at length she againe interchanged new
114. frightfully [1, 1621, Lady M. Wroth] 63 as if she had fearefully or frightfully espied somewhat hagging about her [a 1 cit]
115. gain [1c, 1648, *Eikon Bas.*] 53 he would ... gaine him to forgiue her
116. generous [2b, 1623, Cockeram] 117 more or lesse of generose desire and ingenuous exercise
117. golden [5, 1674, Godfrey] 125 ancient golden rules of truth
118. gratification [1d, 1669, Stillingfleet *Serm*] 70 the diuell doth vsually beguile ... perswading oft times those actions and euents to be his gratification of their malicious affections, which are indeed the very works of nature
119. gush [1,1682, P. Walker] 26 See **diruption**, anted.
120. habitually [2, 1682, Browne] 109 that which reason doth demo[n]strate, & art habitually performe
121. hermetical [2, 1664, Boyle] 83 See **monopoly**, anted.
122. high-coloured [1664, Pepys] 91 an vrine high-coloured, red, and thicke [fpl]
123. hoodwinked [1640, Bp. Hall] 97 for hoodwinked happe may sometimes light vpon truth [a 1 cit]
124. hydra-like [1666, Dryden] much more monstrous and Hydra-like [a 1 cit] [fpl]
125. hydropical [*a*, 3, 1649, Taylor, J.] 100 in some heuenly coniunctions or combinations there may arise an hydropicall constellation
126. hypochondriac [A, 1a, 1615, Crooke] 15 The other accused the hypochondriaca passio [a 1 cit]
127. illumination [1c, 1646, Browne] 121 all knowledge cometh either by the ordinarie light of nature, or the extraordinarie illumination of the Creator of nature
128. imaginary [B, 1, 1709, Mrs Manley] 51 by the iuglings of the imaginarie, are so liuely framed resemblances and counterfets

129. imminence [1, 1655, Fuller] 90 the danger and imminence of a Marasme
130. imperceptibility [1, Gilpin *Demonol.*] 13 It was imagined by some learned dissenting fro my first howres dislike, that it was no other but an imperceptibilitie of his pulse [a 1 cit]
131. impression [6a, 1632, J. Hayward] 69 the abusiue impression of some indiscreete whispering about the sicke
132. incumbence [1677, Hale *Contempl.*] 48 the businesse lesse, and the diligence and incumbence equall [a 1 cit]
133. incur [II, 5, 1627, Hakewill *Apol.*] 80 Great wounds and cuts of the head ... procure and incurre feauers
134. indefatigable [*a*, b, 1621, Burton *Anat. Mel.*] 120 long dayes and time carefully spent, indefatigable studie [a 1 cit]
135. indication [2, 1660, H. More] 104 the vrine is truly of it selfe and properly indication of no other immediate dispositions
136. indifference [6, 1644, Milton] 99 the body ... in the most different constellations doth comonly find indifference of alteration
137. individual [*a*, A, 3b, 1613, Jackson *Creed*] 118 For as all particulars do euer participate the nature and kind of the generall, and are there comprehended so besides that which vnto euerie indiuiduall nature is specially proper, there is an essentiall propertie in it belonging vnto the generall
138. inestimate [*a*, 1614, Rowlands *Fooles Bolt*] 123 so doth the generall slightnesse and lightnesse herein of most, sprinkle a common disgrace and ignomie vpon all, casting the excellent facultie it selfe inestimate almost behind the most inferiour science [a 1 cit]
139. infirmity [1b, 1614, Donne] 41 there is, and euer must be sometimes mistaking and infirmities
140. influence [5, 1652, Heylin] 53 some secret power or influence
141. inherent [*a*, 3b, 1622, Malynes, *Anc. Law-Mer.*] 108 The first is the action or function proper and inherent in the partie
142. institutor [2, 1675, Walker, A.] 129 The hope and opinion of good precept, doth vnto the most ignorant giue prudent guesse, either by the particular knowledge, or at least inquisition of precedent timely institution and likely institutors
143. intellection [1, 1614, Jackson] 126 frequent oft after reuiew of their former seuerall notions, reflecting the vnderstanding vpon it selfe in the recognition of his passed intellection
144. intelligible [2b, 1655, Fuller] 64 a mumbling ... vnto those that were thereto accustomed, oft intelligible
145. intermit [*v*[1], 2b, 1626, *Art ag. Dk. Buck.*] 15 a woman vexed with a palpitation of her heart, together with an oft intermission of her pulse, by an inward presentation mouing from a sodaine troubled agitation of her minde, would vsually vnto my selfe ... foretell when her pulse should stand and intermit [a 1 cit]

146. interposition [1b, 1650, Cromwell *Lett.*] 56 That the Sunne should stand still in the firmament, the Moone be ecclipsed in no interposition ... these and the like are miracles
147. intrusion [1, 1639, Woodall] 87 As for those that are of meane literature in their owne professions, their intrusion in others ... must needs preach their insufficiencie
148. inured [1619, Fotherby] See **bigamy**, anted. [a 1 cit]
149. jovial [2, 1665, Hooke] 99 many in the most Saturnine and deadly constellations liue, as the contrary also cause that many in the most faire and Iouiall die
150. judicate [*v*, 1638, Whitaker, T.] 3 some iudicate the constitution of the sicke [a 1 cit]
151. judication [1625, Hart] 3 significations, iudications and prognostications [a 1 cit]
152. marasm [1625, Hart] 6 Hence toward declining age (if not before) some fall into consumptions and marasmes [a 1 cit]
153. mastership [5b, 1697, Aubrey] 47 the pride and maister-ship of the medicine
154. maturation [5c, 1818, Thompson, E. *Cullen's*] 107 distractions of the naturall heate & spirits, by criticall intentions, concoctions, & maturations of diseases
155. medication [1b, 1626, Bacon] 4 dangerous diseases ... in short time grow too proud for any medication
156. medicine-monger [6a, 1651, Wittie *Prim. Pop. Err.*] 8 And hereby not onely the simple and vnlettered, but oft times men of better sort and qualitie, casting their eyes vpon some attempts of these barbarous medicine-mongers ... desirously oft times entertaine the messengers and ministers of vnrecoverable miserie [a 1 cit] [fpl]
157. meditated [1736, Gray] 80 without meditated differences and exceptions [a 1 cit]
158. membrane [1a, 1615, Crooke] 14 the skin or membrane of her belly
159. mercurial [5, 1657, Starkey] 37 he gaue vnto him a Ladanum pill of Paracelsus, and after Mercuriall pilles for another supposed end
160. mixed [8, 1767, Gooch] 14 a mixt and diuers coloured iaundies
161. monopolize [2, 1628, Prynne] 3 the monopolizing of cures vnto the prerogatiue of this or that secret
162. monopoly [3a, 1643, Browne *Relig. Med.*] 83 A third and more commendable sort differeth from both these, and leauing in the one his learned morositie and disdainfull impatience of different hearing, and in the other his ignorant and peruerse Hermeticall monopoly, with impartiall and ingenuous desire ... doth from both draw whatsoeuer may in either seeme good [a 1 cit]
163. mourn [1e, 1626, Bacon] 97 all things mourne, wither, fall and droupe
164. moving [2a, 1659, Leak] 68 See **compose**, anted.

165. nicotian [A, 1825, Scott *Diary*] 5 And fro[m] this Nicotian fume grow now adaies, doubtlesly, many our frequent complaints [a 1 cit]
166. obscure [4b, 1757, Foote] 3 sometimes the accident doth obscure the disease
167. obvious [4, 1635, Quarles] 42 her smiles are obuious to any one
168. occasion [4, 1634, Sir T. Herbert] 11 occasioned and helped by bookes and reading
169. oracle [III, 6, 1625, Hart] 53 Women oft times out of their sleepes haue foreseene and foretold many things ... but this doth make their dreames no oracles
170. originally [3, 1654, Bramhall] 112 If therefore the vnderstanding be either in it selfe originally defectiue, or by want of time vnsetled
171. over-use [1862, Ansted] 6 their ignorant and rash ouervse [a 1 cit]
172. overrun [10, 1633, Bp. Hall] 132 euer either ouerrunne or come short of that happie and safe issue
173. parity [3, 1620, Venner] 17 by mistaking parities for imparities disioyne helpes better vnited
174. parson-physician [1625, Hart] 14 (margin) A Parson-Physition [a 1 cit] [fpl]
175. percolation [a, 1613, Purchas *Pilg.*] 105 and the thinne aquositie oft onely issueth by so straight a percolation, as can carrie no signe [a 1 cit]
176. permistion [1615, Crooke *Body*] 37 as also by the more perfect permistion thereof with the substance of the vrine [a 1 cit]
177. perpension [1646, Browne *Pseud. Ep.*] 10 The Empericke is he who reiecteth the disquisition of diseases and remedies, their causes, natures & qualities according to iudgement and vnderstanding, and the carefull perpension and ballancing of his action [a 1 cit]
178. perplex [1b, 1686, tr. *Chardin's Coron*] 14 She was miserably perplexed with the doubtfull deliuery of a dangerously begunne abortion
179. personal [4, 1614, T. Lorkin] 29 to exchange reasonable likelihood, for personall confidence
180. perspective [5, 1620, Shelton] 112 thence accomplished brightness of his beames doth seasonably breake forth, and soly giue the rectified perspectiue of particular objects
181. pinching [1, 1693, Evelyn] 63 Hereof was oft made triall by pinching and the like
182. pin-head [1, 1662, R. Mathew] 38 See **fluctuate**, anted. [a 1 cit]
183. potent [2, 1715, Rowe] 53 a wandring Surgeon, whom fame, it seemeth, had magnified for charmed and potent cures of such as were bewitched
184. precipitate [III, 5, 1644, Digby] 39 Barbers and Surgeons, who precipitate commonly euery one alike
185. preconsult [*v*, 1620, Wotton, *Reliq.*] 71 Euery one in these cases is not fit or competent arbiter: it requireth the learned ... whom euer to preconsult in these occasions is onely safe [a 1 cit]

186. preparation [6, 1646, Browne] 108 the ordinary recrements of concoctions, or other preparatio[n]s
187. prevalence [2, 1631, Power] 25 See **tax**, anted.
188. privatively [*adv*, 1, 1659, More, H. *Imm. Soul*] 105 neither is the iudgement by the vrine euer infallible ... diuers impediments both positiuely and priuatiuely forestalling his right estimate: positiuely either by assumption of diuers meates, drinkes or medicines, or when diuers diseases ... together send downe their seuerall or contrary recrements into the vrine, and thereby confound the true iudgement of any of them therein; or thereby priuatiuely, when ... by stoppages ... the substance, colour and contents of the vrine are intercepted
189. proclivity [1b, 1649, J. Taylor] 56 to be blasted by the stupiditie of euery idle feare ... must needs be base procliuitie and vnlearned lightnesse
190. profane [1b, 1616, Jonson] 4 wholesome remedies in vulgar and prophane hands
191. propension [1c, 1626, Bacon] 32 In any propension thereto in the constitution or other disposition of the child, was nothing which might apparently be accused
192. proving [1620, *Form of Service*] 5 vntill this prouing time [a 1 cit]
193. pulsation [1b, 1645, Howell] 15 her pulse should stand and intermit ... sometimes three or foure pulsations
194. radiation [1, 1626, Bacon *Sylva*] 97 No man can deny the heauens as generall and superiour causes to haue power ouer all things created vnder heauen, by whose influence and radiation all things increase
195. reasonlessly [1889, *Harper's*] 90 endlessly and reasonlesly vaine [a 1 cit] [fpl]
196. reception [3b, 1850, Maurice] 126 prompt apprehension and reception of generall rules
197. recrement [2, 1615, Crooke] 108 See **preparation**, anted. [a 1 cit]
198. regularly [3, 1668, Dryden] 120 regularly purge the right and proper humor
199. relaxation [3, 1626, Bacon] 17 a rupture and a relaxation ... dissemble themselues
200. remainder [3c, 1641, Milton] 62 her pulse or breathing onely witnessing a remainder of life
201. repented [1660, Hickeringill] 33 Carelesse attempts draw harmfull and repented issues [a 1 cit]
202. revelation [2b, 1862, Spencer] 94 they hooke simple credulitie to worship and admire their lying revelations
203. saturnine [2, 1862, G. Wilson] 99 a maligne and saturnine aspect
204. sense [11, 1684, Roscommon] 50 idle words and sentences, which all that haue sense, know to be voide of sense
205. sensibleness [5, 1888, Spectator] 131 Thus with a plaine sensiblenesse vnto vulgar capacitie

206. shape [9, 1667, Milton] 65 the fits and accidents which befell this gentlewoman ... with the seuerall shapes of some diseases before mentioned
207. simplicity [2c, 1633, Ford] 104 It is a common practise ... to foretell casualities ... which while impudence doth gloriously set forth, the common simplicitie doth worship and reuere
208. socratically [*adv*, 1641, Smectymnus *Answ.*] 96 Of this sort haue bene not onely one Socrates and the great Philosophers, but many common men Socratically disposed [a 1 cit] [fpl]
209. solicit [7, 1732, Arbuthnot] 63 After I had ... by some quicke medicines solicited nature to a better remembrance of her selfe
210. sphacelate [*a*, 1634, Johnson, T. *Parey's*] 36 These men for the most part esteeming themselues deseruing well for the operary vses of a skilfull and well exercised hands in wounds, incisions, amputations of sphacelate parts and the like [a 1 cit]
211. spurge-comfit [1619, Dalton] 32 her ordinary vse of spurge-comfits [a 1 cit] [fpl]
212. stamp [8d, 1780, Bentham] 77 their imperfect parts stamped and expressed in their daily conuersation
213. stamp [13d, 1652, J. Smith] 123 any ... liuely stampe of iudicious disposition
214. stertor [b ||, 1849, *Blackwood's Mag.*] 37 foming, gnashing his teeth, loud stertors and the like [a 1 cit]
215. structure [3a, 1615, Chapman] 120 the structure and great frame of heauen and earth
216. stupefied [1639, J. Taylor] 69 other parts be stupified or asleepe [a 1 cit]
217. susceptibility [1, 1803, Beddoes] 101 See **congruity**, anted. [a 1 cit]
218. tax [7, 1614, Sir R. Dudley] 25 We may iustly here taxe their dangerous whisperings about the sicke, wherein their preualence oft being too great, they abuse the weake sense of the diseased
219. termination [5b, 1806, V. Knox] 65 the ordinarie terminations of an Apoplexie
220. unchewed [1646, Quarles] 77 they may in haste and greedily swallow vp whole sentences, yea & volumes vnchewed [a 1 cit]
221. uncontroversed [*ppl a*, 1634, Jackson, *Creed*] 95 yet doth the generall concordant consent of most Diuines grant as vncontrouersed, a libertie and freedome of mans will [a 1 cit] [fpl]
222. undiscoverable [1642, Quarles] 106 finding it thereby vndiscouerable, searcheth it by another disquisition
223. undissolved [3, 1674, Scheffer's *Lapland*] 38 one whole pill vndissolued
224. unexperienced [2, 1698, Norris] 11 vntried & vnexperienced truths
225. unfold [1d, 1779, *Mirror*] 56 the cause and reason thereof doth vnfold it selfe to few

226. unheeded [b, 1682, Creech] 40 the harmes vnheeded [a 1 cit]
227. uninterrupted [2, 1657, Cromwell] 105 an vninterrupted certaine iudgement
228. unjudging [1679, J. Goodman] 128 childhood ... in whose vniudging youth their hidden vertue stealeth roote [a 1 cit] [fpl]
229. unjustifiable [1641, Clarendon] 27 euer vniustifiable in the ignorant counsellor [a 1 cit]
230. unlicensed [2b, 1649, J. Taylor] 45 an vnlicenced friendship
231. unobservedly [1656, Earl Orrery] 4 vnobseruedly confirmed in mens bodies [a 1 cit]
232. unsettle [1b, 1649, Milton] 129 there is no goodnesse by time vnsetled hath euer bene after well confirmed
233. urinary [4b, 1822, Good] 108 The expulsiue faculty of the seminarie vessels, mouing sometimes with the vrinarie
234. urinary [*a*, 2, 1646, Browne *Pseud. Ep.*] 106 Concerning the looking of vnborne babes in an vrinarie glasse, and the making of old fooles in loue with their owne reflexion
235. vendication [1658, Phillips] 94 The vnlimited expatiation of so foule wrongs, do challenge all men, not onely the learned, but all honest or ingenuous, vnto the vendication of art and truth from oppression
236. ventilate [8a, 1706, Phillips] 120 ventilate or euacuate the corrupt bloud from the bruised part
237. verbally [2b, 1855, T. Lynch] 80 He that simply and verbally onely vnderstandeth
238. vicissitude [4, 1616, Jonson] 99 the heauens by their motion varying, bring vnto all things vicissitudes, changes, and alterations

2. *New senses*

1. absolved 78 Therefore those that are perfect and absolued artists in their owne facultie, and will impaire their dignitie by engaging it in another
2. advantaged 130 The first haue therefore more certaine vnderstanding, the second somewhat more aduantaged coniecture
3. after-review 126 See **intellection**, anted.
4. condition 7 Rhabarb is said to be the life of the liuer, yet in some conditions thereof it is an enemie
5. consent 108 neither doth their raritie in their motion alwaies then meete or consent with the vrine
6. contemper 99 an equall contemper of all the humors
7. diseased 19 needelesly hazarding the diseased
8. dispent 133 by his ... study and industry well knowne, commendably formerly, and euer dispent
9. estate 7 Purgatio[n]s in some estates with preparatiues ... are harmefull
10. facility 128 Compare the fecilitie of soyle with capacitie in nature
11. indian 5 Since the riotous vse of this strange Indian [tobacco]

12. intention 106 partly by the consequent stoppages of the body, and partly by distracting the naturall heate and spirits from other parts vnto that new intentio[n]
13. interchange 62 With these fits ... at length she againe interchanged new
14. mercurial 6 See **silver-salve**, unrec.
15. recalculate 70 let also be recalculate and cast the strange and slie suggestions of the fancie
16. removed 98 the heauens are outward causes, and remoued causes
17. stertor 37 See **stertor**, anted.
18. undergrowth 36 Some also venture farther ... to educate & institute Physitions, as an vnder-growth vnto themselves, by lying promises

3. Unrecorded

1. after-health 44 the happinesse of after-health
2. after-repented 134 so many lucklesse euents of after-repented choices
3. after-time 131 after-time hath still otherwise proued it
4. animal faculty 67 The power of voluntary motion, which is the animall facultie
5. apted 47 the maine and continuall exercise therein, doth therein also make the meaner iudgement better apted and more prompt
6. both-hand 87 their double and both-hand emploiment
7. cast upon 34 Now seeing we are cast vpon the mention of the former sort of men
8. common-visiting 14 common-uisiting counsellors
9. counsel table 102 a famous Ephemerides-master ... not knowing ... from the counsel table of his Ephemerides pronounced, that ... he made no doubt of his recouerie
10. day-habit 68 The sense and incumbrance of the day-habite is euer an hinderance of perfect sleepes
11. deigning 82 yet did he with humble and daigning desire search & entertaine from any sort of people
12. easie deceiued 94 the common and easie deceiued vulgars
13. ephemerides-master See **counsel-table**, unrec.
14. ever-reasonable 126 See **artificer**, anted.
15. exenterate 88 they exenterate and eate out the bowels of poore mens purses
16. foredoubt 65 a generall stupiditie of one side of her bodie, being the ordinarie terminations of an Apoplexie, and therefore foredoubted
17. funeral feast 33 It was then her feare that he had tasted his owne funeral feast before his death
18. hypochondriaca passio 15 The other accused the hypochondriaca passio
19. indistracted 79 indistracted vigilance and circumspection
20. italian disease 12 The French, Spanish, Neapolitane, Italian disease was a stranger sometime in old Albion

21. lenocination 93 the spirit of flattering intrusion and secret lenocination of false hopes
22. make against 66 It maketh yet farther against the opinion of witchcraft
23. marvelled 62 in a much maruelled fashion
24. never-deceiving 117 the neuer deceiuing generall grounds in the generall dispensation in the nature of all things
25. night-weeds 67 prepared at the night for bed, and vnclothed into her night-weeds
26. over-religious 101 the ouer religious esteeme thereof
27. oversute 42 these men ... may hap luckily to ouersute the danger
28. paper-apothecary-shop 23 paper-Apothecary-shoppes of secrets and medicines
29. pergamene 82 the thrise worthy and renowmed Pergamene Claudius Galen
30. presention 15 an inward presention mouing from a sodaine troubled agitation of her minde
31. seminary vessel 108 The expulsiue facultie of the seminarie vessels
32. sense-informing 114 all other sense-informing meanes and inquisitions of knowledge and science
33. silver-salve 6 such a rottennes ... as suffreth few of our Mercurials to liue, to know their age in health, especially who throughly knew the siluer-salue in their youth
34. Solomon's fly 46 men ... with safe discretion refuse them, fearing lest with Solomons fly being taken in the Apothecaries boxe, they also in like manner make a stinke of the medicine
35. spelling school 49 bad scholers were still at spelling schoole
36. strange seeming 58 their strange seeming formes
37. suck-giving 16 the breasts of a suck-giuing nurse
38. uncontroversed 95 yet doth the generall concordant consent of most Diuines grant as vncontrouersed, a libertie and freedome of mans will
39. undazedly 86 the eagle-eye of cleare & sincere iudgement, seldome vndazedly, or without winking, fixed vpon the perfect brightnesse
40. ungusted 134 In the wise ... succeedeth euer for the sometimes deceiued issue, ordinarily redoubled recompence, of fooles vngusted, but vnto the end deseruing it
41. unwotting 8 numbers of vnwotting innocents
42. unwottingly 9 vnwottingly to the poore patient, vnwittingly to the vnskilfull workeman
43. urinary glass 106 See **urinary**, anted.
44. weale-advising [To the reader] Thy weale-aduising friend

4. Postdatings

1. divine [*sb*, 1, 1587, Holinshed] 95 yet doth the generall concordant consent of most Diuines grant as vncontrouersed, a libertie and freedome of mans will

2. election [2b, 1602, Fulbecke] 9 none almost labour to know with election and according to reason
3. event [2, 1602, Fulbecke] 53 the strange operation of the medicine foretold by the Surgeon, caused the friends about her still to expect some admirable euent of recouerie
4. exequious [1603, Drayton] 18 Hence the vnconsiderate and vnlearned to distinguish, are easily induced, sometimes by vaine hope deceiued to physicke death, sometime too fearefully despairing with exequious offices to comber life and the recouerie of death
5. material [3d, 1541, Copland] 20 There are no materiall diseases wherein the common remedies are not requisite
6. reference [2, 1604, Shakespeare] 67 To the first doth satisfie the former manifest reference of all accidents befalling the gentlewoman mentioned, vnto the prevalence and power of diseases before related
7. roundness [1572, Jones] 71 drawing his head and heeles violently backward, and in that sort carrying his whole body into a roundnesse
8. ructuation [1539, Elyot] 91 painfull distentions and ructuations
9. scour [1584, Munday] 34 scouring vp before them goodly store of harnesse wherewith men of all sorts may arme themselues against all diseases
10. unscanted [1599, Daniel] 135 vnscanted counsell in all occurrents
11. vary [1570, Levins] 3 So that according to the kindes, places, changes and courses of accidents, varie significations, iudications and prognostications
12. verified [1594, Carew] 4 It is a verified and true saying

5. Other

1. after-settling [ncit] 79 they admitted not so true and right after-setling of the second

HESTER, JOHN, *A short discourse*, 1580

1. Antedatings

1. accused [*sb*, 1593, Shakespeare] Aii[r] The good Prince notwithstanding being offered the medicine by the accused, first tooke it, and dranke it vp, and then gaue the Phisition the letter of his accuser to reade [a 1 cit]
2. anatomist [B, 1594, B. T. *La Prim.*] Biii[r] he that wil know the composition of mans body, must of necessitie haue some science, and be Anatomist
3. aperitive [*a*, 2, 1582, Hester, *Secr. Ph.*] Fiii[v] To cure the third cause it were necessary to purge with aperatiue things [a 1 cit]
4. application [2, 1601, Shakespeare] Riv[r] bicause many good and profitable things thorow the want of perfect applycation in time and place many times do hurt

5. aromatized [1661, Lovell *Hist. An.*] Hii^{r} I ordayned a colde Sirope ... and Aromatised it with Muske and Rose water [a 1 cit]
6. cancrenated [1582, Hester *Secr. Ph.*] Biv^{r} wounds ... beeing impostumated, or cancrenated [a 1 cit]
7. captain [3, 1590, Cope] Aii^{r} a worthye and famous Capitaine, called Signior LEONARDO PHIORAVANTI
8. cattarhous [*a*, 1651, Biggs *New Disp.*] Niii^{v} The Cough is caused of a cattarus humor [a 1 cit]
9. caustic [*sb*, 1582, Hester *Secr. Ph.*] Di^{r} The cure of these kindes of vlcers is to apply quickly our *Caustike* to mortifie the euill [a 1 cit]
10. centipede [1601, Holland, and ns] Fiii^{v} See **hog lice** anted. [a 1 cit]
11. cicatrize [1582, Hester *Secr. Ph.*] Biv^{v} All manner of sores that doe not cicatrize perfectly and haue communication with the inward partes, are called Fistoloes
12. clutter [*v*, 1601, Holland *Pliny*] Ri^{v} Rec. Antimoni and calcine it vntill it will smoke no more ... and al wayes as it cluttereth, stampe it agayne
13. communication [6, B, 1715, Desaguliers] Biv^{v} See **cicatrize**, anted.
14. complexionated [1654, Ashmole] Mii^{v} which water is ... giuen to drinke to any that is infirmed or euil complexcionated [a 1 cit]
15. contusion [2, 1593, Shakespeare] Biv^{v} There is an other kinde of Imposthume, that is ingendered of a contusion or broose ...
16. desperate [3a, 1586, Mulcaster] Iiv^{v} in short time the most part were holpe, and there dyed none so desperate as they did afore
17. diapalma [1, 1646, Browne] Dii^{r} lay theron the *Cerote Diapalma* [a 1 cit]
18. difficulty [b, 1747, *Coll. Rec. Penn.*] Li^{r} the which was troubled with a difficultie of vrine
19. discourse [*sb*, 5, 1581, Pettie] tp A short discours of the excellent Doctour and knight
20. dissension [2, 1582, Hester *Secr. Ph.*] Fii^{r} To helpe the tooth atch, that is caused of rotten teeth, or that commeth of a dissention of the heade
21. divinely [2, 1582, Hester *Secr. Ph.*] Ei^{r} this digestiue being applied to a putrified vlcer, worketh diuers effects, for it healeth it diuinely
22. dose [1, 1600, Vaughan, W.] ¶iv^{r} a dose of our imperial powder [a 1 cit]
23. embassador [1603, Shakespeare] Kiv^{v} a certaine Gentleman of the Imbassadours of *Portingall* [a 1 cit]
24. epiderma [1582, Hester *Secr. Ph.*] Hiii^{v} in that extreme part of the toes, that skinne that is called *Epiderma*, is hard, and wil not suffer it to passe or exalare, and there many times it ingendreth a tumor [a 1 cit]
25. expense [3, 1632, Hayward] Mi^{r} and [everyone] shall not neede to seeke the naturall Balme, with so much expenses and daunger of the life
26. fantastical [6, 1599, Shakespeare] Gi^{r} This *Pellaria* is a certeine kinde of fantasticall infirmity the which we ... do know [th]e cause, the which is by vsing company with women corrupted with the pockes

27. fistulated [*ppl a*, 1612, Woodall] Ci^{r} those sores that are vpon the bone ... many times remaine fistolated [a 1 cit]
28. gild [1b, 1674, Boyle] Piii^{r} the quantitie is from one dram to two drams in the morning fasting, but ye may not guild them in anye wise, but drincke after them a cup of water or wine
29. hog lice [1587, Mascall] Fiii^{v} giue him to drinke the powder of Hogge lyce or *Centum pedes* [a 1 cit]
30. horsefish [1723, Morland] Hiv^{v} There is also a great secret in the tooth of a Horsefish if it be worne on a mans finger [a 1 cit]
31. impostumate [*v*, 2, 1607, Markham] Eii^{v} When that woundes are euel healed and that they impostumate, and that the arme, or legge, or other partes where they were wounded is indurated and full of paine [a 1 cit]
32. indisposition [2, 1598, Florio] Dii^{r} as for those Imposthumes that come by indisposition of Nature [a 1 cit]
33. indisposition [3, 1598, Holland] Kiv^{v} these foure remedies may help against al indispositions inwardly [a 1 cit]
34. indurated [1, 1594, Plat *Jewel-ho.*] Eii^{v} See **impostumate**, anted. [a 1 cit]
35. infistolated [*ppl a*, 1706, Phillips ed. Kersey] Kiii^{v} a man ... the which had a Fistoloe in the lower parts ... with .xi. holes infistolated at the which .xi. he made water [a 1 cit]
36. inflame [*v*, 7, 1607, Topsell] Kii^{r} there was a certeine kinde of fish [tha]t as soone as they touched the flesh of a man, presentlye it inflamed
37. install [b, 1647, Ward] Aii^{v} God ... enstall you among his chosen
38. intestinall [1599, A. M. *Gabel.*] Miii^{v} it draweth from al parts, and euacuateth the humours intestinall [a 1 cit]
39. inveterated [1597, Lowe] Ci^{v} the same [scabbe] is also of the french poxe Inueterated [a 1 cit]
40. ligament [1, 1599, A. M. *Gabel.*] Eiii^{v} binde the wounde with ligaments very straight
41. luted [1601, Holland *Pliny*] Fi^{r} Take a retort of glasse, wel luted [a 1 cit]
42. magistral [2, 1605, Bacon *Adv. Learn.*] Eiv^{v} Of our magistral Vnguent that helpeth diuers sortes of sores
43. meatus [1665, Glanvill] Fiii^{v} the stone that inge[n]dreth in the bladder ... stoppeth the *Meati* or powers that the vryne can not passe [a 1 cit]
44. mineral [*a*, 3, 1581, *Tr. Jew. Hist. Soc. Eng.*] Mii^{v} this is the stone that the Philosophers haue long sought to fixe their medicine mynerall [a 1 cit]
45. neapolitan [*a*, A, 1596, Shakespeare] Iii^{r} There was a certeine Gentleman Neapolitan [a 1 cit]
46. operation [3b, 1605, Bacon] Aii^{r} by that same medecine (although extreame in operation) presently recouered his former health
47. oxycroceum [1646, Browne] Dii^{r} the Cerote of *Oxycrocij* is excellent [a 1 cit]

48. pellagra [1811, Hooper] Gi^r To helpe Pellaria, that is a disease which causeth the haire and bearde to fall away [a 1 cit]
49. penetrating [1, 1598, Florio] Oi^v it will helpe the rupture, and all sortes of woundes penetrating and vlcers of the longes [a 1 cit]
50. presently [6, 1634, Tyrwhit] Aii^r See **operation**, anted.
51. projection [2, 1594, Plat *Jewel-ho.*] Mii^v so that making the proiection they ioyne the medicine with metalling bodyes, and not to go away in fume [a 1 cit]
52. questioning [1, 1635, Sibbes] Lii^v There hath alwayes beene a greate questioning among the Philosophers [a 1 cit]
53. rasped [1599, A. M. *Gabel.*] Ni^r *Rec.* One pounde of *Lignum sanctum, Raspead* [*sic*] [a 1 cit]
54. rectified [2, 1605, Timme *Quersit.*] Eiii^r *Aqua vitæ* rectified, pou[n]d
55. refriscative [1582, Hester, *Secr. Ph*, and ns] Riii^r a delycate Vnguent, an refriscatiue, which cicatrizeth vlcers with great speede [a 1 cit]
56. relax [1b, 1620, Venner *Via Recta*] Fiii^r the powers are too much relaxed or opened
57. restriction [3b, cf. 3a, 1758, Sparrow, J. *Le Dran*] Fiii^v The third is caused of an obstruction or restriction of the powers
58. restringe [2, 1604, Wright, T.] Fiii^r ye shall giue … halfe a dram of Masticke with a little Plantaine water, for this is hot and restringeth the powers [a 1 cit]
59. sarcocolla [1599, Hakluyt] Hiv^v Rosen of the Pine tree that is drye, *Olibanum, Masticke, Sarcocolla* [a 1 cit]
60. scolopendra [2, 1608, Topsell *Ff. B.*] Ii^r *Scolopendria*, one ounce [a 1 cit]
61. signior [1a, 1584, Greene] Aii^r a worthye and famous Capitaine, called Signior LEONARDO PHIORAVANTI
62. specie [II, 5, 1644, *Doc. Lett. Pat. at Ox.*] ¶iv^r these medicines … *Quintaessencia solutiua, Specie Imperiale*
63. stocado [1582, Hester *Secr. Ph.*] Iiii^r That being done, the sayde Generall ryse [*sic*] from the table … & gaue him 5. stocados in the breast [a 1 cit]
64. stomachal [2, 1599, A. M. *Gabel.*] Niv^r [th]e cinamon is stomacall [a 1 cit]
65. stove [4, 1640, Brugis, T.] Lii^r The remedies that helpe the pockes are … *Oriola* … a stoue of hearbes
66. stow [*sb*, 3, 1599, A. M. *Gabel.*] Fiii^{r-v} keepe them warme in bedde vntill ye haue ended to anoynt him, and then go to the stowe, and he shall be helpt of that infirmitie
67. talpa [2, 1693, *Blancard's*] Biv^v In the head there grow certeine kindes of sores that are called *Talpa* or *Topinare*
68. tenting [*v*, 4, 1597, A. M. *Guill.*] Ci^r such sores as tary long before they be incarnated come to fistoloes, & many times it commeth through long

curing, by tenting with their tentes, the which are cause that nature maketh a *Callow* [a 1 cit]

69. unglazed [1599, A. M. *Gabel.*] Riii^{v} an earthen panne vnglased [a 1 cit]

70. varnish [*sb*, 1e, 1899, Allbutt *Syst. Med.*] Eiii^{r} *Rec.* Lyquid Vernish, pound .3

71. vegetable stone [1d, 1652, Ashmole] Mii^{r} The way to make the vigitable stone is rare [a 1 cit]

72. viscousness [1594, Plat *Jewel-ho.*] Fiv^{r} The third cause is a certein viscousnesse the which holdeth to the botome of the Vrinal [a 1 cit]

73. wind furnace [30d, 1651, French] Liii^{r} distill it in a winde furnace, so that ye maye make fire with woode [a 1 cit]

74. youthfully [1581, Mulcaster] Liv^{r} The first water ... the face being washed ther-with ... preserueth it youthfully [a 1 cit]

2. *New senses*

1. caret Miii^{r} aromatise it with two caretes of Muske

2. centipede Fiii^{v} See **hog lice**, anted.

3. disunited Iiv^{r} this order of curing is very naturall, for Nature doth shew it in hearbes, plantes, and stones, how that they cannot stande dis vnited [*sic*]

4. intestinals Hiv^{r} The Hemerhodes are a certeine kind of euil tumor, caused of the bloud in the veynes Emorodiale and these come alwayes in the extremitie of the Intestinals

5. metalling Mii^{v} See **projection**, anted.

6. mundification Ei^{r} Of the mundification vnguent wherewith they dresse the woundes

7. refriscative Riii^{r} a delycate Vnguent, an refriscatiue, which cicatrizeth vlcers with great speede

8. spina Niv^{r} a certeine kinde of frute called of some, *Spina merula*, of other *Spini ceruino*, with his bery they make a kinde of sap greene

3. *Unrecorded*

1. affectioned Aii^{v} The moste affectioned of all those, which owe your L. dutifull seruice

2. aqua celestis Eii^{v} wash it with our *Aqua celestis*

3. aqua realle Lii^{r} those remedies that helpe the scabbes are *Aqua realle*

4. aromatico Li^{v} I gave him a quantitie of our *Aromatico*

5. assutiliate Civ^{v} this medicine doth assuttiliate the matter that runneth vnto the wound

6. caruoli Gii^{v} Those *caruoli* that come vppon the yarde, are of diuerse kindes

7. citrach Diii^{r} hearbes that coole the lyuer and purifie the bloud, as ... Citrach

8. dictamus albus Lii^{r} those that are troubled with paines in the bodye, may vse … *Dictamus albus*
9. distemperament Giv^{v} The other is caused of great heat, Feuer, and distemperament of Nature, and this is called *Disenteria*
10. epitemum Miii^{v} Rec. … Epitemu[m]
11. fess Mii^{v} grinde them … distill them … and alwayes at the last giue it a stronge fire that the fesses may remaine well burnt
12. fest[13] Hi^{v} and his common drinke was wine and water boyled on the festes of the same [decoction]
13. fistola lacrimosa Ci^{v} The fistoloes that come in the eyes, are called *fistola lacrimosa*
14. formicola Cii^{r} Of Formicola and his effects
15. imperial powder ¶iv^{r} See **dose**, anted.
16. mal di formica Hii^{r} his disease came of the Pockes, and those sores are commonly called *Mal di formica*
17. marte militare Hiii^{r} it wer necessary to extinguish the heat … which thou shalt doe with the rednesse of Marte Militare … for that is the most souereigne remedie
18. mathematica Bi^{v} Other vnderstand the *Mathematica*, whereby they measure land and all other thinges
19. mesue Mii^{r} two ounces *Electuario de succo rosarum, Mesue*
20. oleum Oiii^{v} To make our oleum benedictum
21. oleum benedictum Oiii^{v} See **oleum**, unrec.
22. olivella Lii^{r} The remedies that helpe the pockes are these … *Olivella*
23. petigine Diii^{v} Ther is an other kinde of scabbe that goeth creeping with a dry crust like vnto petigine
24. petra philosophalla ¶ii^{r} And first to make our petra philosophalla
25. plaintain water Fiii^{r} See **restringe**, anted.
26. rottory Qi^{r} a sore is mortified with a rottorye made of Subblimate, or Arsenicke
27. sine Lii^{r} those remedies that helpe the feuers of all sortes, the which are these, the sirope of Burrage … Sine
28. specie imperiale ¶iv^{r} See **specie**, anted.
29. squamma ferri Ii^{r} *Rec. squamma ferri* one ounce
30. stocate Biii^{v} some [woundes] are thrusts or stocate
31. testinals Cii^{v} Woundes … in the stomacke or belly or in *Testinalles*, in the bladder
32. topinare Biv^{v} In the head there grow certeine kindes of sores that are called *Talpa* or *Topinare*
33. ulcera Biv^{r} when it is cancrenated, it is called *Vlcera corasiva* bicause it goeth eating and creeping on the flesh
34. ulcera corasiva Biv^{r} See **ulcera**, unrec.
35. ulcera putrida Biv^{r} But when the wou[n]d is impostumated and full of matter, it is called, *Vlcera putrida*

36. ulcera sordida Biv[r] But when it is neither cancrenated nor yet apostumated, but that through some euill disposition the wound is closed ... then it is called *Vlcera sordida*

4. Postdatings

1. consolida [1480, Caxton] Oi[v] This *Consolida magore* is a herbe
2. inspecially [1557, North] Liv[v] The Oyle of Balme, doth serue ... inspecially for woundes in the heade [fpl]
3. orielle [1400, Mandeville] See **stove**, anted.
4. repercute [1578, Banister] Li[v] *Aromatico* with Plantayne water ... euacuate the stomacke, repercute and mittigateth [th]e alteration

HILL, THOMAS, *A ioyfull iewel*, 1579

1. Antedatings

1. absterse [1646, Browne] Hiii[v] the *Oyle of Roses* is absterge [*sic*] and molificatiue [a 1 cit]
2. aforenamed [D, 1603, Knolles] Ci[v] All the aforenamed deuices were left of, and euery man did as it liked him best [a 1 cit]
3. aperitive [*a*, 2, 1582, Hester] Eiiii[v] This Oyle of Sulfur is ... aperative [a 1 cit]
4. benjamin [1, 1580, Hollyband] Cii[v] Receiue *Tigname*, which is a sweet wood, *white Sau[n]ders, Storax calamite, Bengimine* [a 1 cit]
5. calx [2, 1581, Styward] Hii[v] Receiue red hens dung, the dung of an Oule, quick Snailes *Calux vise*
6. catarrhal [1651, Biggs] Hi[r] appropriat vnto that kinde of catterall pestile[n]ce that raigneth with colde [a 1 cit]
7. centre [2b, 1606, Shakespeare] Biii[v] Often times the Water is corrupted by the cause of the center aswel as by the other causes of planets
8. common vein [18a, 1842, Wilson] Ciii[v] hee tooke blood of the common vain
9. consequent [*a*, 7, 1692, Locke] Gi[v] Our *Quintæssence* by nature preserueth all things that is put therein, and by consquent beeing in the stomack: it preserueth all the body inwardly
10. dishabit [1595, Shakespeare] Biii[v] and for that cause many places are dishabited [a 1 cit]
11. divinely [2, 1582, Hester] Diiii[v] ye shall put therin our *Cowstick* once only, because it purgeth it deuinely
12. dose [1, 1600, Vaughan] Eiii[v] the dose is half an ounce [a 1 cit]
13. expel [b, 1669, Sturmy] Aiiii[r] A meruelous fumigation to expell the euil aire out of the house
14. experiment [1b, 1586, Cogan] Ci[r] if it happen that a Phisition doo practise in the time of pestilence, and findeth some exellent experiment

15. magistrall [2a, 1605, Bacon] Hiii^{v} put therto as much of our *Cerate magistrall*
16. melrose [1790, Fordyce] Ciii^{v} three ounces of *Mel rosarum* [a 1 cit]
17. mollificative [a, 1590, Barrough] Hiii^{v} the *Oyle of Roses* is absterge [*sic*] and molificatiue
18. mordicative [1603, Holland] Hii^{v} the *Lilly root* draweth and openeth, & is mordicatiue [a 1 cit]
19. pellagra [1811, Hooper] Fiiii^{r} If any haue Pellaria, anoint him with our *Magno Licore* [a 1 cit]
20. poet [1d, 1839, tr. *Lamartine*] Aiii^{r} the excellent Philosopher & rare Poet in all sciences
21. rectified [2, 1605, Timme *Quersit.*] Ciii^{v} put them into fiue powndes, of rectified *Aqua vite*
22. refine [*v*, 1a, 1582, Stanyhurst] Diii^{r} as in melting or refining metalls
23. restringe [1,1597, A. M. *Guill.*] Hii^{v} it is restrictiue, & in restringing it draweth the humors to it [a 1 cit]
24. sarcocolla [1599, Hakluyt] Eiiii^{r} put therin ... *Sarcocola* [a 1 cit]
25. solution [I, 1c, 1851, Dunglison] Gi^{r} The second remedy to vse, is to take medecins appropriat to the solution of that disease
26. stomachal [2, 1599, A. M. *Gabel.*] Aiii^{r} A confection cordiall and stomacall [a 1 cit]
27. terrestrial [*a*, 5a, 1638, Rawley] Gi^{v} beware of eati[n]g those things that are nurished of [th]e earth, as all sorts of herbs and fruits, and Animalles terrestrialls

2. *New senses*

1. motion Bii^{r} The principall ... cause why the pestilence doth come: is a motion of the deuine goodness ... as ... God is the true moouer of al things created
2. penetrative Eiii^{v} it is a mervelous Penetratiue

3. *Unrecorded*

1. alterated Gii^{r} our *Quintæssence Soluti[u]e* ... expelleth the corrupt and alterated matter in our Bodyes
2. aromatius Ciii^{v} Receiue *Boll armoniake, Valerian, Carlina, Zedoaria, mirra, Gentiane, Aristolochia, Rotunda, Calamus, Aromatius, Camphir*, white *Ditany*, ana ... put them into fiue powndes of rectfied [*sic*] *Aqua vitæ*
3. camedrios Eii^{v} Receiue ... *Camedrios, Stecados, Channepiteos*
4. cantarides Diiii^{r} straw theron [th]e pouder of *Ca[n]tarides* and binde it streight for it wil draw foorth great quantitie of water
5. catta patre Hi^{r} Receiue ... *catta patre*
6. channepiteos Eii^{v} See **camedrios**, unrec.
7. dia aromatico Fii^{r} *Of our Dia Aromatico of our invention, and the order to make it*

8. diamarinato Di^r Receiue … *diamarinato*
9. fes Eii^r take it out … uery softly for feare of mixing, for it will be seperated from his feses, and that abooue will be of a heaue[n]ly colour
10. imperatoria Ciii^r put therto … *Imperatoria*
11. imperatoria of mercury Fii^v Receiue … *Imperatoria of Mercury*
12. lua artetica Ciii^v take … *lua artetica*
13. mal di formica Fi^r all malign sores, as *mal di formica*
14. muscardini Aiiii^r To make Muscardini [th]e which are meruelous good against the pestilence
15. oriola Dii^v Receiue … *Oriola*
16. prefruit Hi^v ye may call them the pre-fruit of life … and they haue certified me of wunderfull things of their operation
17. rotunda Ciii^v Receive … *Rotunda*
18. sandraea Ciii^v Put therto … Sa[n]draea
19. tamaro Eiiii^r put therin … *Tamaro, Vitecella*
20. tigname Cii^v See **benjamin**, anted.
21. trosis Giii^v There is a kinde of *Trosis* made, the which are called *Moscardina* … Beat the aforesaid matters very finely and make therof *trosis*, with *Dragant* and *Rosewater*, and then dry them in the Sun
22. vitecella Eiiii^r See **tamaro**, unrec.
23. wine furnace Eiii^v set it on a wine Furnace, & giue it fire[14]

4. Postdatings

1. medicine [2c, 1575, Laneham] Fiii^r meruell not that I write this medicin, because the earth is our mother, and that which purifieth all things
2. putrefying [1500, *Melasine*] Gii^r it will preserue him from putrifying

LANGTON, CHRISTOPHER, *An introduction into physicke*, 1547

1. Antedatings

1. accordingly [4, 1599, Shakespeare] Av^r And I praye you, haue I not rewarded both Hypocrates & Gallene accordynglye? seinge that … they are glorifyed in fame as moche as eyther Alexander Magnus, or any other notable prince
2. adhesion [1, 1645, Howell *Lett.*] Gv^v See **assimilation**, anted. [a 1 cit]
3. adjunction [1, 1618, Raleigh] Gvi^r in nutrition, there muste fyrste be adiunction, and then agglutination [a 1 cit]
4. affirmation [2, 1611, Shakespeare] Miii^v Dreames of the seconde kynde, although they be coniectures, yet there ought to be no affirmation of them
5. ambiguity [4, 1591, Horsey *Trav.*] Miii^v we ought to gyue no credit vnto them [dreams], and for the mooste parte, they be full of ambiguitie
6. annex [*v*, II, 2, 1605, Bacon *Adv. L.*] 55 the splene … doth drawe vnto it melancholye or blacke choler, by a veyne whyche commeth from the lyuer,

receyuyng heat of the heart, to digest the forsaid blacke choler, by certayne pulses annexed vnto it

7. arithmetician [1557, Recorde *Whets.*] Bvi^{r} And this is that whyche Arithmetricions call *Temperamentu[m] ad pondus* [a 1 cit]

8. assimilation [4, 1626, Bacon *Sylva*] Gv^{v} the assimilation or makynge lyke of that that norysheth, to that which is nouryshed, the whyche to be done as these must nedes go before, agglutination or adhesio[n], so before agglutination, there must of necessitie, be apposition, or puttynge to of the nouryshment, to that that is noryshed [a 1 cit]

9. auction [*sb*, 1, 1692, Ray *Misc. Dis.*] Gi^{v} an other natural worke is to bryng the same to their ful groweth, whiche is done by the facultie called auction [a 1 cit]

10. avoid [*v*, 4b, 1562, Cooper *Answ. Priv.*] Cvi^{r} auoydeth no excrementes at hys fundament

11. bastard rib [a, *sb*, 11, 1594, T. B. *La Prim.*] Ev^{v} the splene ... is tyed vnto the backe aboute the myddes of the bastard ryb

12. brine [*v*, 1552, Huolet] 2 Also all fyshes [tha]t can not well suffre salte, nor can be bryned hole [a 1 cit]

13. cerebellum [Hall, 1565] Diii^{r} in Latyne it is called *Cerebellum* [a 1 cit]

14. cognation [4, 1555, Bradford *Wks.*] Cviii^{v} there is a certayne cognation or kynderede betwene the sky, and mannes brayne

15. concoctive [*a*, 1, 1578, Banister *Hist. Man*] 56^{v} There be .iiii. powers or faculties ... of the whyche the fyrst is named attractife, the seconde retentyue, the thyrd concoctyue, and the fowerth and last expulsyue [a 1 cit]

16. consist [*v*, 1c, 1576, Baker *J. Health*] Cviii^{v} the brayn by a certayne diuine nature [tha]t it hath doth consist wythout any stay or fortresse that can be perceyued by sence

17. constitute [*v*, 5, 1646, Browne] 96 But he that wyl knowe perfectly howe to iudge the differences of bodies in temperature by comparison, must constitute in euery kynde of thynges, that same temperate meane

18. continual [*a*, 5b, 1578, Banister *Hist. Man*] Cviii^{v} the skulle ... is made lyke an helmet ... and it is not one hole continual bone but is deuyded by certayne semes in to seuen bones

19. contrary [*v*, 1b, 1586, Day, A. *Eng. Secr.*] Biiii^{v} This definition is taken both out of Gallen and Aristotle: therefore I truste, no man wyll be so impudent to contrary or impugne it

20. deliver [*v*^{1}, I, 3b, 1581, Pettie *Guazzo's*] Cvi^{r} The infant ... after he is delyuered

21. dialect [3, 1551, Wilson *Logicke*] Ciii^{r} begynners as yet verye rawe in Physycke, whose bryngynge vp hath not ben amongest learned men of the vniuersityes, wherby they are destitute, bothe of dialecte, naturall Philosophye, and other artes [a 1 cit]

22. dogmatic [B, 1b, 1605, Timme] Avii^{r} phisitions ... were deuyded into .iii. sectes ... the last and best were called dogmatici [a 1 cit]

23. domestical [A, *adj*, 3, 1562, Bulleyn *Bk. Simpl.*] Ivi^{r} of domestical beastes

24. emulgent [A, 1578, Banister] Evi^{r} two veynes, whyche be called *Mulgentes*, and in oure tongue sucking veynes [a 1 cit]

25. encouragement [1568, Grafton *Chron.*] 18 See **provokement**, anted. [a 1 cit]

26. equally [4, 1599, Hakluyt *Voy.*] Dvi^{r} Nature hath prouyded the hart to be set so egallye in the middest of the brest, as is possyble to be deuyded, by al the mathematikes in the worlde

27. exagitation [1603, Holland *Plutarch*] Kiiii^{r} the vyolence of the greate heate, whych exercyse and the veheme[n]t exagitation causeth [a 1 cit]

28. excrement [1, 1588, Shakespeare] Cvii^{r} begynnyng in the heares thogh they be but excrementes

29. exitious [*a*, 1563, *Homilies*] 13 Wherefore youth ought ... so muche the lesse to haunt banketynge and drynkynge tyl mydnyght no not to spend the tyme in exitious labour [a 1 cit]

30. experiment [2, 1594, Carew *Huarte's*] Avii^{r} Than after that they had gathered after thys fasshion, a great many of experie[n]tes, they did vtterly abolyshe, and condempne all reason as voyde

31. flame [1f, 1706, Phillips] Fvii^{v} vitall spirite is a flambe in the heart

32. frame [*v*, 5a, 1553, Eden *Treat New Ind.*] Hvi^{r} thys maye be euidently perceyued in the example aforesayde of the woman goynge wyth chylde, for so longe as euerye thynge aboute the chylde frameth well, so longe the power expulsiue resteth

33. impudent [*a*, 2, 1563, Foxe] Biiii^{v} See **contrary**, anted.

34. infundibulum [2, 1799, Hooper] Diii^{v} See **infusorium**, anted. [a 1 cit]

35. infusorium [1876, Lankester, and ns] Diii^{r} a holow cauitie, which receyueth the excreme[n]tes ... of the brayne ... the Grekes cal this cauitie /S/χοαν(?)μ/S/, the Latyn men *infusorium*, or *infundibulum*, we haue no proper name for it: nowe it maye be called a droppynge pan [a 1 cit]

36. instauration [1, 1603, Cartwright *Confut. Rem.*] 53 preceptes be gyuen of the phisitions for the conseruation and instauratio[n] of spirites [a 1 cit]

37. internal [A, *adj*, 1590, Spenser] Bi^{v} he muste knowe also ... the internall partes, by dyligent searche, and cuttynges of bodyes [a 1 cit]

38. janitor [2, 1584, Grant and ns] Ei^{v} the mouthe that letteth oute the meate ... called in Greke /S/*Πιλισοσ*/S/, in Latyne *Ianitor* [a 1 cit]

39. laboursome [*a*, 2, 1577, Holinshed] Kvi^{v} If he be cholerycke, and strong of nature ledynge a laboursume life, then he may fede of grosse and strong meates

40. larynx [1578, Banister] Diii^{v} See **nodus gutturis**, unrec. [a 1 cit]

41. mathematics [*sb pl*, 1581, Mulcaster] Dvi^{r} See **equally**, anted. [a 1 cit]

42. nasturtium [1, 1570, Foxe] Cii^{r} nasturtiu[m] is hotte [a 1 cit]

43. nates [2, 1681, Willis] Dii^{v} two lumpes, whych of the verye similitude of buttockes be called *Nates* [a 1 cit]

44. parencephalon [1704, Harris, J.] Diii^{r} a greate part of the brayne, whiche the Grecians call /S/παρενκεφαλιζ/S/, in latyne it is called *Cerebellum* [a 1 cit]

45. parricide [1554, Prat, *Africa*] Av^{r} I am ... also a mayntayner of Paricides [a 1 cit]

46. provokement [1553, Brende *Q. Curtius*] Miiii^{r} the encouragementes and provokementes of Domitius Lentulus and Labienus ... counsayled hym to fyght [a 1 cit]

47. pylorus [1615, Crooke] Ei^{v} See **janitor**, anted. [a 1 cit]

48. redound [*v*, 1b, 1568, Skene *The Pest*] Fv^{v} Vnnaturall flegme is a rawe wateryshe humour, colde and moyste, redoundynge in that body, where as is a weake concoction

49. scrupulous [*a*, 5, 1638, Junius *Paint. Anc.*] Cvi^{v} See **situation**, anted.

50. section [*sb*, 1, 1559, Geminius] Avi^{v} the section of the body, with all the faculties and actions of the same [a 1 cit]

51. sensible [*a*, I, 1c, 1642, Milton *Ap. Smect.*] Biii^{r} The Phisitions also do call the veynes pulses, and bones, w[ith] all other suche partes as the Latyne men call similares, sensible elementes: bycause they are the fyrst beginners of mannes bodye

52. similar [1, 1626, Bacon] Biii^{r} See **sensible**, anted. [a 1 cit]

53. situation [3a, 1600, Shakespeare] Cvi^{v} I wyll not be so scrupulous, as to reherse euery lytle part or the scituation or fygure of euery bone and vayne

54. society [I, 1b, 1588, Shakespeare] Aiii^{r} [th]e hole course of our lyfe, consysteth in [th]e societie and mutuall doinge one for another [a 1 cit]

55. sorbition [1623, Cockeram] Hiiii^{r} all maner of decoctions & sorbitions, as mylke wyne, meath, with such other [a 1 cit]

56. suffocate [*v*, 1, 1599, A. M. *Gabel.*] Eviii^{r} if that same superfluouse water, shoulde not be caryed awaye, but be permitted to runne togyther in the vaynes, with the blood ... man shoulde be suffocated or choked [a 1 cit]

57. terrestrial [*a*, 3, 1594, Plat *Jewell-Ho.*] Fiiii^{r} Blacke choler or melancholie is a thycke terrestrial humour

58. trump [v^2, II, 3a, 1553, Bale, *Gardiner's De Vera*] Av^{r} trumpyng eftsones in my waye

59. unconcoct [*a*, 1591, Sylvester *Du B.*] Hiii^{v} take a dog, or any other brute beast, & fede him, & than after he hath rest an houre, nyp his mawe, for loke what ye fedde him w[ith], ye shal fynde it there vnconcoct [a 1 cit]

60. vena cava [1598, Florio] Eiiii^{v} th[e] veyne which is called *Porta*, & also of th[at], that is called *Caua vena*, we haue no names in our tungue whych be propre or peculier to them onely, but muste be fayne to call them master veynes, and in dede so that we vnderstande the thynge, it shall make but lytle matter for names [a 1 cit] [fpl]

2. *New senses*

1. divider Diii[v] Nexte vndernethe be the iawes, furnyshed wyth xxxii teeth: the foure formost of eche syde be called deuiders, bycause they teare the meate
2. feeder Iiii[r] Of drynkes, ale is the stro[n]gest feder: and tha[n] mylke
3. infusorium Diii[r] See **infusorium**, anted.
4. janitor Ei[v] See **janitor**, anted.
5. underset Cviii[v] the skye beynge a great & heauye substance without any proppes, or vndersettes

3. *Unrecorded*

1. complexioned Bviii[r] a complexio[n]ed body
2. crassum Cvii[v] *Dura mater*, which Galen calleth *Crassum*
3. elementum Biii[r] The signification of this worde Elementum
4. eucraton Bvii[v] the meane whiche is named Eucraton
5. grossed Ciiii[v] a veyne ... dothe drawe vp the grossed bloode
6. nodus gutturis Diiii[v] laronyx, in latyn *Nodus gutturis*, which in Englysh is the knotte of the throte
7. nutrimentum Gvii[v] properlye that is named *nutrimentum* and in our tonge, nouryshment
8. papaver Cii[r] Mandragora, Salamandra or Papauer is colde
9. partes similares Cv[v] *Partes similares* ... sensible elementes
10. pessule Dii[v] the mydle cha[m]bre ... is shut w[ith] a pessule or barre
11. sanguis menstruis Cvi[r] that bloud whyche is called *Sanguis menstruis*
12. transversum septum Ei[r] which the Latyne men call *Transuersum septu[m]*, or *p[er]cordia*
13. vitilina bilis Fv[v] choler ... called of [th]e Latynes *Vitilina bilis* bycause it is lyke in coloure, to the yolke of an egge

LANGTON, CHRISTOPHER, *A uery brefe treatise, ordrely declaring the principal partes of phisick*, 1547

1. *Antedatings*

1. absurd [2, 1557, Recorde *Whetstone*] Ki[r] obsurde and vnnaturall sauores, belonging to the taste [a 1 cit]
2. accident [I, 3, 1563, Gale] Iii[r] The third is the accidentes folowyng the disease
3. accomplishing [*sb*, 1581, Marbecke] Kiii[r] Therfore first of all to the accomplysshynge, or gettyng of this knowlege [a 1 cit]
4. adhesion [1645, Howell *Lett.*] Dviii[r] Nutrition, is the assimilation, or makyng lyke, of the nurishment to that, that is nurished: to the whiche, apposition, and agglutination or adhesio[n] be necessary [a 1 cit]

5. affected [III, 1, 1619, Donne] Av^{r} they transfer one medicine to dyuers euyls, and from one place affected to another
6. agitation [1, 1573, Cooper] Liii^{v} great trouble and agitation [a 1 cit]
7. alterative [A, *adj*, 1, 1605, Bacon] Dv^{v} See **concoctive**, anted. [a 1 cit]
8. appetition [1603, Holland] Dviii^{r} See **auction**, anted. [a 1 cit]
9. assimilation Dviii^{r} See **adhesion**, anted. [a 1 cit]
10. auction [1, 1692, Ray] Dviii^{r} Amongest the naturall actions, be reckened, generation, Auction, nutrition, Formation, Alteration, appeticion, attraction, concoction, retention, distribution, excretion [a 1 cit]
11. avulsion [1622, Peacham] Ivii^{r} The thirde kynde of disease ... is the deuision of that that is hole ... which diuision yf it be in the tiynges or byndynges it is called auulsio[n] ... in the bone, a broken crevise: in the senowes, a conuulsion, or crampe [a 1 cit]
12. barrenness [3, 1568, Thynne] Div^{v} the sterilitie and baraynes of the english tong
13. boxing [1562, Turner] Gvi^{r} & these be light boxing glasses, which be vsed w[ith]out scarifiyng
14. colliquation [2, 1605, Bacon] Lv^{v} The .iii. cause is the collyquation of such thynges, as consume and melt in the body [a 1 cit]
15. composition [2, 1555, Eden] Ivi^{v} The disease ... of co[m]posicion [is] whan [some parts] be put in wronge places, or wha[n] they that shoulde agre together, doe not
16. concoctive [1, 1578, Banister] Dv^{v} the power alteratiue, or concoctiue [a 1 cit]
17. concurring [*sb*, 1594, T. B.] Aiv^{r} the whyche in Lattyn is called *Congeries*, and *concursus*, and in Englishe a heape, and concurryng, or runnynge together [a 1 cit]
18. conformation [3, 1646, Browne] Ivi^{v} The disease of conformation happeneth of the vncumly figure, as whan summe part is holowe from the natiuitie, or elles after by casualitie, which shoulde not
19. congerie [1619, Fotherby] See **concurring**, anted.
20. continual [5, 1570, Billingsley] Lvii^{v} They be called light, which be continuall & of one pece, not rough, nor broken in any part
21. convulsion [2, 1585, Lloyd *Treas. Health*] Ivii^{r} See **avulsion**, anted. [a 1 cit]
22. corruptible [2, 1586, Cogan] Bvi^{r} but after these elementes be once mixte in the body ... that [tha]t is made of them, is a body mixt, and corruptible
23. crevice [3, 1580, Baret] See **avulsion**, anted.
24. dainty [a, 5, 1576, Fleming] Cvi^{r} I thinke these sufficient, for suche as be not to deynty, and exquisite
25. detention [1b, 1650, Fuller] Ki^{v} vnnaturall inanitions, or detentions ... as ... the emorroydes ... wemens flowres [a 1 cit]

26. disperse [6, 1576, Fleming] Ei^{r} spirit ... being dispersed in the senewes
27. dissipate [*ppl a*, 1606, Woodcocke] Fviii^{v} the strength of theyre bodyes whiche dwell in [th]e hote contrey, is afterwarde dissolued or dissipate, w[ith] ouermuche heate
28. distemperate [*a*, 2, 1548, Recorde] Ci^{v} And hereof it is euident, that sumtyme one temperament is equall and temperate in one opposicion, and distemperate, and not equall in an other
29. distribute [*v*, 4, 1664, Evelyn] Biii^{v} Oure forfathers have distributed, and deuided Phisicke, into thre formes
30. distribution [3, 1605, Bacon] Biii^{v} The distribution of Phisicke in to thre formes
31. evaporation [3b, 1551, Turner] Fvi^{v} the differences of emptinesse, or euacuatio[n], which may cum many wayes ... by the Hemorroides, by carnal copulation, by insensible euaporatio[n]
32. excretion [1, 1605, Timme] Dviii^{r} See **auction**, anted. [a 1 cit]
33. excretive [1666, Harvey] Lvii^{r} the weaknesse of the excretiue power, both in the raynes & other partes [a 1 cit]
34. expectation [2, 1552, Hamilton, Apb.] Miv^{v} wherfore gentyll readers accept my good wyll though I have not satisfied youre expectation
35. external [A, 1, 1599, Shakespeare] Iiii^{v} There be .ii. manner of causes of diseases: one is externall so called, because it is outwardly receiued, and was not before within the body [a 1 cit]
36. fortifying [*sb*, 1580, Hollyband] Lviii^{v} the fortifiynge of the excretiue facultie
37. fret [*sb*^{2}, 2, 1600, Surflet] Hii^{r} for in such [abstinence] bredeth chollar & causeth feuers with many frettes and pinchinges both in the belly & also in the mouth of the mawe
38. function [*sb*, 2, 1579, Lyly] Bviii^{r} it may be knowen of hys functions, and officis, who is hole according to hys nature
39. getting [*ppl a*, 1634, Rainbow] Aiii^{r} The fowerth [art] in Latyn is called *comparans*, which in our tong may be called a gettyng arte, for it doeth make nothynge, but by studye [a 1 cit]
40. hawking [*sb*, 1583, Stanyhurst] Dii^{r} The second kynde [flewme], is that which after [th]e hawking out, hath a swete taste [a 1 cit]
41. incide [2, 1612, *Enchir. Med.*] Gii^{v} suche decoctions & syrupes as doe incyde grosse matter [a 1 cit]
42. incline [*v*, 12b, 1589, Cogan] Dii^{v} The forth [kynde] inclineth sumwhat towardes grene
43. internal [A, 1, 1590, Spenser] Iiii^{v} The tother, is called internall, which is within the body, as humors putrified within the body [a 1 cit]
44. intestines [*sb*, 1a, 1597, A. M. *Guill.*] Di^{r} yelow choller clenseth the intestines of their flewme and filthe [a 1 cit]
45. invasion [1b, 1566, Alday] Kiv^{r} the first inuasion of the disease is the firste beginnynge

46. involuntary [b, 1840, Wilson, E.] Kv^{v} signes, and causes both together, as ... involuntary teares

47. judging day [1550, Lloyd] Gviii^{v} those sweates in feruent and hote diseases, which co[m]meth in the iudgyng dayes, & doe ende the feuer

48. mitigate [6, 1611, Tourneur] Cvii^{v} flewme ... mittigateth the greate ferment, and outragious heat of [th]e bloud [a 1 cit]

49. nutrition [1, 1615, Crooke] Dviii^{r} See **auction**, anted.

50. observation [5, 1557, N. T.] Av^{r} suche thynges as they have noted and observed ... which is to saye an obseruacion made by chaunce

51. opposition [4, 1581, Mulcaster] Ci^{v} See **distemperate**, anted.

52. plentifully [1, 1553, Mulcaster] Kviii^{r} it is necessary that whan *crisis* happeneth, chollar ple[n]tifully to be voyded

53. preposterous [1, 1552, Huolet] Evii^{v} it is a preposterous ordar, to beginne with quynces or orynges and ende with sallades

54. prescribing [*vbl sb*, 1618, Baret *M. Horsemanship*] Evi^{r} Therfore the Phisicio[n] in prescribing of diet, must marke well the strength of hys pacient

55. quivering [1562, Turner *Herbal*] Kv^{v} quiuerynge of [th]e neyther lippe

56. redound [1c, 1590, Jonson] Ai^{v} that whyche is superfluous, & redoundeth

57. remedying [*vbl sb*, 1570, Foxe] Bi^{v} Hippocrates wrot thre great bokes of the remediynge of all feruent diseases

58. so-called [1, 1657, Howell *Londinop.*] Iiii^{v} See **external**, anted.

59. sterility [3, 1665, Glanville] Bv^{r} the sterillite of my simple wyt

60. superstition [4, 1794, Hutton *Philos. Light*] Kvii^{r} ther is in them, more error then truthe, more superstition, then knowlege

61. suppress [7, 1621, Burton] Hv^{r} if the floures be suppressed at any tyme, excepte that tyme that the woman goethe with childe ... it decayeth health vtterly

62. tinct [1579, Spenser] Liv^{r} After whyte they be next, that be sum deale pale, the which because they be a littell tincte, they ar not extreme crude

63. turbulent [2, 1573, Harvey, G.] Liii^{v} sum inequall turbulent matter remayning behynde in the vaynes

64. tying [*sb*, 2, 1548, Udall] Diii^{v} ther is nether oxe, horse, ne dogge, but they haue pulses, vaynes, senewes, tiinges, gristilles

65. universal [11, 1551, T. Wilson] Kiv^{v} These be the vniuersall tymes in diseases, besydes whiche there is other called particular

2. *New senses*

1. agglutination Dviii^{r} nutritions, is the assimilation, or makyng lyke, of the nurishment to that, that is nurished: to the whiche, apposition, and agglutination or adhesio[n] be necessary

2. binding [*vbl sb*] See **avulsion**, anted.

3. distemperate [not as *vbl sb*] Ciii^{v} The second is whan [th]e distemperate is compared to the temperate of the same kynde

4. **judgement** Kiii^{v} this worde *Crisis*, which the lattyns call *iudicium*, & in english it may be called iudgement: but at this present time it signifieth any sudde[n] mutation in euery disease
5. **neezing** [*vbl sb*] Hiv^{v} the puttyng of medicines in to the nose called nisynge
6. **occation** Lv^{r} oftentymes, with euery light occation, the cullar of the vrine dothe alter
7. **submission** Miii^{v} the submission, or contraction of the forenamed Arteries

3. Unrecorded

1. **agoggle** Iviii^{r} a man of force, seeth thinges which he did not beholde with hys common sense, as they do which loke a goggell
2. **bolum** Lvi^{v} a light red, whiche is [th]e cullar of a certayne drug, called bolum
3. **cartamus** Liv^{r} a cullar like the floures of cartamus, which is commonly called the gardyn saffaron
4. **dryeth** Evii^{r} it must be brought in temper ... yf they be ouer moyst, by dryeth
5. **finition** Aii^{r} Gallen vseth thys finition, in hys boke
6. **hectica** Ivi^{r} in all kynde of feuers, excepte the before named hectica

MORE, PHILLIP, *The hope of helth*, 1564

1. Antedatings

1. **afore-named** [*adv*, D, 1b, 1603, Stubbes] Aiiii^{r} takyng example at the life of the first sorte of phisitio[n]s aforenamed [a 1 cit]
2. **agglutinate** [*v*, 2, 1620, Venner] Bi^{v} and by the same power also it is aglutinate and ioyned to the member whiche is to be nourished [a 1 cit]
3. **allium** [1807, Crabbe] Evi^{r} Garlike. *Allium* [a 1 cit]
4. **annex** [*v*, II, 2, 1605, Bacon] *iii^{v} certain rules of Astronomy, wherof the most part are annexed vnto Phisicke
5. **brassica** [1832, *Veg. Subst. Food*] Dv^{r} Coleworte. *Brassica*. Of Colewortes there be foure kindes [a 1 cit]
6. **calendula** [1871, *Mrq. & Merch.*] Eiii^{v} Marigouldes. *Calendulæ* [a 1 cit]
7. **comfrey** [2, 1578, Lyte] Eiiii^{v} Comferie. *Consolida maior*
8. **compass** [1573, Tusser] Dii^{r} laye compasse vppon the grounde [a 1 cit]
9. **conjunction** [2b, 1567, Maplet] Ai^{v} yet it tooke soche effecte that all mankinde ... haue proceded of them and their posteritee, beyng ingendred by the coniunction of their pare[n]tes
10. **contention** [1, 1580, J. Rogers] Gvii^{v} but let him kepe himselfe quiet & watche, auoydyng all contention and exercise of bodie and mynde [a 1 cit]
11. **convulsion** [2a, 1585, Lloyd] Eiiii^{r} The herbe ... is good against conuultions [a 1 cit]

12. correct [*v*, 7, 1578, Dodoens] Dviii[r] And also it being burned in a house correcteth pestilent ayre
13. cucurbit [1866, *Treas. Bot.*] Eiii[r] Gourdes. *Cucurbita* [a 1 cit]
14. derive [*v*, I, 2, 1598, Stow] Aviii[r] For in the braine consisteth the facultie and power animall, whiche is deriued & sent from these by synowes that spring there into al partes of the bodie
15. desirous [*a*, 1c, 1601, Shakespeare] vi[v] all soche as bee desirous to preserue their bodies in healthe
16. digesting [*ppl a*, 1605, Timme] Bi[v] See **altering**, ns.
17. discredit [*v*, 3, 1579, Harvey] Aiiii[r] as the vile Renobites and Papistes at this prese[n]t daie, do seke meanes to discredite preachers as muche as they can, by scrupulous serching and examininge of their liuing, which somtime they finde to disagree from their doctrine
18. doctrine [*sb*, 3, 1594, West] Aiii[v] them that searche out the knowlege therof [phisicke] to guide their liues according to the doctrine of it
19. dominical [B, *sb*, 4, 1628, Jackson] Hviii[v] wherein is declared, the rising and going doune of the sunne, and the length of the daie & night with the prime, and Dominicall, and sainctes daies
20. dominical letter [A, I, 2b, 1577-87, Holinshed] *ii[r] First a table to finde out the dominicall letter [a 1 cit]
21. dracunculus [3, Phillips, 1706] Eii[v] Dragons. *Dracunculus maior* [a 1 cit]
22. effect [*sb*, 5, 1668, *Phil. Trans.*] Ai[v] See **conjunction**, anted.
23. egestion [2d, 1607, Topsell] Biii[v] that it might helpe their excrecion (that is) that it might raise and stire vp the vertue expulsiue, to driue out the egestions
24. evaporate [*ppl a*, 1607, Topsell] Ci[v] and therfore the whole bodie would sone bee wasted and consumed, vnlesse the like substau[n]ce to that whiche is euaporate and spredde were daily engendred in the body
25. exactly [*adv*, 2, 1612, Brinsley] Aiii[r] which thinges duely and exactely considered
26. handiwork [2b, 1838, Dickens] Bviii[v] Also thereby he may knowe that he is apte to learning, or to be a Lawier, or to be a Capitaine, or to doe any handie woorke
27. historiographer [3, 1579–80, North] Bvii[v] this one example doth declare, whiche is written of auncient and credible Historiographiers
28. incession [1651, Biggs] Ev[r] it is good to make incessions in the decoction thereof to prouoke secretes [a 1 cit]
29. inflamed [*ppl a*, 3, 1599, Buttes] Dvii[v] It is good for a hote and inflamed stomake, it abateth carnall luste
30. intermittent [*a*, a, 1603, Holland] Gv[r] Also bloudletting is good in feuers, whether they be continual or intermittent [a 1 cit]
31. malignant [A, *a*, 2, 1568, Skene] Hi[r] (margin) Purge none humours but malignaunte to nature
32. melissa [1593, Hester] Fii[v] Balme. *Melissa*. [a 1 cit]

33. **molest** [*v*, 1b, 1576, Fleming] Gvii^{r} Those therefore that doe abounde with bloude & wilbe let bloud to preserue themselfes from the daunger of any disease, that is like shortly to ensue and moleste them
34. **mollifying** [*ppl a*, 1590, Barrough] Cv^{r} and let them eate moiste meates before drie meates, and mollifiyng meates before binding and restrictiue meates [a 1 cit]
35. **nasturtium** [1, 1570, Foxe] Eii^{r} Cresses. *Nasturtium* [a 1 cit]
36. **observation** [8, b, 1593] Ciiii^{v} I thought it worthie of obseruacion, that there bee not a preposterous order vsed in eatyng of diuerse meates
37. **ocyme** [1621, Burton] Fi^{r} Basill. *Ocimum* [a 1 cit]
38. **peculiar** [A, *a*, 3, 1590, Sir J. Smith] Bii^{r} But beside them other me[m]bers that are lesse principall, haue their peculier operations
39. **pestilent** [*a*, 2, 1613, Cawdrey] See **correct**, anted.
40. **princeps** [1, 1809, Ferriar] More Aviii^{r} The thirde action is inwarde sense, and wit, or vnderstanding, and it is called in Latine, *Princeps* [a 1 cit]
41. **raphanus** [1730-6, Bailey] Fii^{r} Radishe. *Raphanus* [a 1 cit]
42. **refer** [*v*, I, 8a, 1601, Moryson] Avii^{v} As for the knowledge of special, or particular differences of eche parte of euery member, I referre the Reader to bookes of Anatomies
43. **sanguisorb** [1846, Lindley] Dviii^{r} Burnet. *Sanguisorba* [a 1 cit]
44. **scouring** [*ppl a*, 2, 1597, Gerarde] Diiii^{v} Thei are of a scouryng and abstersiue qualitie [a 1 cit]
45. **scrupulous** [*a*, 5, 1638, Junius] Aiiii^{r} See **discredit**, anted.
46. **spermatic** [*sb*, 6, 1690] Avii^{r} Note moreouer that to [th]e aforesaid foure principall members, there be foure ministers or ha[n]dmaydes, that is, senues, arteries, vaines, and sparmatike vessels
47. **stumbling-block** [c, 1593, Nashe] Aiiii^{v} God geue them grace to repente in time, that they laye no soche stumbling blockes in weiklinges wayes
48. **suffocate** [3a, 1584, Scot] Ciiii^{r} for excesse of meates doth ouercharge nature, suffocating & quenching naturall heate [a 1 cit]
49. **suppression** [5, 1601, Holland] Ev^{r} It is also good againste the stone and suppression of vrine
50. **try** [*v*, 4, 1582, W. H. Turner] Bi^{r} euen so, whe[n] natural heate will turne the substaunce of meates, receiued into the substaunce of the members of our body, it first boileth them and trieth them, taking so moche of them as is moste apte and mete
51. **untemperate** [*a*, 3, 1589, Puttenham] Gvii^{r} for those whiche be vntemperate & gluttonous in meates or great drinkers
52. **vicious** [*a*, 8, 1615, Crooke] Cii^{v} For so they be of great force, to engender greuous sicnesses, by engendring euill and vitious humours
53. **willing-minded** [*ppl a*, 5, 1648, Hexham] vii^{r} to declare vnto the willyng minded [a 1 cit]

2. *New senses*

1. **alter** *v*, Aii^{v} As the stomack to haue a good appetite, and to digest and alter meates well
2. **altering** Bi^{v} & these two faculties are ministers, or ha[n]dmaides to the altring or disgesting facultie
3. **secret** Ev^{r} See **incession**, anted.
4. **seed** Ev^{r} obstructio[n]s of the liuer and the raynes, specially the rootes and seedes of it
5. **straightway** Gvi^{r} Also it causeth natural heat to haue a larger scope, and a free passage by opening and emptiying the straightwayes & passages of the vaines and arteries

3. *Unrecorded*

1. **abrotonum** Ev^{v} Sothernwood. *Abrotonum*
2. **anethum** Evii^{r} Dill. *Anettrum.* [*sic*]
3. **apium** Ev^{r} Smalache. *Apium*
4. **atriplex** Ev^{v} Orache. *Atriplex*
5. **bellis** Eiiii^{v} Daysies. *Bellis minor*
6. **beta** Diiii^{r} Betes. *Beta*
7. **betonica** Eiiii^{r} Betony. *Betonica*
8. **bismalva** Evii^{r} Great Mallowes. *Bismalua*
9. **bonerite** *vi^{r} abused of many sortes of detestable heretiques, as of Arrians, Anabaptistes, and the damnable, vile, Romishe Papistes, the Darbellites, the Garnarites, the Bonerites, &c
10. **borago** Diii^{v} Borage. *Borago*
11. **buglossum** Diiii^{r} Buglosse. *Buglossum*
12. **cepa** Evi^{r} Onions. *Cepa*
13. **chamedris** Eiiii^{r} Germaunder. *Chamedris*
14. **chamomælon** Dv^{v} Camomyll. *Chamomælon*
15. **chælidonia** Eiii^{r} Selandine. *Chælidonia*
16. **cucumis** Eii^{v} Cucumbers. *Cucumis*
17. **darbellite** vi^{r} See **bonerite**, unrec.
18. **dishevering** Fv^{v} solucion and disheuering of some partes
19. **distempure** Avi^{r} And contrariwyse that disease chaunce to the body by distempure of the said foure qualities of the eleme[n]tes
20. **envacuate** Gv^{v} And note that bloudletting, dothe emptie and enuacuate from the bodie, all humours alike
21. **eruca** Eii^{r} Rocket. *Eruca*
22. **feniculum** Ei^{v} Fenell. *Feniculum*
23. **five-leaved grass** Fiiii^{v} Fiue leaued grasse
24. **fragaria** Ei^{v} Straweberies. *Fragaria*
25. **garnarite** *vi^{r} See **bonerite**, unrec.
26. **harminum** Eiii^{v} Clarie. *Harminum*
27. **hyssopus** Ei^{r} Hysope. *Hyssopus*

28. lactuca Diiii^{v} Letuse. *Lactuca*
29. laurus Evii^{v} Laurell. *Laurus*
30. lavendula Dvii^{v} Lauender. *Lauendula*
31. levisticum Eviii^{r} Louage. *Leuisticum*
32. lilium Eviii^{r} Lilies. *Lilium*
33. linguabovis Eiii^{v} Langue de bief. *Lingua bovis*
34. menta Eviii^{v} Mynthes. *Menta*
35. nepeta Eviii^{v} Neppe. *Nepeta*
36. olusatrum Fi^{r} Alisanders. *Olusatrum*
37. oxyacantha Fi^{v} Berberes. *Oxyacantha*
38. papaver Fii^{r} Poppie. *Papauer*
39. petroselinum Dvi^{r} Percely. *Petroselinum*
40. pionia Fi^{v} Pæonie. *Pionia*
41. pulegium Dvii^{v} Penyroyall. *Pulegium*
42. renobite Avi^{r} See **discredit,** anted.
43. rosa Dviii^{v} Roses. *Rosa*
44. rosmarinus Dviii^{r} Rosemary. *Rosmarinus*
45. ruta Dviii^{v} Rue. *Ruta*
46. saturea Fiii^{v} Sauery. *Saturea*
47. saxifraga Fi^{r} Filipendula. *Saxifraga rubea*
48. tanacetum Ei^{r} Tansey. *Tanacetum*
49. tenderous Fiii^{r} The leaues and te[n]derous vines, are good to be applied for paine of the head
50. thymus Dviii^{v} Time. *Thymus*
51. vitis Fii^{v} Vines. *Vitis vinifera*

4. Postdatings

1. astonied [*ppl a*, 1b, 1398, Trevisa] Dvii^{v} it helpeth the teeth that be astoined [*sic*] if it be chawed
2. consolida [1480, Caxton] Eiiii^{v} Comferie. *Consolida maior*

[PLUTARCH], *The governaunce of good helth*, 1549

1. Antedatings

1. affect [*v*, 2, 1550, *Robin Hood*] Biiii^{r} many nobleme[n] be affected agaynst theyr wyues
2. avoid [II, 4b, 1562, Cooper *Ans. Priv. Masse.*] Diiii^{r} medycynes … auoyde superfluyte of fleume
3. blanch [3, 1747, Hooson] Diii^{v} Also of blanca .iii. drammes [a 1 cit]
4. depravedly [1643, Browne *Rel. Med.*] Aii^{v} bycause that he is amongest other best learned, he hath of all other ben moste deprauedly handled [a 1 cit]

5. diaprune [1625, Hart *Anat. Ur*] Diii^{v} [th]e electuary called diaprunis [a 1 cit]
6. disperse [*v*, 6, 1576, Fleming *Pan. Epist.*] Aiiii^{v} disperse matter throughe all the body
7. disperse [*v*, 7, 1563, Fulke *Meteors*] Ci^{r} there is moche ease in warme bathes, for they ... disparse such thynges as otherwyse can not be dysgested
8. freshly [1b, 1613, Purchas] Bii^{r} But in case that after any feast when we be suffysed, that necessyte constrayneth vs in the co[m]pany of great men ... by straunger [*sic*], fresshely approchynge
9. inwardly [II, 4a, 1667, *Obs. Burn. Lond.*] Aiiii^{v} an ague or feuer causeth vtter partes of the body customably to be colde, whe[n] he co[n]strayneth heate all to fle inwardly
10. monstrous [5, 1573-80, Baret *Alv.*] Aii^{v} so sore haue I wrasteled almoste in euery lyne with monsterous lyes
11. moved [*ppl a*, 1, 1592, Shakespeare] Aiii^{r} it is his maner in dysputacyon to be ouer quicke and curious so at that tyme with a moued stomacke, thus rasshely crieng he came to ouercome vs [a 1 cit]
12. overladen [1654, Gayton *Pleas. Notes.*] Di^{r} a Shyp which is ouerladen, that must nedes be dyscharged [a 1 cit] [fpl]
13. physiclike [1581, Mulcaster] Aii^{v} though he teache this not so physycke lyke as doth Galyen [a 1 cit] [fpl]
14. pinched [1649, Daniel, G. *Trinarch. H5*] Dii^{r} he can not co[n]serue his health, for all his pynched lyuynge
15. preservation [2, 1751, Stuart *Lett. Lit. Men*] Aiii^{r} what shulde be good to [th]e state of lyuyng in preseruacion and gouerau[n]ce of good healthe
16. problem [3, 1594, Carew] Aiii^{r} the physicion ... whiche so fayne wolde haue keped a p[ro]bleme with vs in phylosophy
17. quarrelling [1589, Nashe] Aiii^{r} such a quaryllynge felowe [a 1 cit]
18. refreshing [1, 1580, Sidney *Ps.*] Ciii^{r} a refresshing meane betwene lust and laboure [a 1 cit]
19. scrupulous [1b, 1559, Cuningham *Cosm. Gl.*] Bi^{r} let vs put out of our mynde the supersticyous and scrupulous care of such thynges
20. so-called [1, 1657, Howell *Londinop.*] Ciii^{r} many tymes we do wycked sacrifices vnto Bacchus so called [a 1 cit]
21. suspicion [1592, Shakespeare] Dii^{r} when thou doste fele no contagyon or suspycion of syckenes
22. trade [*sb*, 4, 1575, *Recorde's Grt. Artes.*] Bi^{v} And let them so note the co[m]mon trade in quaffynge, which they maye not without dyshonesty refuse such company
23. urgent [2, 1559, *Reg. St. And. Kirk. Sess.*] Biiii^{r} intysement and vrge[n]t desyre
24. usually [2, 1573, Tusser *Husb.*] Cii^{v} it is not mete to drynke mylke vsually, but moderately to vse it

2. New senses

1. ambitious Ci[r] to wasshe in [th]e whothouse is more ambycyous and wanton then wholsome
2. amiable Biiii[v] Euen as the mocyon of tyklynge do styre vp a laughyng whiche is neyther naturall, pleasaunt, nor amiable
3. delay Ciii[r] we had more nede of aswagyng and delay
4. observe Bii[r] it is co[n]venyent that we do obserue our selues from such excessyue bankettes in loking for dayntyes, and kepynge a place for quaffyng

3. Unrecorded

1. agryl Diiii[v] other veymy [*sic*] moystynges and vyolent, as Turpyt, Elebre, Agryl, Euforbie
2. benedicta Diii[v] Also of benedicta maye be .iii. drammes
3. caterica imperiale Diiii[r] Also of Caterica imperiale one dramme
4. diacene Diiii[r] As it is said of Ieraphyny, so we shall say of Diacene, and the gyuynge of the qua[n]tytye shalbe an ounce
5. electuarium dulce Diiii[r] Also of electuarium dulce .ii. drammes
6. esule Diiii[v] medycynes ... sharped ... with Esule
7. ieralododion Diiii[r] Also of ieralododio[n].ii. drammes
8. ieraphini Diii[v] Ieraphini ... is more co[m]pou[n]ded with venymous medycynes & vyole[n]t tha[n] Irapigra
9. over-empty Di[r] to be ouer emptie is as paynfull as be ouer full
10. pallinum Diiii[v] medycynes that auoyde colde humours of the brest, and of his membres ... the fyrste is Pallinum
11. pilularum de euforbie Diiii[r] Also of pilularum de euforbie .iii. dra[m]mes
12. pilularum fetidum Diiii[r] Also of pilularum fetidum
13. sacca Diiii[r] the receyte of sacca rosarum
14. sacca rosarum Diiii[r] See **sacca**, unrec.
15. stomaticum laxitivum Diiii[r] Stomaticum laxatiuum .ii. drammes
16. theodoricon eupisticon Diiii[r] Also of Theodoricon eupisticon .ii. dra[m]mes
17. trifera saracenica Diiii[r] of Trifera saracenica [th]e receite of it is .iiii. dra[m]mes
18. withstop Ci[r] euyll affectyon and hardnes ... in stoppynge the poores, and thyckyng the humours, withstoppeth the vapores

Notes

1. Note that the citation for this from Banister in *OED* is given as a fig. use of 5, which seems quite wrong.
2. Cf. **exility**, but see also spurious words **exiled**.
3. This could be a misspelling, but it occurs twice on this signum and again on Eiiii[r] ff.
4. Perhaps this is the same as **instrie**, *c.*1420, Pallad, q.v.

5. Perhaps a misspelling of **meseraical**.
6. **Beating** *ppl a*³, 1702, Rowe is clearly possible, but I have chosen the earlier date, as in other cases within main lemmas where a clear decision is impossible.
7. The *OED* gives Cotgrave as the source in the preamble, but does not indicate whether the date should be 1611 or 1632.
8. The word is used in the definition of **laser**, q.v.
9. Listed by *OED* as spurious, but this instance may legitimize the word.
10. In the *OED* supplement.
11. Clever's text has two page 39s, but the second is additional to the sequence so that it cannot be notionally renumbered. The antedatings **gracile**, **indivertible**, and **solicit**, as the postdating **bend**, appear on the second.
12. Schäfer (1984) took exception to this antedating, suggesting that it was a misprint for **pinsell** (pencil), but the word is repeated in a marginal note and spelt the same way; it seems unlikely that this would occur twice, in different typefaces, if it were simply a misprint.
13. Probably the same as **fess**, above.
14. Possibly a misprint for 'wind furnace'.

APPENDIX 2

Graphs of the Lengths of Antedatings by Author

In the following graphs, the horizontal axis represents the length in years of the antedatings, while the vertical axis represents the number of antedatings recorded for each length. The date of publication of the work in question has in each case been taken to equal 0.

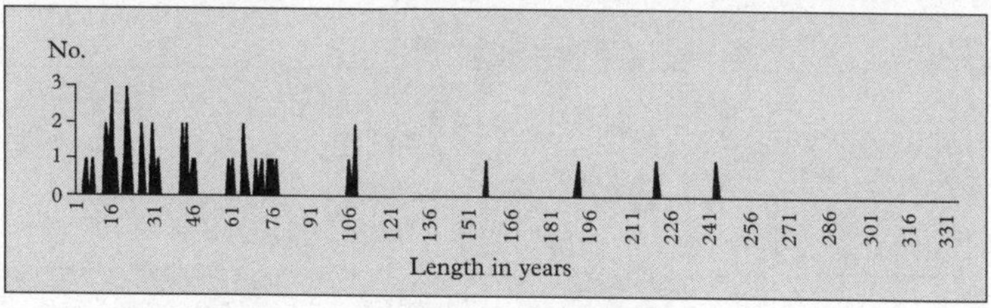

Graph 1. Walter Bailey

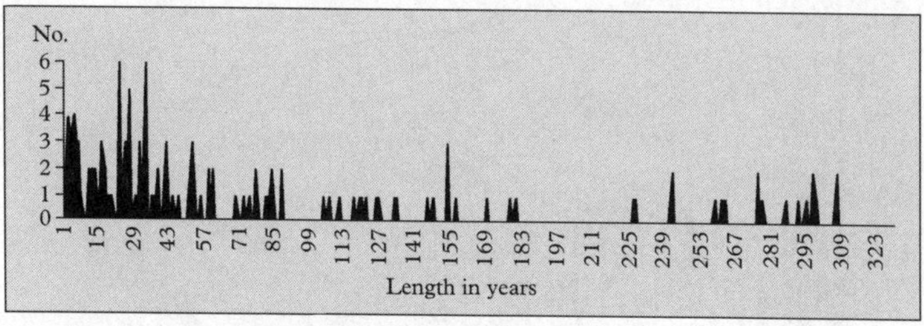

Graph 2. George Baker

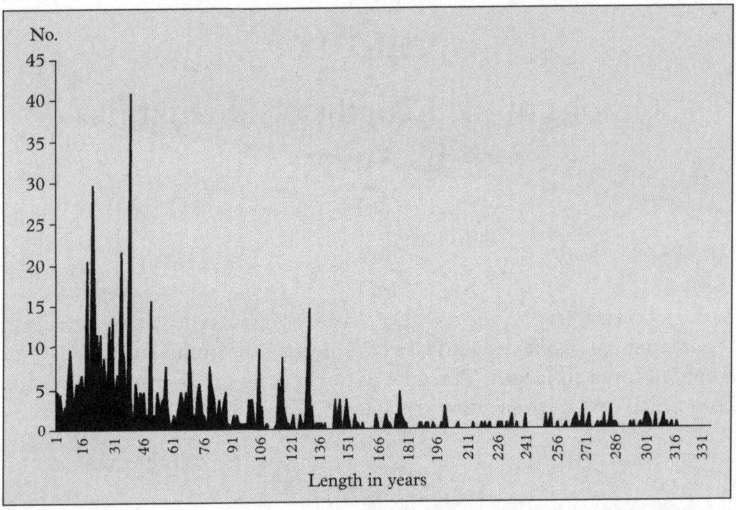

Graph 3. John Banister

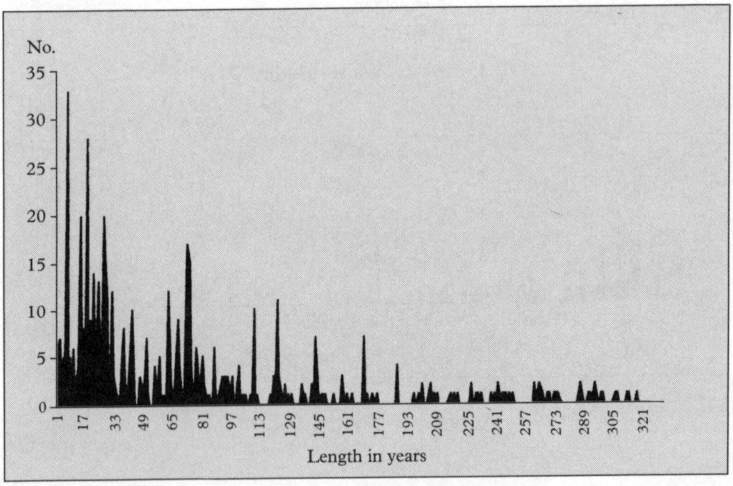

Graph 4. Phillip Barrough

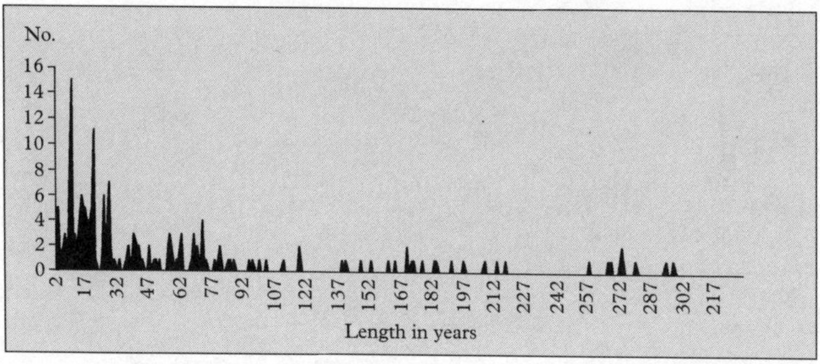

Graph 5. R[obert] B[ostocke]

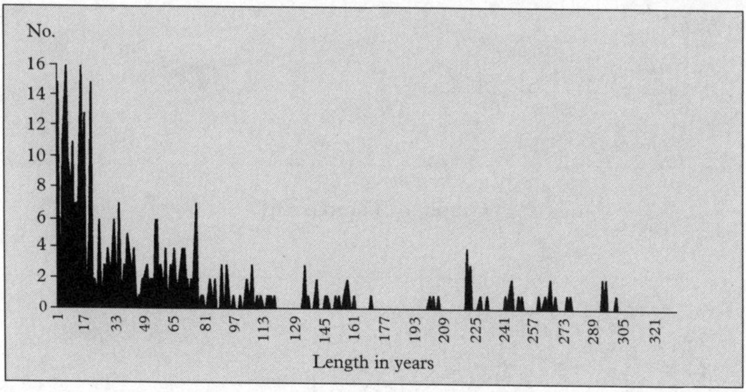

Graph 6. William Clever

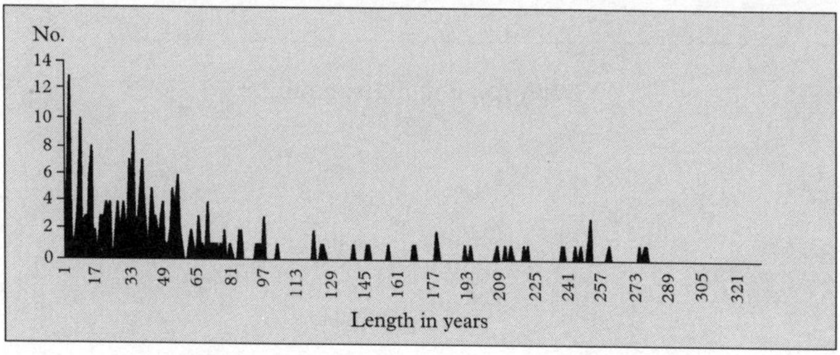

Graph 7. John Cotta

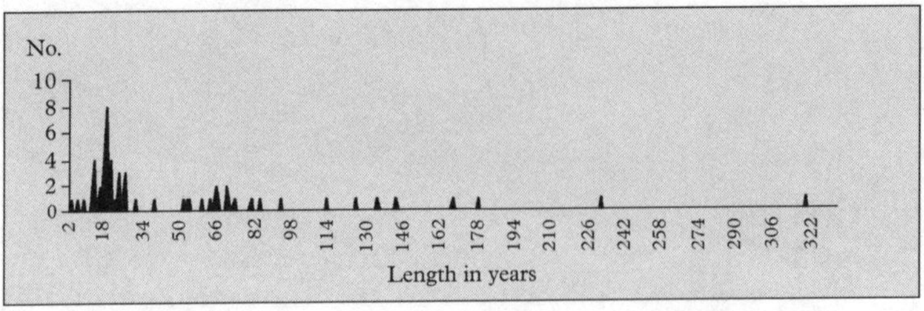

Graph 8. John Hester

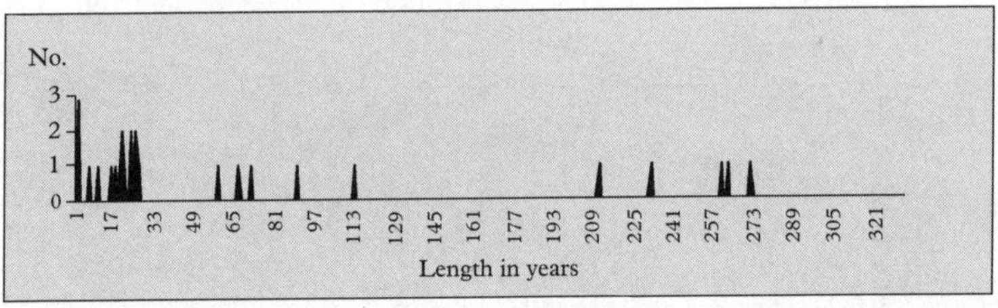

Graph 9. Thomas Hill

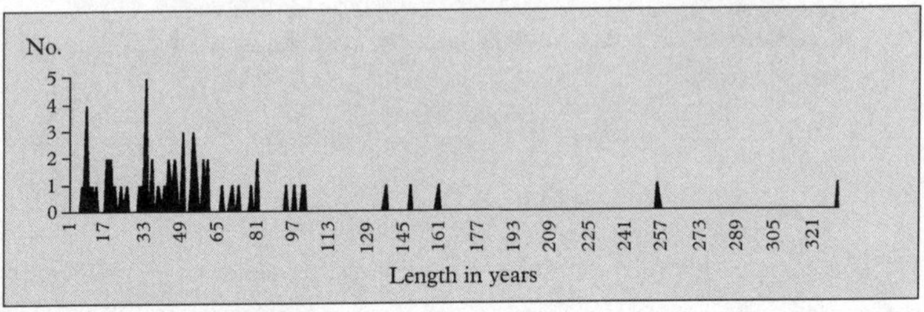

Graph 10. Phillip Langton, *IP*

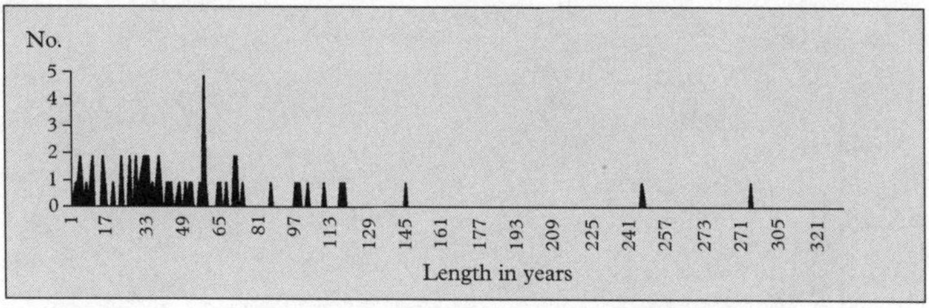

Graph 11. Phillip Langton, *VBT*

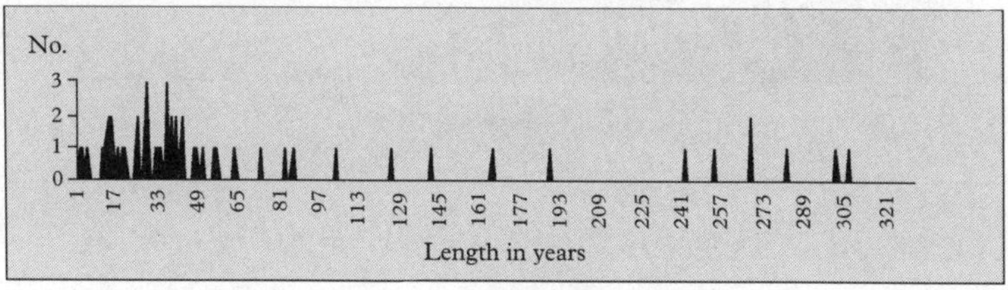

Graph 12. Phillip More

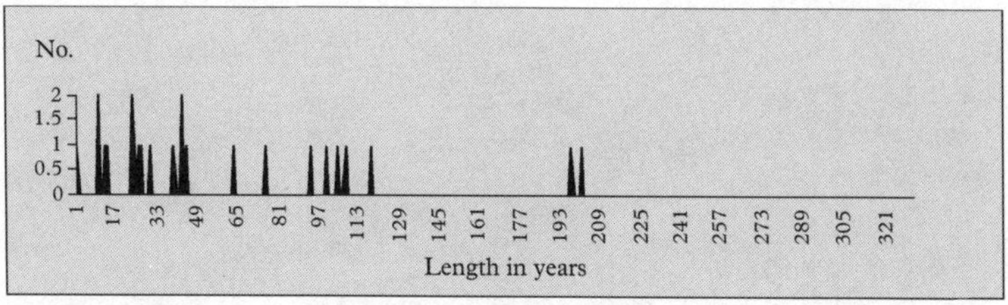

Graph 13. [Plutarch]

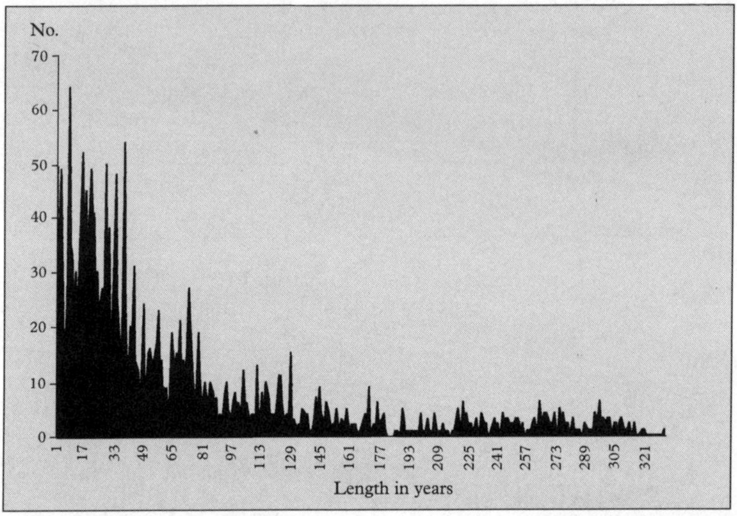

Graph 14. Total antedating lengths

Graph 15 plots the number of antedatings recorded for each letter of the alphabet, expressed as a percentage.

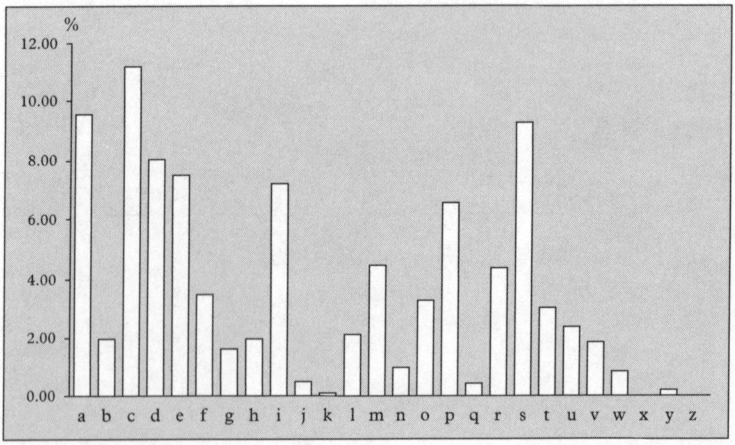

Graph 15. Letter percentages of the present antedatings

Graph 16 plots the percentage of antedatings in this study for each letter of the alphabet against the percentage which each letter of the alphabet represents of the total in the *OED*, including main lemmas, combinations and special combinations, and subordinate words. Letters are represented numerically along the horizontal axis (1 = A). All duplications have been removed in constructing this graph, so that any given antedating is recorded only once.

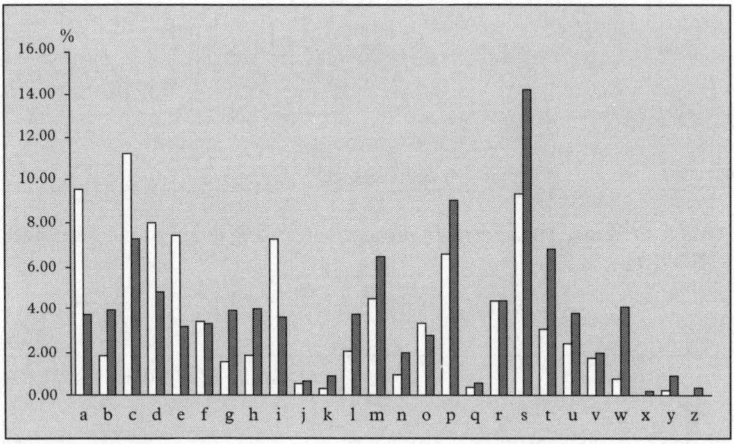

Graph 16. Present letter percentages (white) against *OED* letter percentages (grey)

Graph 17 shows the difference between the percentages for each letter of the alphabet yielded by this study and those for the whole *OED*. The horizontal axis therefore represents parity between the two.

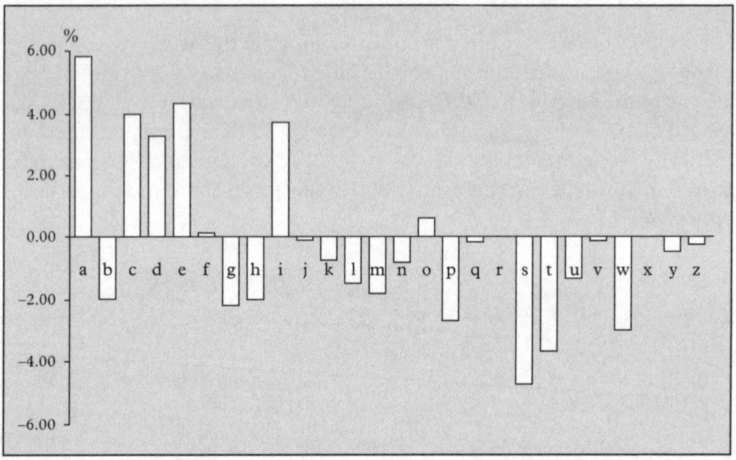

Graph 17. Difference between present antedating letter percentages and *OED* letter percentages

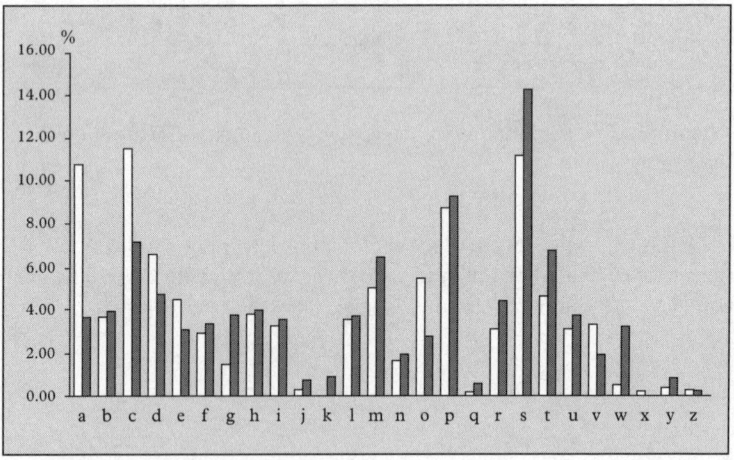

Graph 18. Percentages of present unrecorded (white) against *OED* letter percentages (grey)

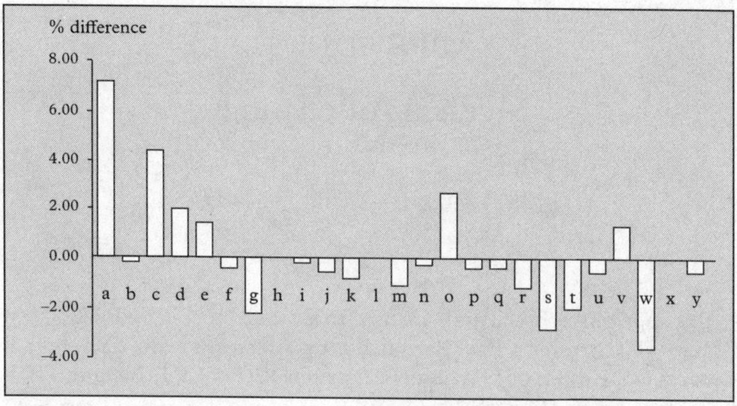

Graph 19. Difference between present unrecorded percentages and *OED* letter percentages

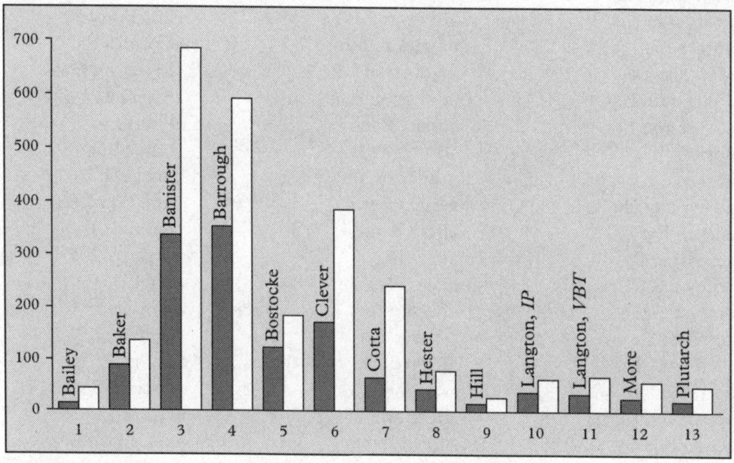

Graph 20. Ratio of a 1 cits for each author. White=total antedatings; black=a 1 cits

APPENDIX 3

Medical Antedatings

In this appendix abbreviations are used to indicate the source: Bailey = By, Baker = Ba, Banister = Ban, Barrough = Bar, Bostocke = Bo, Clever = Cl, Cotta = Co, Hester = He, Hill= Hi, Langton *VBT* = LBT, Langton, *IP* = LIP, More = Mo, [Plutarch] = Pl.

abdomen Ba
abdomen Ban
abdomen Bar
abort Ban
abrase Ban
abrasion Co
abscession Bar
abscession Bar
absinth Bar
absterge Hi
abstergent Bo
acanth Bar
accession By
accession Cl
accession Co
accident Bo
accident LBT
acetable Ban
acetabulum Ban
achanthus Bar
achor Bar
acopon Ba
acorus Bar
acrochordon Bar
action Ban
active Ban
active Cl
acuminate Ban
acuminated Ban
acute Bar
acute Co
aden Bar
adherent Ban
adherent Co
adhesion LIP
adhesion LBT
adiantum Bar
adjunction LIP
admission Ban
adnate Ban
adulterate Bo
aegilops Ban
aerugo Bar
affect Ban
affect Bar
affect Co
affected Ban
affected Bar
affected Cl
affection Co
affection Pl
affixed Ban
afflicted Ba
afflicted Bo
affliction Cl
affluence Cl
affluxion Bar
aforegoing Ban
agglutinate Ba
agglutinate Mo
agglutination Ban
aggravate Cl
aggrieved Bar
alcanna Bar
alienate Ban
alienated Cl
alienation Cl
alimentary Bo
alkermes Bar
alleviation Co
alligate Ban
allium Mo
alphos Bar
alteration Cl
alteration LBT
alterative Ban
alterative LBT
althea Bar
alum-water Bar
ammission Ban
amplitude Ban
anabatic Bar
anastomosis Ban
anatomical Ban
anatomist Bar
anatomist He
anatonist Ban
ancient Bo
ancient Co
ancyroid Ban
anethine Ba
anfractuous Ban
anfractuouse Ban
angina Ban
angina Bar
angular Ban

annex Ban
annular Ban
antecedent Bar
antecedent Bar
anterior Ban
antevert Bar
anthos Bar
antidotary By
aorta Ban
aperitive He
aperitive Hi
apertion Bar
aphtha Bar
apnœa Bar
apophlegmatic Bar
apostemation Ba
apozem Bar
appetition LBT
application Ba
application Ban
application Ban
application He
apposition Ban
apprehension Ban
appropinquate Ban
approve Cl
aqueous Ban
arabia Ban
arabic Co
arachnoides Ban
arcanum Bo
aromatized He
arteriac Cl
arterious Ban
artful Cl
arthrodia Ban
articulate Ban
articulate Ban
articulate Ban
articulation Ban
articulus Ban
artificial Co
artificially Ban
artist Ban
artist Co
arytenoid Ban
asarin Ba
ascendent Ban
ascendent Ban
ascendent Cl
ascending Cl
asclepiad Bo
aspect Ban
aspect Ban
assation Bo
assident Ban
assimilated Co
assimilation LIP
asthmatic Bar
astrological Bo
atheroma Bar
attenuated Ban
attenuation Bar
attractive Ban
auction LBT
auction LIP
augmentation Bar
augmentation Cl
auricle Ban
auricula Ban
aurum potabile Bo
aurum potabile Co
aversion Bar
avoid LIP
avoid Pl
avoiding LBT
avulsion LBT
axillary Ban
balaustine Bar
balneum Bar
balsamum Bo
bark Cl
basilica Ban
basilica Bar
bastard Ban
bastard rib Bar
bastard rib LIP
bastardly Bar
bather Bo
bdellium Bar
beating Ban
beating Bar
belking Bar
belly Ban
benjamin Hi
binary Bo
black Cl
blatta Bar
blind gut Ban
blind gut Bar
bole Bar
boll Ban
bolus Bar
boxing glass LBT
brachial Ban
branching Ban
brassica Bar
brassica Mo
bringing Bo
bronchocele Ba
bronchocele Bar
bruised Ba
bubonocele Ba
burst Bar
cabbalistic Bo
caecum Ban
caked Bar
calastic Bar
calendula Mo
calx vive Hi
calycle Bar
cancer Bar
cancrenated He
canella By
capacity Ban
capsule Ban
carcinoma Bar
cardia Ban
cardiac Ban
carminative Bar
caros Ban
carotid Bar
carus Bar
carvi Ba
castor Bar
castor Bar
catagmatic Ba
catarrhal Hi
catheter Bar
catholicon Bar
catoche Bar
cattarhous He
caustic Ba
caustic He
cava Ban
cave Ban
cavernous Ban

cecily Bar
cedron Ba
cele Ban
cele Bar
cenchrine Bar
cephalic Ban
cerebrum Ban
cerule Bar
chalcite Bar
chemical Bo
cholagogue Bar
cholerous Bar
chorion Ban
choroid Ban
chrysocolla Ba
cicatrix Bar
cicatrize He
cicatrizing Ba
cimolia Bar
circulate Bo
circulate Bo
clavicle Ban
clavus Bar
clutter He
cluttered Ba
coagmentation Ban
coagulate Cl
coagulation Bo
coarticulation Ban
cobweblike Ban
coccyx Ban
cocted By
cohobate Bo
colature Bar
colliquation Bar
colliquation Bar
colliquation Cl
colliquation LBT
collution Bar
columella Ban
columella Bar
coma Bar
combination Ban
comfrey Mo
cominiciall Cl
commixing Bar
commixture Cl
common vein Hi
communication Ba
compact Bar
complexionated He
complicate Ban
complicate Bar
complicate Bar
complication Bar
compositum Bar
compositum LBT
compressed Ban
compression Ban
compressor Ba
conarium Ban
concaved Ban
concoction Bar
concoction Co
concoctive LBT
concoctive LIP
concrete Cl
concreted Ban
concretion Bar
concupiscible faculty Ban
condensate Cl
condite Bar
confecting By
confectioner By
conflate Bar
conflux Cl
confused Ban
confused Ban
confusion Bar
congealment Cl
congest Cl
congested Cl
congested Cl
congestion Bar
conjugated Ban
conjunct Bar
conjunctive Cl
connect Ban
connectively Ban
connexion Bar
connexion Bar
consent Bar
consist LIP
consistence Ba
consistence Ban
consistence Ban
consistence Bar
consistence By
consistence Co
consistency Bar
consisting Co
consolidant Bo
consolidate Bar
consolidating Bar
constitute Cl
constitute LIP
constitution Bar
constitution Cl
constringe Ban
constringe Ban
constringent Bo
construction Bar
consultation Bo
contagion Cl
contagiously Cl
contemper By
contexture Ban
continent Bar
continual LBT
contract Ban
contract Ban
contract Cl
contraction Ba
contraction Ban
contraction Ban
contraction Ban
contraction Bar
contraction Co
contractive Ban
contractive Bar
contrition Bo
contrition Bo
contusion Ban
convexity Ban
convulsion Ba
convulsion Ban
convulsion Bar
convulsion Co
convulsion LBT
convulsion Mo
convulsive Co
cooling Ba
coracoid Ban
corona Ban
coronal Ban
coronal suture Ban
corpulent Ban

corpus Ban
correct Cl
correct Mo
corrosiving Bar
corrugated Cl
cotton-wool Bar
cotyledon Bar
course Cl
course Co
coursing Ban
coxa Bar
coxendix Ban
crab Bar
cremaster Ban
critical Cl
critical Cl
crooked-backed Cl
crud Cl
crudity Bar
crus Ban
crystalloid Ban
cubiform Ban
cucurbit Mo
curd Bar
cuticula Ban
cutis Ban
cyprine Bar
cyst Ban
dacryd Bar
dark Bar
dartos Ba
dartos Ban
dartre Bar
decline By
declining Co
decorticate Bar
deduct Cl
deduction Ban
defect Ban
defect Bar
defedation Bar
defensative Ba
defer Ban
defer Bar
deferent Ban
deferent Ban
deflation Cl
deflux Cl
defluxion Ba
defluxion Cl
degeneration Ba
deglution Ban
dejection Bar
dejection Cl
deleterious Cl
deligature Bar
delineate Bar
deliver LIP
deltoid Ban
demit Bar
denervation Ba
dental Ban
dentition Ban
depascent Bar
depraved Ban
depressed Ban
depression Ban
derivation Ban
derivation Bar
derive Ban
derive Bar
derive Mo
derma Ban
descendent Ban
descendent Ban
descendent Cl
desiccate Ba
desperate He
desudation Bar
detention Bar
detersion Bar
diabotanum Ba
diacalaminthe Bar
diacapparis Bar
diacorallion Bar
diacorum Bar
diacyminon Bar
dialacca Bar
dialthea Bar
diamoschum Bar
dianisum Bar
dianthos Bar
diapalma Bar
diapalma He
diapapaver Bar
diaphœnicon Bar
diapompholygos Bar
diaprune Bar
diaprunis Pl
diarrhodon Bar
diary Bar
diary Bar
diasatyrion Bar
diatragacanth Bar
diduction Bar
differentia Bar
difflate Cl
diffuse Ban
digesting Bar
digesting Mo
digit Ban
diruption Co
discolorate Bar
discussing Bar
discussion Bar
discussive Bar
dislocate Ban
disperse Pl
dispersing Bar
dissect Ban
dissect Ban
dissected Ban
dissecting Ban
dissection Ban
dissection Ban
disseminate Ban
disseminate Ban
dissension He
dissimilar Ban
dissipate Ban
dissipation Bar
dissolution Cl
dissolved Co
dissolver Bar
dissolving Bar
distemperate LBT
distend Ban
distend Bar
distension Bar
distention Ban
distort Co
distracted Co
distraction Ban
distribute Bar
distribution Ban
distribution Ban
distribution Bar

distribution Bar
distribution Bo
diuretical Bar
doctorship Bo
dodeca- Ban
doglike Bar
dogmatic LIP
dormitory By
dorsum Ban
dose He
dose Hi
dracunculus Ba
dracunculus Bar
dracunculus Mo
dragon Cl
dropax Bar
duplex Bar
dura Ban
dynamic Bo
dyspnœa Cl
earthy Ban
eclegme Bar
ecthyma Bar
educe Ban
effectrix Bar
effluxion Bar
egestion Bar
egestion Bar
egestion Mo
egredience Cl
ejaculation Ban
ejaculator Ba
element Bo
elevate Ban
elevate Bar
elevator Ba
elongate Ban
elongated Ban
embrocation Bar
embroch Bar
eminence Ban
eminence Bar
emissary Bar
emission Ban
emission Ban
emission Bar
emphysema Bar
emptying Bar
empyema Ban
empyema Bar
emulgent Ban
emulgent LIP
enarthrosis Ban
enclosure Ban
enema Bar
enfolding Ban
enfreeze Cl
engendered Cl
engross Ban
enterocele Ba
entire Ban
ephialtes Bar
epiderma He
epidermis Ban
epididymus Ban
epiglottis Ban
epileptical Co
epinyctides Bar
epiplocele Ba
equal Ban
equal Bo
equal By
equal Co
erect Ban
erect Ban
erect Bar
erected Ban
erection Ban
erection Ban
erigeron Bar
erosion Bar
errhine Bar
eruption Bar
erysipelatous Bar
erythoid Ban
essera Bar
ethmoid Ban
ethmoida Bar
evaporate Bar
evaporating Bar
evaporation Bar
evaporation LBT
evaporative Bar
exacerbation Bar
exagitation LIP
exalted Bo
exanthema Bar
exasperate Bar
exasperate Cl
excedent Bar
excluding Ban
exclusion Ban
excoriated Cl
excremental Ban
excretion Bar
excretion Co
excretion LBT
excretive LBT
exedent Bar
exhalate Bar
exhaust Cl
exhaust Co
expel Hi
expense He
experiment Ba
experiment Bar
experiment Bo
experiment Hi
experiment LIP
expirate Bar
expiration Ban
expired Ban
expiring Ban
expiring Ban
explicate Ban
explicate Ban
exquisite Ban
exquisite Bar
extension Ban
extension Ban
extension Bar
extenuating Bar
extenuative Bar
external LBT
extract Ban
extrinsical Ban
extrinsical Ban
extrusion Ban
exustion Bar
face Ban
falern Bar
false rib Ban
fatty Bar
fatuity Bar
fatuity Co
fay Bar
feeling Bo

femur Ba
fermentation By
fibre Ban
fibrous Ban
fibula Ban
filament Ban
filling Bar
filmy Bar
fistulated He
fistulous Bar
fit Co
flat Ban
flax-hurd Bar
flux Cl
fluxible Cl
fluxing Cl
foment Ba
foreign Cl
fornix Ban
fotus Bar
foundation Ban
fracture Ban
fragile Ban
fraxin Ba
frequency Bar
frons Ban
frontal Bar
fugitive Bo
fumatic Cl
function Ban
function Bar
fur Bar
furcula Ban
furuncle Bar
galange Bar
galenist Bo
ganglion Bar
ganglion Bar
gargareon Ban
ginglymos Ban
glandule Bar
glans Ban
glans Bar
glene Ban
gluten Bar
glutination Ba
glutinative Ba
gracile Ban
gracile Cl
gravelly Cl
great artery Ban
green dragon Bo
greenness Cl
grossly Cl
grossness Cl
gurgulio Bar
gutta serena Bar
haemorrhoidal He
hairlike Ban
hammer Ban
harmonia Ban
heartburn Bar
heating Bar
helcoid Bar
helm Bo
hemicrania Bar
hemina Ba
hepatic Ban
herb Bar
herbary Bar
hermetical Co
hollow vein Ban
hollowed Ban
homotonous Bar
hoodlike Ban
hopper Ban
humeral Ban
humeral Ban
humid Cl
hurted Ba
hurting Cl
husked Bar
hydrocele Ba
hydropical Co
hyoid Ban
hypochondriac Co
hypsiloid Ban
ilium Ban
ilium Ban
ilium Bar
imbecility Ban
immedicable Cl
immethodical Cl
imminution Bar
immixed Cl
immixtion Cl
impendent Cl
imperceptibility Co
impermixt Cl
impostumate Cl
impostumate He
impure Bo
impurity Bo
inarticulate Ban
incisor Ban
incisory Ban
inclination Cl
inconcocted Cl
incrust Ban
incursion Ban
incursion Bar
indented Ban
indic Bar
indicate Cl
indication By
indication Cl
indication Co
indicatory Bar
indigested Bo
indisposition He
indisposition He
indurate He
indurated Ban
inequality Ban
inequality Bar
inferiour Ban
infirmity Co
infistulated He
inflame Cl
inflamed Bar
inflamed He
inflamed Mo
inflammation Pl
inflict Bo
inflow Cl
influence Co
influx Ban
influxion Bar
infrigidation Bar
infundibulum Ban
infundibulum LIP
ingurge Cl
inherent Co
inherent Co
inhumation Bo
innest Ban
insatiableness Cl

insensible Bar
insert Ban
insession Bar
insinuate Ban
insinuate Ban
insinuate Cl
insulse Cl
insult Cl
intelligent Bo
intend Bar
inter Ban
inter Cl
interception Bar
interceptive Ban
intercostal Ban
intercostal Ban
intercourse Ban
intercourse Cl
intercourse Cl
interjacent Ban
interjected Ban
interjoin Cl
interlay Ban
intermit Bar
intermit Co
intermittent Mo
intermitting Bar
internal Bar
internal LBT
internal LIP
intersect Ban
interseptum Ban
intestinal Ban
intestinal He
intestine Ban
intestine Ban
intestine LBT
intestines Ba
intestines Bar
intrench Ban
invention Bo
inverse Ban
invert Ban
invest Ban
invest Cl
inveterated He
involucrum Bar
involuntary LBT
involution Ban
involution Ban
involvement Ban
inwardly Cl
inwardly Pl
irrigate Ban
irrigate Bar
irrigation Bar
irritation Bar
ischiadic Bar
ischium Ban
ischium Bar
ischuria Bar
issue Bar
janitor Ban
janitor LIP
jovial Co
judging day LBT
judicable Cl
judicate Co
judication Ba
judication Cl
judication Co
jugal Ban
jugal Ban
jugular Ban
jugulum Ban
just age Ban
kernel Cl
knit Cl
labrum Ban
labyrinth Ban
lambdoides Ban
languishing Bar
languishing Cl
lapidous Bar
lapis Bar
lapis hæmatites Bar
lapis indiacus Bar
lappet Bar
larynx LIP
laserpitium Cl
lateral Ban
lateral Ban
lateral Ban
lateral Ban
latitant Ban
latus Bar
lavation Bo
lawful Ban
laxative Pl
leek Bar
lengthways Ban
lenition Pl
lenticular Ba
lenticule Bar
lesion Bo
leucophlegmacy Bar
levigate Ban
lichen Bar
lienary Bar
ligament Bar
ligament He
lithoid Ban
liver Bo
lixivium Ba
loose Bo
loosener Bar
loosening Bar
loosing Bar
lues Ba
lumbal Ban
lunatical Cl
lupulin Bar
luted He
luxate Ban
lymphate Bar
macrocephaly Ban
magisterium Bo
magistral Bar
magistral He
magistral Hi
malefaction Cl
malignity By
mallet Ban
mamilla Ban
mamillar Ban
manchet Bar
mangling Bo
maniple Bar
manual Bar
manus Ban
marasm Co
marasmoid Bar
marasmus Bar
masseter Ban
masticatory Bar
mastoid Ban
mattered Bar

maturation Co
maxillary Ban
measled Cl
meatus He
medicable Cl
medication Co
medicine-monger Co
medium Bo
medulla Ban
medulla Bar
melancholic Cl
melancholiously Cl
melancholiousness Bar
melancholiousness Cl
melancholy Ban
melanthy Bar
melissa Mo
melrose Hi
membrane Ba
membrane Ban
membrane Cl
membrane Co
membraneous Ban
meninx Ban
menstruous Ban
menstruous Bar
mentagra Bar
mentha Bar
mercurial Co
mesaræum Ban
mesentery Bar
mesopleuron Ba
method Bo
methodical Ba
metrenchyte Bar
miliary Bar
millipede Bar
mineral Bo
minoration Cl
minoration Cl
misy Ba
mithridatium By
mithridatum Ba
mithridatum Bar
mitigate LBT
mitigating Bar
mitigating Bo
mitigating Cl
moderating Bar
moistly Cl
mola Bar
mole Bar
molest Mo
mollefaction Cl
mollificative Hi
mollifier Bar
mollifying Ba
mollifying Bar
mollifying Mo
morbilli Bar
mordacity Bar
mordicative Hi
motion Bar
moulting Bar
moving Cl
moving Co
mucilage Ba
mucilaginous Cl
mucous Ban
mucronate Ban
muddy Cl
mundifying Bo
nasal Bar
nasturtium LIP
nates Ban
nates LIP
naviform Ban
neck Ban
necrosis Bar
nefresie Bar
neoteric Bar
nerve Ban
nicotian Co
nitrous Bar
noble Ba
node Ba
nodulus Bar
nutrition Ban
nutrition Ban
nutrition LBT
obdurate Bar
obelion Ban
obligate Ban
oblique Ban
obscurity Ban
obstriction Ban
obstruct Ban
obstruct Cl
obstruction Bar
obstructive Bar
obturation Bar
obtuse Ban
occlude Bar
ocyme Bar
ocyme Mo
odontoides Ban
œdematous Bar
olecranon Ban
operation Ban
operation Bo
operation Cl
operation He
operative Cl
operative Cl
ophioglossum Bar
ophrys Bar
opiate Bar
opistetanos By
orbicular Ban
orthopnic Bar
os hyoides Ban
os ilium Ban
os pubis Ban
os sacrum Ban
outbreathing Ba
outgoing Ban
outstretching Ban
outward Bar
overeat Cl
overfloat Cl
overspreading Ban
overtravel Cl
oxoleon Ba
oxybaphon Ba
oxycratum Bar
oxycroceum He
oxyrrhodin Bar
ozæna Bar
panacea Ba
panax Bar
papule Bar
paracelsical Bo
paracelsist Ba
paracmastic Bar
paraplegia Bar
parastatic Ban
paregoric Bar

parencephalon LIP
parenchyma Ban
parotid Ban
parotis Bar
parson-physician Co
particular Bo
pastil Ba
patella Ban
pectus Ban
pellagra He
pellagra Hi
pelvis Ban
penetrating He
penis Ban
percolation Co
perforated Ban
perforating Ban
perfusion Bar
periosteum Ba
periosteum Ban
permistion Co
persic Bar
perspirable Bar
perspiration Bar
pestilent Bar
pestilent Mo
petasite Bar
petroseline Bar
phagadæna Cl
phagedæna Bar
phlegmagogue Bar
phlegmonoid Bar
phlegmonous Bar
phlogosis Bar
phlyctena Bar
phrenes Ban
phrenitis Bar
phyma Bar
pinching Bar
pinching Co
pineal Ban
pituitous Cl
pituitous Ban
plectrum Ban
plethoric Bar
pleura Ban
pleuritic Bar
plexus Ban
pneumatocele Ba
poisonsome Cl
polygonum Bar
pompholix Ba
pompholyx Bar
pomum Bar
possess Cl
postbrachial Ban
posterior Ban
powdered Cl
præcordia Ban
precipitate Co
pregression Bar
preparation Cl
preparation Co
prepare Bo
prepared Ban
prescission Bar
prescript Bar
pretend Ban
pretergress Bar
priapism Bar
princeps Mo
principium Bo
processus Ban
produced Ban
profluence Bar
profusion Bar
prominence Ban
protuberated Ban
protuberating Ban
psalloid Ban
psoas Ban
psora Bar
psydracium Bar
pterigoid Ban
pubis Ban
puff Ban
pulsation Co
putative Cl
putrefact Bar
pylon Cl
pylorus Ban
pylorus LIP
quadrangular Ban
quadrans Ba
quality Bar
quenched Ba
quilt Bar
radicle Bar
radius Ban
radix Ba
raging Cl
ramex Ban
ramex Bar
raphanus Mo
rare Bar
rarefying Bar
rational Bo
reading Cl
recovery Cl
recrement Ban
recrement Co
rectified Bar
rectified He
rectified Hi
rectus Ban
recurrent Ban
redound LIP
reduce Ba
reduce Cl
reducible Bo
reducible Bo
reducible Bo
reduplication Ban
refined Hi
reflected Ban
reflecting Ban
refrication Bar
refrigerating Bar
refrigerative Bar
refriscative He
regenerant Bo
regenerate Cl
regular Cl
regurgitate Ban
regurgitate Ban
relax Ban
relax He
relaxation Ba
relaxation Cl
relaxation Co
remedying LBT
remission Bar
remit Bar
remit Bar
remitting Bar
remollition Bar
renovant Bo

repel Bar
repellent Bar
repelling Bar
repugnant Bo
repulse Cl
repulsion Bar
repulsion Cl
repulsive Bar
repulsive Bar
resolute Ba
resolution Bar
resonant Ban
respect Ban
restriction Bar
restriction He
restringe He
restringe Hi
reticular Ban
revulsive Ba
rhagades Ba
rheum Bar
rhodium Bar
rhus Bar
ripen Cl
ripening Bar
rooted Bo
rostrum Bar
rotator Ban
rotatory Ban
rotundity Ban
rounded Ban
rove Bar
rubefacient Bar
rubeola Bar
ruff Bar
runged Ban
sacculus Bar
sacrum Ban
sagapenum Ba
salvatrice Bar
salving Cl
sanguisorb Mo
sapa Ba
sapa Bar
saphenus Ba
sarcocele Ba
sarcocolla He
sarcocolla Hi
saturnine Co
satyriasis Bar
scaphoid Ban
scirrhus Bar
scissible Bar
scolopendra He
scope Ban
scope Bar
scope Bo
scourer Bar
scouring Bar
scraped Bar
scrofulose Bar
scrotum Ba
scrotum Ban
scrupulous Ban
scutiform Ban
scutum Bar
seam Ban
seamy Ban
searching Cl
seat Ban
section LIP
seed vein Ban
semicircled Ban
semicupium Bar
seminary Ban
semitertian Bar
sense Cl
sensible LIP
sensibly Cl
separate Bo
separation Ban
septic Bar
septum Ban
sequestration Bar
serous Ban
serous Bar
sesamine Ban
sesamine Ban
settled Cl
sharp Ban
sharp-bellied Ban
shiplike Ban
short-necked Cl
sickly Bo
sideration Bar
sigmoid Ban
similar Ban
similar LIP
simplex Bar
simplex Bo
sinapsism Bar
sinuate Ban
situation Ban
skink Bar
skinning Ba
smoothness Cl
solidity Ban
solution Bar
solution Hi
solutive Ba
somnoriferous Bar
sophistical Cl
sopor Bar
soporiferous Ban
soporiferous Bar
sorbition LIP
sorbus Bar
spather Bar
specie He
speculation Bo
spermatic Mo
spermatic vessels Ba
spew Cl
sphacelate Co
spinal Ban
spinal process Ban
spine Ban
spirit Bo
spleen vein Bar
spontaneous Bar
spur Ban
spur-like Ban
spurge-comfit Co
squeeze Cl
state Ba
state Cl
steady Ban
steatoma Bar
stephanion Ban
sternon Ban
sternutament Bar
stertor Co
stethos Ban
stillicidium Bar
stomachal He
stomachal Hi
stomachic Bar

stomachic Bar
stone-colic Cl
stove He
straight Ban
strain Bar
straining Ba
straitening Ban
strigment Bar
strike Bar
structure Ban
strumous Bar
strumous Bar
struthion Bar
stupefact Bar
stupefied Co
stupefy By
stupefying By
styloid Ban
subduction Ban
sublevated Ban
substract Cl
succus Ba
suckling box Bar
sudamina Bar
suffiment Bar
suffite Bar
suffocate LIP
suffocate Mo
sugar Bo
sulphur vivum Bar
sulphur water Bar
sulphurous Bar
supercilium Ban
superficial Bar
superior Ban
superjacent Ban
suppress Ban
suppression Bar
suppurated Bar
suppuration Bar
susceptibility Co
suspensor Ban
suspensory Ban
sweating Ban
swimming Cl
symptomate Bar
symptomatic Cl
synchondrosis Ban
syndesmo- Ban
syndesmosis Ban
synneurosis Ban
synteresis Bo
synulotic Bar
syssarcosis Ban
tabes Bar
table Ban
tabulate Bar
talpa Bar
talpa He
talus Ban
tardiness Bar
tarsus Ban
taxis Bar
temporal Ban
tend Ban
tendinous Ban
tenebricose Bar
tent Ba
tenting He
terebinthine Ba
termination Co
terra lemnia Bar
terrene Ba
terrestrial Ban
terrestrial LIP
testis Ban
tetrapharmacon Bar
tetrapharmacum Ba
thymus Ban
thymus Bar
thyroid Ban
tibia Ban
timpana Cl
tincture Bo
tonsil Ban
tonsil Bar
tooth Ban
topic Ban
topic medicinis Ban
torcular Ban
tormina Bar
tracheal artery Bar
transplantation Bo
transporter Ban
transversely Ban
tremor Bar
triangle Ban
trochanter Ban
try Mo
tubercle Bar
tuberculome Bar
tunic Bar
turning Ban
twig Ban
typhoid Bar
typic Bar
ulceration Ban
umbilical Ban
umbilical Ban
umbilicus Ban
umbilicus Bar
uncia Ba
unclarified Ba
unconcoct LIP
unction Ba
undissolved Co
ungle Bar
union Ban
union Cl
unite Ban
universal Bo
unnamed Ban
unnourishable Cl
unpure Bar
unsettle Cl
unsettled Cl
unsoundness Cl
untemperate Mo
unulcerate Bar
urinary Co
usnea Bar
ustion Bar
vacuation Bar
vaporous Cl
variola Bar
varnish He
varus Bar
vas Ban
vault Ban
vegetable Bo
vegetable stone He
vehemence Pl
vena axillaris Ban
vena cava Bar
vena porta Ban
venerean Ba
ventilate Co

ventricle Bar
vestigium Ban
vial glass Bar
vicious Bar
vicious Mo
vim Bo
vinculum Ban
virility Ban
viscus Bar
visual Bar
vitelline Bar
vitiligo Bar
vitreous Ban
vitrum Bo
vocal Ban
volatic Bar
volatile Bar
volatile Bo
volvulus Bar
vomiting Ban
vulnerary Bo
vulpine Bar
warmer Bo
waterish Ban
watery Ban
wheeling Ban
white dittany Bar
white line Ban
wind-colic Cl
wing Ban
writhing Ban
wry-necked Cl
xiphoid Ban
yellowish Bar

Index

All words discussed in the text have been cited in the index. These have not been altered from their original forms except that æ–ae, i–j, and v–u have been modernized for convenience.